Nurse's
Quick
Check

Fluids &
Electrolytes

Nurse's Quick Check

Fluids & Electrolytes

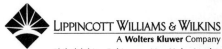

LIPPINCOTT WILLIAMS & WILKINS
A **Wolters Kluwer** Company

Philadelphia • Baltimore • New York • London
Buenos Aires • Hong Kong • Sydney • Tokyo

STAFF

Executive Publisher
Judith A. Schilling McCann, RN, MSN

Editorial Director
William J. Kelly

Clinical Director
Joan M. Robinson, RN, MSN

Senior Art Director
Arlene Putterman

Editorial Project Manager
Catherine E. Harold

Clinical Project Managers
Tamara M. Kear, RN, MSN, CNN;
Beverly Ann Tscheschlog, RN, BS

Editor
Nancy Priff

Clinical Editors
Karen Hamel, RN, BSN; Kate McGovern, RN, MSN

Copy Editor
Jenifer F. Walker

Designers
Will Boehm (book design),
E. Jane Spencer (project manager)

Digital Composition Services
Diane Paluba (manager), Joyce Rossi Biletz,
Donna S. Morris

Manufacturing
Patricia K. Dorshaw (director), Beth J. Welsh

Editorial Assistants
Megan Aldinger, Karen Kirk, Linda Ruhf

Indexer
Barbara Hodgson

The clinical procedures described and recommended in this publication are based on research and consultation with medical and nursing authorities. To the best of our knowledge, these procedures reflect currently accepted clinical practice; nevertheless, they can't be considered absolute and universal recommendations. For individual application, treatment recommendations must be considered in light of the patient's clinical condition and, before administration of new or infrequently used drugs, in light of the latest package-insert information. The authors and the publisher disclaim responsibility for any adverse effects resulting directly or indirectly from the suggested procedures, from any undetected errors, or from the reader's misunderstanding of the text.

Library of Congress Cataloging-in-Publication Data
Nurse's quick check. Fluids & electrolytes.
    p. ; cm.
  Includes bibliographical references and index.
  1. Water-electrolyte imbalances—Nursing—Handbooks,
manuals, etc. 2. Water-electrolyte balance (Physiology)—
Handbooks, manuals, etc. I. Lippincott Williams &
Wilkins. II. Title: Fluids & electrolytes. [DNLM: 1. Water-
Electrolyte Imbalance—nursing—Handbooks. 2. Nursing
Care—Handbooks. WY 49 N97423 2006]
RC630.N87 2006
616.3'9920231—dc22
ISBN 1-58255-414-5 (alk. paper)   2004031001

Contents

Contributors
and consultants

Marguerite Ambrose, RN, DNSc, APRN, BC
Faculty, Department of Nursing
Immaculata University
Immaculata, Pa.

Patricia Laing Arie, RN, BSEd
Coordinator, Practical Nursing
Central Technology Center
Drumright, Okla.

Margaret W. Bellak, RN, MN
Associate Professor
Indiana University of Pennsylvania
Indiana, Pa.

Mary Ann Boucher, RN, ND, APRN, BC
Assistant Professor, Nursing
University of Massachusetts Dartmouth
Dartmouth, Mass.

Cheryl L. Brady, RN, MSN
Adjunct Faculty
Kent State University
East Liverpool, Ohio

Shari Regina Cammon, RN, MSN, CCRN
Clinical Risk Management & Safety Surveillance
  Associate
Merck & Co., Inc.
West Point, Pa.

Lillian Craig, MSN, FNP, CS
Family Nurse Practitioner
Veterans' Administration Medical Center
Amarillo, Texas

Peggy A. Davis, RN, MSN, CNS
Assistant Professor of Nursing
University of Tennessee
Martin, Tenn.

Shelba Durston, RN, MSN, CCRN
Adjunct Faculty
San Joaquin Delta College
Stockton, Calif.
Staff Nurse
San Joaquin General Hospital
French Camp, Calif.

Helen Fu, MSN, FNP
Family Nurse Practitioner
Soteria Family Health Center
Plymouth, Minn.

Margaret M. Gingrich, RN, MSN
Associate Professor
Harrisburg Area Community College
Harrisburg, Pa.

David J. Hartman, MSN, CRNP
Nurse Practitioner
University of Pennsylvania Health System
Philadelphia

Angela R. Irvin, RN, BSN, FNP student
Clinical Instructor
Western Kentucky University
Bowling Green, Ky.

Kathy J. Keister, RN, MS
Assistant Professor
Miami University
Middletown, Ohio

Linda Kucher, RN, MSN
Assistant Professor of Nursing
Gordon College
Barnesville, Ga.

Ellen Marcolongo, RN, MSN, CRNP
Clinical Nurse Specialist
North Philadelphia Health System
Philadelphia, Pa.

Dawna Martich, RN, BSN, MSN
Clinical Trainer
American Healthways
Pittsburgh, Pa.

Lakshmi McRae, RNC, BA
Staff Nurse
Doctor's Outpatient Surgical Center
Pasadena, Texas

Valerie Mignatti, RN, BSN
Cardiovascular Clinical Nurse
University of Pennsylvania Medical Center
Philadelphia

Sharon D. O'Kelley, ADN, OCN
Clinical Nurse III
Duke University Hospital
Durham, N.C.

Sherry A. Parmenter, RD, LD
Clinical Dietitian
Fairfield Medical Center
Lancaster, Ohio

Clare Petrotta, RN, PHN, BSN
Nursing Instructor
Pacific College
Costa Mesa, Calif.

Abby Plambeck, RN, BSN
Freelance Writer
Milwaukee, Wis.

Theresa Pulvano, RN, BSN
Practical Nursing Instructor
Ocean County Vocational Technical School
Lakehurst, N.J.

Monica Narvaez Ramirez, RN, MSN
Instructor
University of the Incarnate Word School of Nursing &
  Health Professions
San Antonio, Texas

Lisa A. Salamon, MSN, RNBC, ET
Clinical Nurse Specialist
Cleveland Clinic Foundation
Cleveland, Ohio

Barbara K. Scheirer, RN, BS, MSN
Assistant Professor
Grambling State University
Grambling, La.

Bruce Austin Scott, MSN, APRN, BC
Instructor
San Joaquin Delta College
Stockton, Calif.
Clinical Nurse
University of California, Davis Medical Center
Sacramento, Calif.

Patricia Weiskittel, RN, MSN, CNN, APRN, BC
Primary Care Nurse Practitioner, Internal Medicine
Veterans Administration Hospital
Cincinnati, Ohio

Sharon Wing, RN, MSN
Assistant Professor
Cleveland State University
Cleveland, Ohio

Denise York, RNC, CNS, MS, MEd
Associate Professor
Columbus State Community College
Columbus, Ohio

Foreword

For students and practicing nurses alike, there's one physiologic concept that intimidates nearly everyone: fluids and electrolytes. Many disorders can cause or influence fluid shifts, electrolyte imbalances, acid-base imbalances, and metabolic problems. In some cases, these changes can be life-threatening.

What's more, many treatments influence fluid and electrolyte status. Take just one example: I.V. therapy. A patient with an I.V. line may be receiving parenteral maintenance to replace fluids, electrolytes, or both. The fluid may be serving as a carrier for parenterally administered drugs. It may contain additives that significantly affect the patient's fluid and electrolyte balance. And it may be running into a patient whose innate ability to maintain homeostasis is compromised by a disease, an injury, or an imbalance.

To care for your patients appropriately, you need a solid foundation of understanding fluids and electrolytes, acids and bases, pH, buffering mechanisms, and more. Plus, you need to be able to weave your knowledge about disorders together with your knowledge about treatments to help predict and manage their combined effects on fluids and electrolytes.

To many nurses, that seems like a tall order. That's why I'm so pleased with *Nurse's Quick Check: Fluids & Electrolytes*. Written by expert nurses, it offers succinct, two-page entries on all the major disorders that affect fluid and electrolyte balance. Each entry includes information designed especially to cover what nurses need to know. You'll find a description of the disorder followed by a brief review of its pathophysiology, causes, prevalence, and complications. You'll find essential elements of assessment, including history, physical findings, and test results. And you'll find a review of nursing diagnoses, outcomes, interventions, patient teaching, and discharge planning.

The best part is that all the material is presented in scan-and-go bulleted lists that spare you the laborious reading most books require.

To provide even more help, the book opens with a quick refresher course in fluid and electrolyte basics that's presented in the same time-saving format as the main part of the book. It covers such crucial topics as fluid movement, volume shifts, major cations and anions, acid-base balance, fluid and electrolyte replacement, parenteral nutrition, and dialysis.

Throughout the book, you'll find special icons designed to direct your attention to important details: An *ALERT* icon highlights crucial information, and an *AGE AWARE* icon points out information particular to certain age groups.

The fact is that nurses are the patient's first and last line of defense when it comes to overall care. Clearly, that care must encompass issues of acid-base balance, fluid volume composition, and interpretation of the laboratory values that reveal the patient's fluid and electrolyte status. I've heard many a nurse say in frustration, head bent over a patient's lab report, "If only I had a quick key or refresher to help me understand the imbalances I'm seeing here, I'd feel so much more confident." Of course, they have laboratory books, medical-surgical books, and pathophysiology books, but not at their fingertips, not on the unit, and not in a format that allows a quick check.

Understanding the intricacies of fluid and electrolyte balance can be intimidating, but it's crucial to good nursing care — not just for patients receiving infusion therapy, but for all patients. In my view, *Nurse's Quick Check: Fluids & Electrolytes* offers practical, time-saving help with this complex area of nursing care. I recommend it highly.

Patricia N. Allen, RN, MSN, APRN
Clinical Instructor, School of Nursing
Indiana University

Part one

Essential concepts

Fluid types

Fluid tonicity

Isotonic solutions

- A solute is a substance that's dissolved in a solvent. Together, they make a solution.
- An isotonic solution has the same solute concentration as another solution to which it's being compared.
- Normal saline solution is an example of an isotonic solution; its concentration of sodium nearly equals the concentration of sodium in blood. (See *Understanding isotonic, hypotonic, and hypertonic solutions.*)
- If two fluids in adjacent compartments have equal concentrations of a certain solute — if they're isotonic, in other words — the fluid in each compartment stays where it is.
- A balanced solute concentration means no net shift in fluid.

Hypotonic solutions

- A hypotonic solution has a lower solute concentration than another solution to which it's being compared.
- If one solution contains only a little sodium and another solution contains more sodium, the first solution is hypotonic compared with the second solution.
- Half-normal saline solution is an example of a hypotonic solution; its concentration of sodium is lower than the concentration of sodium in blood.
- The body constantly seeks to maintain a state of balance, or equilibrium. As a result, fluid from the hypotonic solution shifts into the more concentrated solution until the two solutions have equal concentrations of solutes.

Hypertonic solutions

- A hypertonic solution has a higher solute concentration than another solution to which it's being compared.
- For instance, say one solution contains a large amount of sodium and a second solution contains much less sodium. The first solution is hypertonic compared with the second solution.
- Dextrose 5% in normal saline solution is an example of a hypertonic solution because the concentration of solutes in the solution is greater than the concentration of solutes in blood.
- Because the body seeks equilibrium, fluid from the less concentrated solution will move into the hypertonic solution until the two solutions contain equal concentrations of solutes.

▼ **ALERT** *Fluid shifts can have important implications for your nursing care. For instance, if you give a hypotonic fluid to a patient, it may cause too much fluid to shift out of the veins (where the fluid is delivered) and into the cells, and the cells can swell. Conversely, if you give a hypertonic solution to a patient, it may cause too much fluid to shift out of the cells and into the bloodstream, and the cells can shrink.*

Fluid locations

Intracellular fluid

- Intracellular fluid is the fluid that's inside cells.
- In a typical adult, intracellular fluid averages about 40% of body weight, or about 28 L.

Understanding isotonic, hypotonic, and hypertonic solutions

Isotonic solution	*Hypotonic solution*	*Hypertonic solution*
There's no net fluid shift between isotonic solutions because the solutions contain equal concentrations of solutes.	When a less concentrated, or hypotonic, solution is placed next to a more concentrated solution, fluid shifts from the hypotonic solution into the more concentrated compartment to equalize concentrations.	If one solution has more solutes than an adjacent solution, it has less fluid relative to the adjacent solution. Fluid will move out of the less concentrated solution into the more concentrated, or hypertonic, solution until both solutions have the same amount of solutes and fluid.

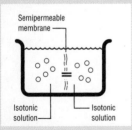

Semipermeable membrane

Isotonic solution — Isotonic solution

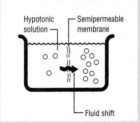

Hypotonic solution — Semipermeable membrane

Fluid shift

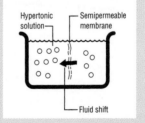

Hypertonic solution — Semipermeable membrane

Fluid shift

Fluid compartments

This illustration shows the main body's fluid compartments: intracellular and extracellular, the latter of which is further divided into interstitial and intravascular. Capillary walls and cell membranes separate intracellular fluids from extracellular fluids.

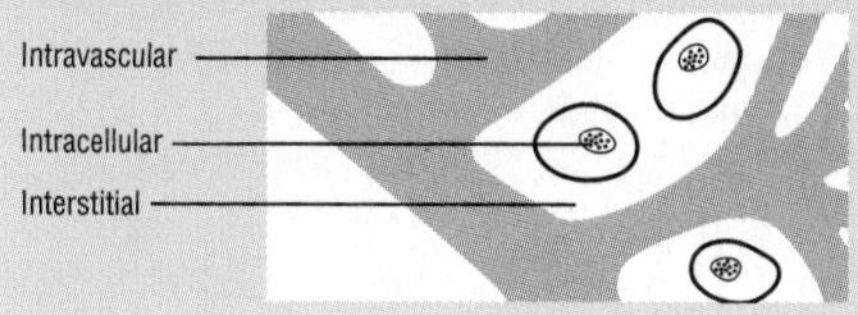

- Capillary walls and cell membranes separate intracellular fluid from fluid that exists outside the cells.
- Fluid inside and outside the cells must stay in balance.

Extracellular fluid

- Extracellular fluid is the fluid that's outside the cells, either in the interstitial space (interstitial fluid) or in blood vessels (intravascular fluid). (See *Fluid compartments*.)
- Interstitial fluid surrounds the cells.
- Intravascular fluid, or plasma, is the liquid portion of blood.
- In a typical adult, extracellular fluid averages about 20% of the person's body weight, or about 14 L.
- Extracellular fluid must be balanced with intracellular fluid.

Transcellular fluid

- Transcellular fluid is found in the cerebrospinal column, pleural cavity, lymph system, joints, and eyes.
- Usually, transcellular fluids don't undergo significant gains and losses throughout the day.

AGE AWARE The distribution of fluid in the body changes with age. In a typical young adult, interstitial fluid makes up about 15% of body weight; that percentage decreases progressively with age. In contrast, plasma makes up about 5% of total fluid volume, a percentage that remains stable throughout life.

Fluid movement

Diffusion

○ In this type of fluid movement, solutes shift from an area of higher concentration to an area of lower concentration.
○ Eventually, solute concentrations equalize between the two areas.
○ Diffusion is a form of passive transport because no energy is needed to make it happen. (See *Understanding diffusion and osmosis*.)

Osmosis

○ Osmosis refers to the movement of fluid across a membrane from an area of lower solute concentration and comparatively more fluid into an area of higher solute concentration and comparatively less fluid.
○ Like diffusion, osmosis is a passive process; it requires no energy expenditure.
○ Osmosis stops when enough fluid has moved through the membrane to equalize the solute concentration on both sides of the membrane.

Active transport

○ In active transport, solutes move from an area of lower concentration to an area of higher concentration.
○ This process requires energy because it goes against the body's natural tendency to equalize concentrations.
○ The energy needed for a solute to move against a concentration gradient comes from a substance called adenosine triphosphate (ATP).

○ ATP is stored in all cells, and it supplies energy for solute movement in and out of cells. (See *Understanding active transport*.)
○ Some solutes, such as sodium and potassium, use ATP to move in and out of cells in a form of active transport called the sodium-potassium pump.
○ Other solutes that cross cell membranes by active transport include calcium ions, hydrogen ions, amino acids, and certain sugars.

▶ **ALERT** *In the vascular system, only capillaries have walls thin enough to let solutes pass through. The movement of fluids and solutes through the capillary walls plays a critical role in fluid balance.*

Capillary filtration

○ The movement of fluids through capillaries — a process called capillary filtration — results from blood pushing against the walls of the capillary. That pressure, called hydrostatic (or fluid-pushing) pressure, forces fluids and solutes through the capillary wall.
○ When the hydrostatic pressure inside a capillary exceeds the pressure in the surrounding interstitial space, fluids and solutes inside the capillary are forced out into the interstitial space.
○ When pressure outside of a capillary exceeds pressure inside it, fluids and solutes move back into the capillary.

Reabsorption

○ Reabsorption prevents too much fluid from leaving the capillaries no matter how much hydrostatic pressure is inside them.
○ When fluid filters through a capillary, the protein albumin stays behind in the shrinking volume of water.

Understanding diffusion and osmosis

In diffusion, solutes move from an area of higher concentration to an area of lower concentration, as shown on the left, until the concentration is equal in both areas. In osmosis, fluid moves from an area of lower solute concentration to an area of higher solute concentration, as shown on the right, until the concentration is equal in both areas. Both processes are passive; that is, they need no energy. Just remember that, in diffusion, solutes move; in osmosis, fluid moves.

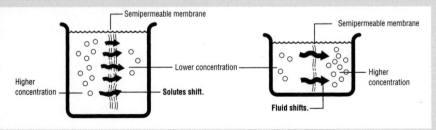

Understanding active transport

During active transport, energy from a molecule called adenosine triphosphate (ATP) moves solutes against the gradient, from an area of lower concentration to an area of higher concentration. Sodium and potassium are examples of two solutes moved by active transport.

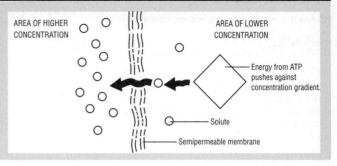

○ Albumin is a large molecule that normally can't pass through capillary membranes.

○ As the concentration of albumin inside a capillary increases, fluid begins to move back into the capillaries by osmosis.

○ The osmotic, or pulling, force of albumin in the intravascular space is called plasma colloid osmotic pressure.

○ Plasma colloid osmotic pressure in capillaries averages about 25 mm Hg.

○ As long as hydrostatic pressure exceeds plasma colloid osmotic pressure, water and solutes can leave the capillaries and enter interstitial fluid. If hydrostatic pressure falls below plasma colloid osmotic pressure, water and diffusible solutes return to the capillaries.

○ Normally, hydrostatic pressure exceeds plasma colloid osmotic pressure in the arteriole end and falls below it in the venule end. As a result, capillary filtration occurs along the first half of the vessel and reabsorption occurs along the second half.

○ As long as hydrostatic pressure and plasma albumin levels remain normal, the amount of water moving into the capillaries equals the amount moving out.

○ Occasionally, extra fluid filters out of the capillary. When that happens, excess fluid shifts into lymphatic vessels located just outside the capillaries and eventually returns to the heart for recirculation.

Fluid balance

Types of fluid loss

Sensible loss

○ Sensible loss is fluid loss that can be measured.
○ It includes fluid lost through urination, defecation, bleeding, wound drainage, gastric drainage, and vomiting. (See *Tracking fluid intake and output*.)
○ A typical adult loses 100 to 200 ml/day of fluid through defecation. In severe diarrhea, losses may exceed 5,000 ml/day.
○ Gastric, intestinal, pancreatic, and biliary secretions are almost completely reabsorbed and aren't usually counted in daily fluid gains and losses.

Insensible loss

○ Insensible loss is fluid loss that can't be measured.
○ It includes fluid lost through skin (perspiration) and lungs (respiration).

✿ AGE AWARE *The body surface area of an infant is greater than that of an adult relative to their respective weights. As a result, infants typically lose a greater proportion of water from their skin than adults do.*

○ Changes in humidity levels affect the amount of fluid lost through the skin.
○ Changes in respiratory rate and depth affect the amount of fluid lost through the lungs. In tachypnea, for example, water loss increases; in bradypnea, it decreases.
○ Fever increases insensible losses from both the skin and lungs.

Tracking fluid intake and output

Each day the body gains and loses fluid through several processes. The main ones are shown here. The body's processes work together to balance output with intake.

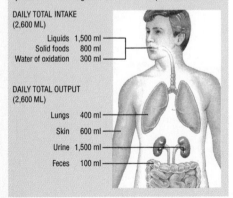

DAILY TOTAL INTAKE
(2,600 ML)

Liquids 1,500 ml
Solid foods 800 ml
Water of oxidation 300 ml

DAILY TOTAL OUTPUT
(2,600 ML)

Lungs 400 ml
Skin 600 ml
Urine 1,500 ml
Feces 100 ml

Balancing systems

Renal system

○ The kidneys play a vital role in fluid balance. If they aren't working properly, the body has great difficulty controlling fluid balance.
○ The nephron is the part of the kidney that forms urine. (See *Parts of a nephron.*)
○ A nephron consists of a glomerulus and a tubule.
  – The glomerulus is a cluster of capillaries that filters blood.
  – Surrounding the glomerulus like a vascular cradle is Bowman's capsule.
  – The tubule, sometimes convoluted, ends in a collecting duct.
○ Capillary blood pressure forces fluid through the capillary walls and into Bowman's capsule at the proximal end of the tubule.
○ Along the tubule, water and electrolytes are either excreted or retained according to the body's needs.
  – If the body needs more fluid, it retains more.
  – If the body needs less fluid, less is reabsorbed and more is excreted.
○ Electrolytes, such as sodium and potassium, are either filtered or reabsorbed throughout the same area. The resulting filtrate, which eventually becomes urine, flows through the tubule into the collecting ducts and eventually into the bladder as urine.
○ Nephrons filter about 125 ml of blood every minute, or about 180 L/day. That rate, called the glomerular filtration rate, leads to the production of 1 to 2 L of urine per day. The nephrons reabsorb the remaining 178 L or more of fluid.

✿ AGE AWARE *Infants and young children excrete urine at a higher rate than adults because their higher metabolic rates produce more waste. Also, an infant's kidneys can't concentrate urine until about age 3 months, and they remain less efficient than an adult's kidney until about age 2 years.*

Antidiuretic hormone

○ Antidiuretic hormone (ADH) is a water-retaining hormone also known as vasopressin.
○ When the hypothalamus senses a low blood volume and increased serum osmolality, it signals the pituitary gland.
○ The posterior pituitary gland, which stores ADH, secretes it into the bloodstream.
○ ADH prompts the kidneys to retain water, which increases blood volume, decreases serum osmolality, and increases the concentration of urine.
○ Decreased serum osmolality or increased blood volume inhibits the release of ADH and causes less water to be reabsorbed, making the urine less concentrated.

○ The amount of ADH released varies throughout the day, depending on the body's needs.

Renin-angiotensin-aldosterone system

○ Juxtaglomerular cells near each glomerulus secrete renin to help balance sodium and water and maintain blood volume and pressure.
- Renin is an enzyme.
- Through a complex series of steps, renin leads to production of angiotensin II.
○ Angiotensin II causes peripheral vasoconstriction, which increases blood pressure.
○ Angiotensin II also stimulates the adrenal glands to produce aldosterone.
- Aldosterone is a hormone.
- It cues the kidneys to retain sodium and water, thus increasing blood pressure and volume.
○ As soon as blood pressure reaches a normal level, the body stops releasing renin, and this feedback loop of renin to angiotensin to aldosterone stops.
○ The amount of renin secreted depends on blood flow and the level of sodium in the bloodstream.
- If blood flow to the kidneys declines (as in a hemorrhage) or the amount of sodium reaching the glomerulus drops, juxtaglomerular cells secrete more renin, which causes vasoconstriction and increases blood pressure.
- If blood flow to the kidneys increases or the amount of sodium reaching the glomerulus increases, juxtaglomerular cells secrete less renin, which reduces vasoconstriction and keeps blood pressure from rising.
○ Aldosterone acts as well when blood volume drops.
- It starts the active transport of sodium from the distal tubules and the collecting ducts into the bloodstream.
- When sodium is forced into the bloodstream, more water is reabsorbed and blood volume expands.

Atrial natriuretic peptide

○ A cardiac hormone called atrial natriuretic peptide (ANP) also helps maintain fluid balance.
- ANP is stored in the cells of the atria.
- It's released when atrial pressure increases.
○ ANP opposes the renin-angiotensin-aldosterone system.
- If blood volume and pressure rise, the atrial walls stretch, prompting release of ANP.
- ANP shuts off the renin-angiotensin-aldosterone system, thus decreasing blood pressure and reducing intravascular blood volume.
○ ANP has several key functions:
- suppressing serum renin levels
- decreasing aldosterone release from the adrenal glands
- increasing glomerular filtration, which increases urinary excretion of sodium and water
- decreasing ADH release from the posterior pituitary gland

Parts of a nephron

The nephron filters blood, produces urine, and excretes excess solutes, electrolytes, fluids, and metabolic waste products while keeping the blood composition and volume constant.

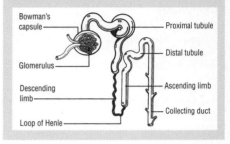

- decreasing vascular resistance by causing vasodilation.
○ The amount of ANP that atria release rises in response to many conditions, including chronic renal failure and heart failure.

ALERT Anything that causes atrial stretching can increase ANP release, including orthostatic changes, atrial tachycardia, high sodium intake, sodium chloride infusions, and use of drugs that cause vasoconstriction.

Thirst

○ Perhaps the simplest mechanism for maintaining fluid balance is the thirst mechanism.
○ Thirst arises after even small fluid losses.
○ Losing body fluids or eating salty foods leads to an increase in extracellular fluid osmolality.
○ This increase dries the mucus membranes in the mouth, which stimulates the thirst center in the hypothalamus.

AGE AWARE In an elderly person, the thirst mechanism is less effective than it is in a younger person, leaving the older person more prone to dehydration.

Hypovolemia

Overview

Description
○ Isotonic fluid loss (which includes loss of fluids and solutes) from the extracellular space
○ Subtle initial signs and symptoms as the body tries to compensate for reduced circulating blood volume

Pathophysiology
○ Fluid circulating in the blood decreases, lowering cardiac output and leading to hypotension and impaired tissue perfusion.
○ Tissue anoxia prompts a shift in cellular metabolism from aerobic to anaerobic pathways; lactic acid accumulates, and metabolic acidosis may develop.
○ Third-space fluid shifts may occur from increased permeability of the capillary membrane or decreased plasma colloid osmotic pressure.

Risk factors
○ Adrenal insufficiency
○ Coma
○ Diabetes insipidus
○ Hemorrhage
○ Osmotic diuresis
○ Third-space fluid shift

Causes
○ Fluid loss from the extracellular compartment
  – Abdominal surgery
  – Diabetes mellitus (with increased urination)
  – Diarrhea
  – Excessive diuretic therapy
  – Excessive laxative use
  – Excessive sweating
  – Fever
  – Fistula
  – Hemorrhage (frank or occult)
  – Nasogastric drainage
  – Renal failure (with increased urination)
  – Vomiting
○ Third-space fluid shifts
  – Acute intestinal obstruction
  – Acute peritonitis
  – Burns (during the initial phase)
  – Crush injuries
  – Hip fracture
  – Hypoalbuminemia
  – Pleural effusion

Complications
○ Acute respiratory distress syndrome
○ Acute tubular necrosis and renal failure
○ Disseminated intravascular coagulation
○ Multiple organ dysfunction

Assessment

History
○ Presence of one of the above causes
○ Restlessness
○ Anxiety
○ Confusion
○ Thirst
○ Weight loss

Physical assessment
○ Increased heart rate
○ Orthostatic hypotension
○ Delayed capillary refill
○ Cool, pale, clammy skin over the arms and legs
○ Decreased urine output (See *Danger signs of hypovolemia.*)

Test results
Laboratory
○ Decreased hemoglobin level, hematocrit, and red blood cell count
○ Increased serum potassium, sodium, lactic dehydrogenase, creatinine, and blood urea nitrogen levels
○ Increased urine specific gravity and urine osmolality
○ Positive occult blood test (if the patient has gastrointestinal bleeding)
Diagnostic procedures
○ Invasive hemodynamic monitoring shows reduced central venous pressure (CVP), pulmonary artery pressure (PAP), right atrial pressure, pulmonary artery wedge pressure (PAWP), and cardiac output.
○ Gastroscopy may identify an internal bleeding site.

Nursing diagnoses
○ Decreased cardiac output
○ Ineffective tissue perfusion: cardiopulmonary, renal, cerebral

---

Danger signs of hypovolemia

Watch for these signs and symptoms of hypovolemia and impending hypovolemic shock:
● deterioration in mental status (from restlessness and anxiety to unconsciousness)
● thirst
● tachycardia
● delayed capillary refill
● orthostatic hypotension progressing to marked hypotension
● urine output initially more than 30 ml/minute and then dropping below 10 ml/hour
● cool, pale skin over arms and legs
● weight loss
● flat jugular veins
● decreased central venous pressure
● weak or absent peripheral pulses.

○ Impaired gas exchange
○ Deficient fluid volume

Key outcomes

The patient will:
○ maintain adequate cardiac output
○ maintain hemodynamic stability
○ maintain adequate ventilation
○ regain adequate fluid volume.

Interventions

General

○ Identification of cause of fluid loss
○ Oxygen administration
○ Bed rest
○ Isotonic I.V. fluids, such as normal saline solution or Ringer's solution
○ Surgery (possibly) to control underlying problem

Nursing

○ Maintain the patient's airway.
○ Give prescribed I.V. fluids or blood products.
○ Insert an indwelling urinary catheter.
○ Provide emotional support to the patient and family.

Drug therapy

○ Oxygen
○ Vasopressors

Monitoring

○ Vital signs
○ Airway patency
○ Intake and output
○ Weight
○ I.V. site patency
○ Hemodynamic values (cardiac output, CVP, PAP, PAWP)
○ Cardiac rhythm
○ Signs of bleeding
○ Signs of transfusion reaction if giving blood products
○ Signs of impeding shock
○ Laboratory values: complete blood count, electrolyte levels, blood urea nitrogen level, creatinine level
○ Arterial blood gas levels

Patient teaching

Be sure to cover:
○ the disorder, diagnosis, and treatment plan
○ all procedures and their purposes
○ the risks of blood transfusion
○ the purpose of all equipment, including cardiac monitoring
○ warning signs of hypovolemia and when to report them
○ prescribed drugs and their possible adverse effects.

Hypervolemia

Overview

Description
○ Excess isotonic fluid (water and sodium) in the extracellular compartment
○ Fluid and solutes gained in equal proportion, leaving osmolality unaffected
○ Signs and symptoms if compensatory mechanisms fail

Pathophysiology

○ Increased extracellular fluid volume in either the interstitial or intravascular compartments prompts the body to try to compensate and restore fluid balance.
○ It adjusts circulating levels of aldosterone, antidiuretic hormone, and atrial natriuretic peptide to make the kidneys release additional water and sodium.
○ If hypervolemia is prolonged or severe or the patient has poor heart function, the body can't compensate for the extra volume.
○ Fluid is forced out of the blood vessels and into the interstitial space, causing edema.

▶ ALERT *Elderly patients and patients with impaired renal or cardiovascular function are especially prone to hypervolemia.*

Causes
○ Excessive sodium or fluid intake
 – I.V. replacement therapy using normal saline solution or lactated Ringer's solution
 – Blood or plasma replacement
 – Excessive intake of dietary sodium
○ Fluid or sodium retention
 – Heart failure
 – Cirrhosis of the liver
 – Nephrotic syndrome
 – Corticosteroid therapy
 – Hyperaldosteronism
 – Low intake of dietary protein
○ Fluid shift from interstitial to intravascular space
 – Remobilization of fluids after burn treatment
 – Delivery of hypertonic fluids, such as mannitol or hypertonic saline solution
 – Use of plasma proteins, such as albumin
 – Acute or chronic renal failure with low urine output

Complications
○ Heart failure
○ Pulmonary edema

Assessment

History
○ Weight gain
○ Edema of limbs
○ Shortness of breath

Physical assessment
○ Rapid and bounding pulse
○ Increased blood pressure, central venous pressure (CVP), pulmonary artery pressure (PAP), and pulmonary artery wedge pressure (PAWP)
○ Decreased blood pressure and cardiac output as the heart fails
○ An S_3 gallop with heart failure
○ Distended veins, especially in the hands and neck
○ Edema
 – Visible first in dependent areas, such as sacrum and buttocks when the patient is lying down and legs and feet when the patient is standing
 – Becomes generalized (See *Evaluating pitting edema.*)
○ Crackles with lung auscultation
○ Tachypnea
○ Frothy cough

Test results
Laboratory
○ Decreased hematocrit

Evaluating pitting edema

Edema can be evaluated using a scale of +1 to +4. Press your fingertip firmly into the skin over a bony surface for a few seconds. Then note the depth of the imprint your finger leaves. A slight imprint indicates +1 pitting edema, as shown on the left. A deep imprint, with the skin slow to return to its original contour, indicates +4 pitting edema, as shown in the center. If you leave no imprint because the skin is distended so much that fluid can't be displaced, the patient has brawny edema, as shown on the right.

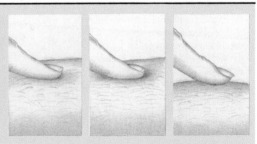

○ Normal serum sodium level but decreased serum potassium and blood urea nitrogen levels
○ Decreased oxygen level (with early tachypnea, possible decreased partial pressure of arterial carbon dioxide, decreased pH, and respiratory alkalosis)

Imaging
○ Chest X-rays reveal pulmonary congestion.

Diagnostic procedures
○ Invasive hemodynamic monitoring shows increased CVP, PAP, right atrial pressure, PAWP, and cardiac output.

Nursing diagnoses

○ Impaired gas exchange
○ Ineffective airway clearance
○ Excess fluid volume
○ Anxiety

Key outcomes
The patient will:
○ maintain adequate ventilation
○ maintain a patent airway
○ regain fluid balance
○ verbalize decreased anxiety and fear.

Interventions

General
○ Restriction of sodium and fluid intake
○ Oxygen therapy
○ Identification and treatment of cause
○ Bed rest

Nursing
○ Give prescribed drugs.
○ Maintain the patient's airway and ventilation.
○ Watch for distended veins in the neck and hands.
○ Restrict fluids.
○ Offer emotional support to the patient and family.

Drug therapy
○ Digoxin
○ Diuretics
○ Morphine
○ Nitroglycerin
○ Oxygen

Monitoring
○ Arterial blood gas values
○ Heart sounds (for an S_3)
○ Intake and output
○ Oxygenation
○ Respiratory status
○ Serum potassium level
○ Vital signs
○ Weight

Patient teaching
Be sure to cover:
○ the disorder, diagnosis, and treatment plan
○ all procedures and their purposes
○ the purpose of all equipment, including cardiac monitoring
○ prescribed drugs and their possible adverse effects
○ fluid and sodium restrictions
○ warning signs of hypervolemia and when to report them.

Electrolyte basics

Charges

Ions

○ Electrolytes are substances that, when in solution, separate (or dissociate) into electrically charged particles called ions.
○ Some ions carry a positive charge. Others carry a negative charge.
○ Several pairs of oppositely charged ions are so closely linked that a problem with one ion causes a problem with the other. Examples include the sodium-chloride pair and the calcium-phosphorus pair.

Anions and cations

○ Anions are electrolytes that generate a negative charge.
○ Chloride, phosphorus, and bicarbonate are anions. (See *Understanding electrolytes*.)
○ Cations are electrolytes that generate a positive charge.
○ Sodium, potassium, calcium, and magnesium are cations.

▽ **ALERT** *The anion gap is a useful test for distinguishing types and causes of acid-base imbalances because it reflects the serum anion-cation balance.*

○ An electrical charge makes cells function normally.
○ Electrolytes exist in extracellular and intracellular fluid compartments.
○ Individual electrolytes differ in concentration, but the totals balance to reach a neutral electrical charge. This balance is called electroneutrality.
○ Most electrolytes interact with hydrogen ions to maintain acid-base balance. The major electrolytes also have specialized functions that contribute to metabolism and fluid and electrolyte balance.

Electrolyte locations

Extracellular electrolytes

○ Sodium, chloride, calcium, and bicarbonate are mainly in extracellular fluid.
○ Sodium affects serum osmolality (solute concentration in 1 L of water) and extracellular fluid volume. It also helps nerve and muscle cells interact.

Understanding electrolytes

Electrolytes help regulate water distribution, govern acid-base balance, and transmit nerve impulses. They also contribute to energy generation and blood clotting. You'll find summaries of the body's major electrolytes below. Check the illustration to see how electrolytes are distributed in and around the cell.

Potassium (K+)
● The main intracellular fluid (ICF) cation
● Regulates cell excitability
● Permeates cell membranes, thereby affecting the cell's electrical status
● Helps control ICF osmolality and, consequently, ICF osmotic pressure

Magnesium (Mg++)
● A leading ICF cation
● Contributes to many enzymatic and metabolic processes, particularly protein synthesis
● Modifies nerve impulse transmission and skeletal muscle response (unbalanced Mg++ concentrations dramatically affect neuromuscular processes)

Phosphorus (P+)
● The main ICF anion
● Promotes energy storage and carbohydrate, protein, and fat metabolism
● Acts as a hydrogen buffer

Sodium (Na+)
● The main extracellular fluid (ECF) cation
● Helps govern normal ECF osmolality (A shift in Na+ concentration triggers a fluid volume change to restore normal solute and water ratios.)
● Helps maintain acid-base balance
● Activates nerve and muscle cells
● Influences water distribution (with chloride)

Chloride (Cl−)
● The main ECF anion
● Helps maintain normal ECF osmolality
● Affects the body's pH
● Plays a vital role in maintaining acid-base balance; combines with hydrogen ions to produce hydrochloric acid

Calcium (Ca+)
● A major cation in teeth and bones
● Found in fairly equal concentrations in ICF and ECF
● Also found in cell membranes, where it helps cells adhere to one another and maintain their shape
● Acts as an enzyme activator in cells (muscles must have Ca+ to contract)
● Aids coagulation
● Affects cell membrane permeability and firing level

Bicarbonate (HCO3−)
● Present in ECF
● Functions mainly to regulate acid-base balance

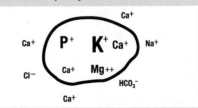

- Chloride helps maintain osmotic (water-pulling) pressure. Gastric mucosal cells need chloride to produce hydrochloric acid.
- Calcium is the major cation involved in the structure and function of bones and teeth and also helps to:
  - stabilize the cell membrane and reduce its permeability to sodium
  - transmit nerve impulses
  - contract muscles
  - coagulate blood.
- Bicarbonate plays a vital role in acid-base balance.

Intracellular electrolytes

- Potassium, phosphate, and magnesium are among the most abundant electrolytes inside the cell.
- Potassium plays an important role in several processes:
  - cell excitability regulation
  - nerve impulse conduction
  - resting membrane potential
  - muscle contraction and myocardial membrane responsiveness
  - intracellular osmolality control.
- Phosphorus occurs in the body as phosphate salts. Sometimes the words phosphorus and phosphate are used interchangeably. Phosphate is essential for energy metabolism. Combined with calcium, it plays a key role in bone and tooth mineralization. It also helps maintain acid-base balance.
- Magnesium acts as a catalyst for enzyme reactions. It also:
  - regulates neuromuscular contraction
  - promotes normal functioning of the nervous and cardiovascular systems
  - aids in protein synthesis and sodium and potassium ion transportation.

Electrolyte movement and balance

- Although electrolytes are concentrated in one compartment or another, they aren't locked or frozen in these areas. Like fluids, electrolytes move about trying to maintain balance and electroneutrality.
- Fluid intake and output, acid-base balance, hormone secretion, and normal cell functioning all influence electrolyte balance.
- Because electrolytes function both with other electrolytes and individually, imbalances in one electrolyte can affect the balance of others.

Electrolyte measurement

- Only levels of extracellular electrolytes are measured.
- The patient's condition determines how often electrolyte levels are checked.

- Results for many laboratory tests are reported in milliequivalents per liter (mEq/L), which is a measure of the ion's chemical activity or its power.

▶ **ALERT** *Although serum electrolyte levels remain fairly stable throughout a person's life span, understanding which levels are normal and which are abnormal is critical to reacting quickly and appropriately to an imbalance. If you see an abnormal laboratory test result, consider it in the context of what you know about the patient. For instance, a serum potassium level of 7 mEq/L for a patient with previously normal serum potassium levels and no apparent reason for the increase may be an inaccurate result. Perhaps the patient's blood sample was hemolyzed from trauma to the cells.*

Potassium

Overview

○ Potassium is the major cation (ion with a positive charge) in intracellular fluid.
○ About 98% of the body's potassium is found in intracellular fluid; about 2% is found in extracellular fluid.

ALERT Potassium levels are affected by disease, injury, drugs, and treatments. Small untreated changes in the serum potassium level can seriously affect neuromuscular and cardiac functioning.

○ Potassium directly affects cell, nerve, and muscle function by:
  – maintaining the electrical neutrality and osmolality of cells
  – aiding neuromuscular transmission of nerve impulses
  – assisting skeletal and cardiac muscle contraction and electrical conductivity
  – affecting acid-base balance in relationship to hydrogen, another cation. (See *Potassium's role in acid-base balance.*)
○ Potassium levels normally range from 3.5 to 5 mEq/L in serum and typically are 140 mEq/L in cells (a level usually not measured).
○ Potassium must be ingested daily because the body can't conserve it.
○ Recommended daily potassium requirement for adults is about 40 mEq; average daily intake is 60 to 100 mEq.

○ Extracellular fluid also gains potassium when cells are destroyed and release intracellular potassium and when potassium shifts out of intracellular fluid and into extracellular fluid.
○ About 80% of ingested potassium is excreted in urine, with each liter of urine containing 20 to 40 mEq of potassium. Any remaining potassium is excreted in feces and sweat.
○ Extracellular potassium also is lost when it moves from extracellular fluid into intracellular fluid and when cells undergo anabolism.
○ Three more factors that affect potassium levels include the sodium-potassium pump, renal regulation, and pH level.

Balance

○ The sodium-potassium pump is an active transport mechanism that moves ions across cell membranes against a concentration gradient.
○ The pump moves sodium from the cell into extracellular fluid and maintains high intracellular potassium levels by pumping potassium into the cell.
○ The body discards excess potassium via the kidneys. As serum potassium levels rise, the renal tubules excrete more of it, leading to increased potassium loss in the urine.
○ Sodium and potassium have a reciprocal relationship. The kidneys reabsorb sodium and excrete potassium when the hormone aldosterone is secreted.
○ The kidneys have no effective way to combat potassium loss and may excrete it even when the serum potassium level is low.

Potassium's role in acid-base balance

Normal balance
Under normal conditions, the potassium ion (K+) content in intracellular fluid is much greater than in extracellular fluid. Hydrogen ion (H+) concentration is low in both compartments.

Acidosis
In acidosis, the hydrogen ion content in extracellular fluid increases and the ions move into the intracellular fluid. To keep the intracellular fluid electrically neutral, an equal number of potassium ions leave the cell, which causes hyperkalemia.

Alkalosis
In alkalosis, more hydrogen ions are present in intracellular fluid than in the extracellular fluid. Therefore, hydrogen ions move from the intracellular fluid into the extracellular fluid. To keep the intracellular fluid electrically neutral, potassium ions move from the extracellular fluid into the intracellular fluid, which causes hypokalemia.

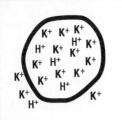

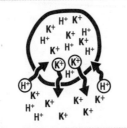

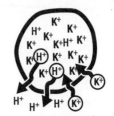

○ A change in pH may affect serum potassium levels because hydrogen ions and potassium ions freely exchange across plasma cell membranes.
○ In acidosis, excess hydrogen ions move into cells and push potassium into the extracellular fluid, which may lead to hyperkalemia as potassium moves out of the cell to maintain balance.
○ In alkalosis, potassium moves into the cell to maintain balance, which may lead to hypokalemia.

▼ **ALERT** *Potassium is gained by intake and lost by excretion. If either is altered, hyperkalemia or hypokalemia may result.*

Dietary sources

○ The Food and Nutrition Board of the National Academy of Sciences recommends 2,000 mg as the minimum daily potassium requirement for men and women older than age 18.
○ A good food source of potassium contains at least 200 mg of potassium in a serving size.
○ Potassium is lost in cooking; therefore, foods should be cooked in a minimum of water and for the shortest possible time.
○ Major sources of potassium include:
  – bread, cereals, and other grain products
  – chocolate
  – dried fruit
  – fruits, such as oranges, bananas, apricots, cantaloupe, watermelon, peaches, and prunes
  – meat and fish
  – milk
  – nuts
  – seeds
  – vegetables, such as squash, potatoes, mushrooms, tomatoes, lima beans, and cauliflower.

Sodium

Overview

○ Sodium is one of the most important elements in the body.

○ It accounts for 90% of extracellular fluid cations (positively charged ions) and is the most abundant solute in extracellular fluid. Almost all sodium in the body is found in this fluid.

○ Sodium attracts fluid and helps preserve the extracellular fluid volume and fluid distribution in the body. It's needed to maintain proper extracellular fluid osmolality (concentration).

○ Sodium helps transmit impulses in nerve and muscle fibers and combines with chloride and bicarbonate to regulate acid-base balance.

○ Because the electrolyte compositions of serum and interstitial fluid are essentially equal, the sodium concentration in extracellular fluid is measured in serum levels.

○ Normally, the sodium level ranges from 135 to 145 mEq/L. The amount of sodium inside the cells is 10 mEq/L.

Balance

○ Sodium levels stay fairly constant because the more sodium a person takes in, the more sodium the kidneys excrete.

○ Sodium is also excreted through the gastrointestinal tract and in sweat.

○ The normal range of serum sodium levels reflects the relationship between sodium and water. If sodium intake suddenly increases, extracellular fluid concentration also rises, and vice versa.

○ The body makes adjustments when the sodium level rises. Increased serum sodium levels cause thirst and prompt the posterior pituitary gland to release antidiuretic hormone (ADH).

○ ADH cues the kidneys to retain water, which dilutes the blood and normalizes serum osmolality.

○ When serum osmolality decreases and thirst and ADH secretion decline, the kidneys excrete more water to maintain normal osmolality. (See *Regulating sodium and water balance.*)

○ Aldosterone also regulates extracellular sodium balance via a feedback loop. The adrenal cortex secretes aldosterone, which stimulates the renal tubules to conserve water and sodium when the sodium level is low, thus helping to normalize extracellular fluid sodium levels.

Regulating sodium and water balance

This flowchart show two of the body's mechanisms for maintaining and restoring sodium and water balance.

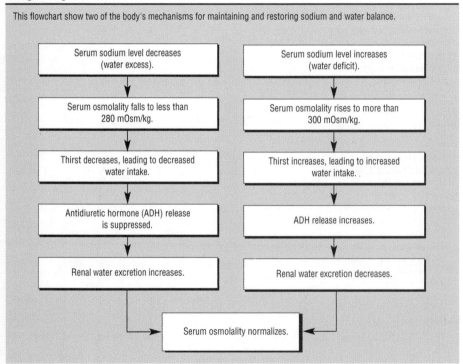

Sodium-potassium pump

Here's how the sodium-potassium pump works. Normally, more sodium (Na+) ions exist outside cells than inside, and more potassium (K+) ions exist inside the cells than outside, as shown on the left. When something increases the membrane's permeability, sodium ions diffuse inward and potassium ions diffuse outward, as shown in the middle. Ions return to their original positions through the cell wall by being linked with a carrier molecule, as shown on the right. Energy for the ions' return trip comes from adenosine triphosphate (ATP), magnesium (Mg++), and an enzyme commonly found in cells.

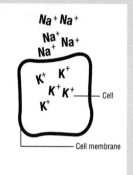

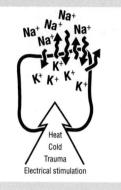

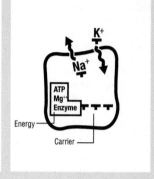

○ Normally, extracellular sodium levels are much higher than intracellular levels. An active transport mechanism called the sodium-potassium pump helps maintain normal sodium levels. (See *Sodium-potassium pump.*)

○ The sodium-potassium pump allows the body to carry out its essential functions and helps prevent cellular swelling from too many ions inside the cell attracting excessive amounts of water. The pump also creates an electrical charge in the cell from the movement of ions, permitting transmission of neuromuscular impulses.

Dietary sources

○ The Food and Nutrition Board of the National Academy of Sciences recommends a minimum daily sodium requirement of 2,300 mg for men and women older than age 18.

○ Sodium may need to be restricted because the average American diet provides at least 6 g of sodium daily. Dietary restrictions should be recommended by a doctor.

○ Salt is 40% sodium by weight. One teaspoon of salt contains 2,400 mg of sodium.

○ Major sources of sodium:
  – butter
  – cheese
  – cold cuts
  – ketchup
  – margarine
  – nuts
  – processed foods to which sodium chloride (salt), benzoate, or phosphate has been added
  – salt added while cooking or eating
  – salted meats.

Magnesium

Overview

- After potassium, magnesium is the most abundant cation (positively charged ion) in intracellular fluid.
- About 60% of the body's magnesium is contained in bones, less than 1% in extracellular fluid, and the rest in intracellular fluid.
- Magnesium performs the following functions in the body:
  – It promotes enzyme reactions in the cells during carbohydrate metabolism.
  – It helps the body produce and use adenosine triphosphate for energy.
  – It takes part in protein synthesis.
  – It influences vasodilation, helping the cardiovascular system function normally.
  – It helps sodium and potassium ions cross cell membranes (which explains why magnesium affects sodium and potassium ion levels both inside and outside the cell).
  – It regulates muscle contractions by acting on the myoneural junctions — the sites where nerve and muscle fibers meet — and affecting the irritability and contractility of cardiac and skeletal muscle.
  – It influences the body's calcium level through its effect on parathyroid hormone, which maintains a constant calcium level in extracellular fluid.
- Normally, the total serum magnesium level is 1.6 to 2.6 mEq/L. However, the measured level may not accurately reflect magnesium stores. That's because most magnesium is found in cells, where it measures about 40 mEq/L. In serum, magnesium levels are relatively low.

Effects of hypomagnesmia

Dysfunction	Effects
Cardiovascular	Arrhythmias Hypertension (occasionally) Vasomotor changes (vasodilation and hypotension)
Neurologic	Confusion Delusions Hallucinations Seizures
Neuromuscular	Chvostek's sign (facial muscle spasms when branches of the facial nerve are tapped) Hyperirritability Leg and foot cramps Tetany

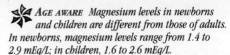 *AGE AWARE Magnesium levels in newborns and children are different from those of adults. In newborns, magnesium levels range from 1.4 to 2.9 mEq/L; in children, 1.6 to 2.6 mEq/L.*

- More than half of circulating magnesium moves in a free, ionized form. Another 30% binds with a protein (mostly albumin), and the remainder binds with other substances.
- Ionized magnesium is physiologically active and must be regulated to maintain homeostasis. However, this form alone can't be measured, so the measured level reflects the total amount of circulating magnesium.

ALERT Magnesium levels are linked to albumin levels. A patient with a low serum albumin level will have a low total serum magnesium level — even if the level of ionized magnesium remains unchanged. That's why serum albumin levels need to be measured with serum magnesium levels.

- Serum calcium and certain other laboratory values also come into play when assessing and treating magnesium imbalances. Because magnesium is mainly an intracellular electrolyte, changes in the levels of other intracellular electrolytes, such as potassium and phosphorus, can affect serum magnesium levels, too.

Balance

- The gastrointestinal (GI) and urinary systems regulate magnesium through absorption, excretion, and retention — that is, through dietary intake and output in urine and feces.
- The body tries to adjust to any changes in magnesium level.
  – If the serum magnesium level drops, the GI tract may absorb more magnesium.
  – If the serum magnesium level rises, the GI tract excretes more magnesium in the feces.
- The kidneys balance magnesium by altering its reabsorption at the proximal tubule and loop of Henle.
  – If serum magnesium levels climb, the kidneys excrete the excess in the urine. Diuretics heighten this effect.
  – If serum magnesium levels fall, the kidneys conserve magnesium. That conservation is so efficient that the daily loss of circulating ionized magnesium may be no more than 1 mEq.
- If magnesium levels become deficient, a range of clinical effects results. (See *Effects of hypomagnesemia.*)

Dietary sources

- The Food and Nutrition Board of the National Academy of Sciences recommends a minimum daily magnesium requirement of 310 to 420 mg for men and women older than age 18.

○ Major sources of magnesium include:
  – chocolate
  – dry beans and peas
  – fruits, such as avocados, bananas, and kiwi
  – green vegetables, such as spinach
  – meats
  – nuts
  – seafood
  – seeds
  – whole grains.

Calcium

Overview

- Calcium is a positively charged ion, or cation, found in both extracellular fluid and intracellular fluid.
- About 99% of the body's calcium is found in the bones and the teeth. Only 1% is found in serum and soft tissue. That 1% is what matters when measuring calcium levels in the blood.
- Calcium functions in the following ways:
  - It's responsible for the formation and structure of bones and teeth.
  - It helps maintain cell structure and function.
  - It plays a role in cell membrane permeability and impulse transmission.
  - It affects the contraction of cardiac muscle, smooth muscle, and skeletal muscle.
  - It participates in the blood-clotting process.
- Calcium can be measured in two ways:
  - total serum calcium level, which measures the total amount of calcium in the blood
  - ionized calcium level, which measures the various forms of calcium in extracellular fluid.
- The normal range for total serum calcium level is 8.9 to 10.1 mg/dl.
- The normal range for ionized calcium level is 4.5 to 5.1 mg/dl.
- Ionized calcium carries out most of the ion's physiologic functions.
- About 41% of extracellular calcium is bound to protein; 9% is bound to citrate or other organic ions.

Calculating calcium and albumin levels

For every 1 g/dl that a noncritically ill patient's serum albumin level drops, his total calcium level decreases by 0.8 mg/dl. To see what your patient's calcium level would be if his serum albumin level were normal—and to help determine if treatment is justified—just do a little math.

Correcting a level
The normal albumin level is 4 g/dl. The formula for correcting a patient's calcium level is:

Total serum calcium level + 0.8 (4 – albumin level) = corrected calcium level

Sample problem
For example, if a patient's serum calcium level is 8.2 mg/dl and his albumin level is 3 g/dl, what would his corrected calcium be?

8.2 + 0.8 (4 – 3) = 9 mg/dl

The corrected calcium level is in the normal range and probably wouldn't be treated.

About half is ionized (or free) calcium, the only active form of calcium.

AGE AWARE Children have higher serum calcium levels than adults. These levels can rise as high as 7 mg/dl during periods of increased growth. In contrast, elderly people have a decreased normal range. For elderly men, the range is 2.3 to 3.7 mg/dl; for elderly women, it's 2.8 to 4.1 mg/dl.

ALERT Because nearly half of all calcium is bound to the protein albumin, serum protein abnormalities can influence total serum calcium levels. For example, in hypoalbuminemia, the total serum calcium level decreases. However, ionized calcium levels—the more important of the two—remain unchanged. So when considering total serum calcium levels, you should also consider serum albumin levels. (See Calculating calcium and albumin levels.)

Balance

- Both intake of dietary calcium and existing stores of calcium affect calcium levels in the body.
- Calcium is absorbed in the small intestine and is excreted in the urine and feces.
- When serum calcium levels are low, the parathyroid glands release parathyroid hormone (PTH).
  - PTH draws calcium from the bones and promotes the transfer of calcium (and phosphorus) into the plasma, a process that increases serum calcium levels.
  - PTH also promotes reabsorption of calcium by the kidneys and stimulates absorption by the intestines. Phosphorus is excreted at the same time. In hypercalcemia, the body suppresses PTH release.
- Calcitonin also helps to regulate calcium levels. A hormone, calcitonin is produced in the thyroid gland and acts as an antagonist to PTH.
  - High levels of calcitonin inhibit bone resorption, which decreases the amount of calcium available from bone and, in turn, decreases the serum calcium level.
  - Calcitonin also decreases absorption of calcium and enhances its excretion by the kidneys.
- Vitamin D also influences calcium levels.
  - Vitamin D is ingested with foods, particularly dairy products.
  - Skin exposed to ultraviolet light synthesizes vitamin D.
  - The active form of vitamin D promotes calcium absorption through the intestines, resorption from bone, and kidney reabsorption, all of which raise the serum calcium level. (See *Calcium in balance.*)
- Phosphorus also affects serum calcium levels.
  - Phosphorus inhibits calcium absorption in the intestines, the opposite effect of vitamin D.

– When calcium levels are low and the kidneys retain calcium, phosphorus is excreted.

ALERT *Calcium and phosphorus exist in inverse relationship. When calcium levels rise, phosphorus levels drop. When calcium levels drop, phosphorus levels rise.*

○ Serum pH has an inverse relationship with the ionized calcium level. If serum pH level rises (the blood becomes alkaline), more calcium binds with protein and the ionized calcium level drops. Thus, a patient with alkalosis typically has hypocalcemia.
○ The opposite is true for acidosis. When the pH level drops, less calcium binds to protein, and the ionized calcium level rises. When all those regulatory efforts fail to control the level of calcium in the body, one of two conditions may result: hypocalcemia or hypercalcemia.

Dietary sources

○ For adults, the recommended daily calcium requirement is 800 to 1,200 mg. Recommendations vary for children, pregnant women, and patients being treated for osteoporosis.
○ Major sources of calcium include:
   – beans
   – bonemeal
   – dairy products, such as milk, cheese, and yogurt
   – fish with edible bones, such as sardines
   – green, leafy vegetables
   – legumes
   – molasses
   – nuts
   – orange juice fortified with calcium
   – whole grains.

Calcium in balance

Normally, several interrelated processes maintain extracellular calcium levels by moving calcium ions into and out of extracellular fluid. Calcium enters the extracellular space through resorption of calcium ions from bone, absorption of dietary calcium in the gastrointestinal (GI) tract, and reabsorption of calcium by the kidneys. Calcium leaves extracellular fluid by being excreted in feces and urine and deposited in bone. This illustration shows how calcium moves through the body.

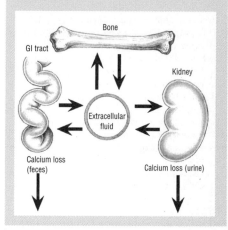

Phosphorus

Overview

○ Phosphorus is the main anion, or negatively charged ion, in intracellular fluid.
○ It's also known as phosphate.
○ About 85% of phosphorus is in bone and teeth, combined in a 1:2 ratio with calcium. About 14% is in soft tissue, and less than 1% is in extracellular fluid.
○ An essential element of all body tissues, phosphorus is vital to various body functions. It plays a crucial role in:
  – cell membrane integrity (phospholipids make up cell membranes)
  – muscle function
  – neurologic function
  – metabolism of carbohydrate, fat, and protein
  – buffering of acids and bases
  – promotion of energy transfer to cells through the formation of energy-storing substances such as adenosine triphosphate
  – white blood cell phagocytosis
  – platelet function.
○ Phosphorus is a primary ingredient in 2,3-diphosphoglycerate, a compound in red blood cells (RBCs) that facilitates oxygen delivery from RBCs to the tissues.
○ Normally, serum phosphorus levels range from 2.5 to 4.5 mg/dl (or 1.8 to 2.6 mEq/L) in adults. The normal cellular level is 100 mEq/L.
○ Because phosphorus is located mainly inside the cells, serum levels may not always reflect the total amount of phosphorus in the body.

Balance

○ The total amount of phosphorus in the body is related to dietary intake, hormonal regulation, kidney excretion, and transcellular shifts.

○ Most ingested phosphorus is absorbed through the jejunum.
○ The kidneys excrete about 90% of phosphorus as they regulate serum levels. The gastrointestinal (GI) tract excretes the rest.
○ If dietary intake of phosphorus increases, the kidneys increase excretion to maintain normal levels of phosphorus. A low-phosphorus diet causes the kidneys to reabsorb more phosphorus in the proximal tubules in order to conserve it.
○ The parathyroid gland controls hormonal regulation of phosphorus levels by affecting the activity of parathyroid hormone (PTH). (See *Parathyroid hormone and phosphorus.*)
  – Changes in calcium levels, rather than changes in phosphorus levels, affect the release of PTH.
  – Normally, calcium and phosphorus have an inverse relationship: If one is elevated, the other is decreased.
  – When the serum calcium level is low, the phosphorus level is high.
  – PTH release increases calcium and phosphorus resorption from bone, raising both calcium and phosphorus levels. Phosphorus absorption from the intestines is also increased. (Activated vitamin D — calcitriol — also enhances its absorption in the intestines.)
  – PTH then acts on the kidneys to increase excretion of phosphorus.
  – Reduced PTH levels allow for phosphorus reabsorption by the kidneys. As a result, serum levels rise.
○ Certain conditions cause phosphorus to shift in and out of cells.
  – Insulin moves not only glucose but also phosphorus into the cell.
  – Alkalosis results in the same kind of phosphorus shift.

✴ *AGE AWARE Elderly patients are at risk for altered electrolyte levels for two main reasons. First, they have a lower ratio of lean body weight to total body weight, which places them at risk for water deficits. Second, their thirst response and renal function are decreased, which makes maintaining elec-*

Parathyroid hormone and phosphorus

This illustration shows how parathyroid hormone (PTH) affects serum phosphorus (P+) levels — by increasing phosphorus release from bone, increasing phosphorus absorption from the intestines, and decreasing phosphorus reabsorption in the renal tubules.

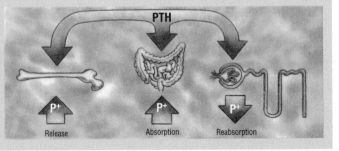

PTH

Release   Absorption   Reabsorption

trolyte balance more difficult. Age-related renal changes affects renal blood flow and glomerular filtration rate. Drugs also may alter electrolyte levels by affecting phosphate absorption. Ask all elderly patients if they take over-the-counter medications, such as antacids, laxatives, herbs, and teas.

Dietary sources

○ The recommended daily phosphorus requirement is 800 to 1,200 mg for adults.
○ Phosphorus is readily absorbed through the GI tract, and the amount absorbed is proportional to the amount ingested.
○ Major dietary sources of phosphorous include:
  – cheese
  – dried beans
  – eggs
  – fish
  – milk products
  – nuts
  – organ meats, such as brain and liver
  – poultry
  – seeds
  – whole grains.

Chloride

Overview

- Chloride is the most abundant anion (negatively charged ion) in extracellular fluid.
- High chloride levels are found in cerebrospinal fluid (CSF), but the anion can also be found in bile and in gastric and pancreatic juices.
- It moves into and out of cells with sodium and potassium.
- Chloride combines with major cations (positively charged ions) to form sodium chloride, hydrochloric acid, potassium chloride, calcium chloride, and other important compounds.
- Because of its negative charge, chloride travels with positively charged sodium and helps maintain serum osmolality and water balance.
- Chloride and sodium also work together to form CSF. The choroid plexus, a tangled mass of tiny blood vessels in the ventricles of the brain, depends on these two electrolytes to attract water and to form the fluid component of CSF.
- In the stomach, chloride is secreted by the gastric mucosa as hydrochloric acid, creating the acid environment conducive to digestion and enzyme activation.
- Chloride helps maintain acid-base balance and assists in carbon dioxide transport in red blood cells.
- Serum chloride levels have a normal range of 96 to 106 mEq/L. The chloride level in cells is 4 mEq/L.

✻ *AGE AWARE Patients between ages 60 and 90 have chloride levels between 98 and 107 mEq/L; patients age 90 and older, between 98 and 111 mEq/L.*

Chloride and bicarbonate

Chloride and bicarbonate have an inverse relationship. When the level of one goes up, the level of the other goes down.

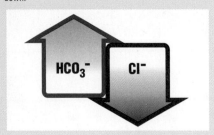

- Chloride levels remain relatively stable with age. Because chloride balance relates closely to sodium balance, the levels of both electrolytes usually change in direct proportion to one another.
- Three types of diuretics increase the risk of chloride deficiency:
  - loop diuretics, such as furosemide
  - osmotic diuretics, such as mannitol
  - thiazide diuretics, such as hydrochlorothiazide.

Balance

- Chloride regulation depends on intake and excretion of chloride and reabsorption of chloride ions in the kidneys.
- Most chloride is absorbed in the intestines, with only a small portion lost in the feces.
- Chloride is produced mainly in the stomach as hydrochloric acid, so chloride levels can be influenced by gastrointestinal disorders.
- Because chloride and sodium are closely linked, a change in one electrolyte level causes a comparable change in the other.
- Chloride levels can be indirectly affected by aldosterone secretion, which causes the renal tubules to reabsorb sodium.
  - As positively charged sodium ions are reabsorbed, negatively charged chloride ions are passively reabsorbed because of their electrical attraction to sodium.
- Regulation of chloride levels also involves acid-base balance.
  - Chloride is reabsorbed and excreted in direct opposition to bicarbonate.
  - When chloride levels change, the body attempts to keep its positive-negative balance by making corresponding changes in levels of bicarbonate (another negatively charged ion) in the kidneys.
  - When chloride levels decrease, the kidneys retain bicarbonate, and bicarbonate levels increase.
  - When chloride levels increase, the kidneys excrete bicarbonate, and bicarbonate levels decrease.
  - Changes in chloride and bicarbonate levels can lead to acidosis or alkalosis. (See *Chloride and bicarbonate*.)

Dietary sources

- The daily chloride requirement for adults is 750 mg.
- Most diets provide sufficient chloride, usually as sodium chloride (table salt) in the same foods that contain sodium.

○ Major sources of chloride include:
  – canned vegetables
  – fruits
  – processed meats
  – salty foods
  – table salt
  – vegetables.

Acid-base balance

Overview

pH

○ pH is a calculation based on the percentage of hydrogen ions in a solution and the amount of acids and bases in the solution. (See *Normal pH.*)
○ A solution with a pH below 7 is an acid.
○ A solution with a pH above 7 is a base.
○ A patient's acid-base balance can be assessed if you know the pH of his blood.
○ Arterial blood is usually used to measure pH.
○ If the hydrogen ion concentration of the blood increases or the bicarbonate level decreases, pH may decrease. A decrease in pH below 7.35 signals acidosis.
○ If the bicarbonate level increases or the hydrogen ion concentration of the blood decreases, pH may increase. An increase in pH above 7.45 signals alkalosis.

Acids

○ Acids are molecules that can give up hydrogen ions to other molecules.
○ Carbonic acid is an acid that occurs naturally in the body.
○ A solution that contains more acid than base has more hydrogen ions, so it has a lower pH.

Bases

○ Bases are molecules that can accept hydrogen ions
○ Bicarbonate is one example of a base.
○ A solution that contains more base than acid has fewer hydrogen ions, so it has a higher pH.

▲ **ALERT** *A change in pH can compromise essential body processes, including electrolyte balance, the activity of critical enzymes, muscle contraction, and basic cellular function.*

Regulatory systems

○ The body responds to acid-base imbalances by activating compensatory mechanisms that minimize pH changes.
○ If the body compensates only partially for an imbalance, pH will still be outside the normal range. If the body compensates fully or completely, pH will be back to normal.
○ Returning the pH to a normal or near-normal level mainly involves changes in the component — metabolic or respiratory — not primarily affected by the imbalance.
○ When pH rises or falls, three regulatory systems come into play:
  – Chemical buffers act immediately to protect tissues and cells. They combine with the offending acid or base, neutralizing harmful effects until other regulators take over.
  – The respiratory system uses hypoventilation or hyperventilation to regulate excretion or retention of acids within minutes of a change in pH.
  – The kidneys excrete or retain more acids or bases as needed to restore a normal hydrogen ion concentration within hours or days.

Chemical buffers

○ The bicarbonate-buffer system is the body's primary buffer system and works mainly in blood and interstitial fluid.
  – This system relies on a series of chemical reactions in which pairs of weak acids and bases (such as carbonic acid and bicarbonate) combine with stronger acids (such as hydrochloric acid) and bases to weaken them.
  – Decreasing the strength of potentially damaging acids and bases reduces the danger those chemicals pose to pH balance.
  – The kidneys assist the bicarbonate-buffer system in regulating production of bicarbonate.
  – The lungs assist by regulating production of carbonic acid, which results from combining carbon dioxide and water.
○ Like the bicarbonate-buffer system, the phosphate-buffer system also depends on a series of chemical reactions to minimize pH changes.
  – Phosphate buffers react with either acids or bases to form compounds that slightly alter pH, which can provide extremely effective buffering.
  – This system proves especially effective in renal tubules, where phosphates exist in greater concentrations.
○ Protein buffers, the most plentiful buffers in the body, work inside and outside cells.
  – These buffers are made up of hemoglobin and other proteins.
  – Protein buffers bind with acids and bases to neutralize them. In red blood cells, for instance, hemoglobin combines with hydrogen ions to act as a buffer.

Respiratory buffers

○ The respiratory system serves as the second line of defense against acid-base imbalances.
○ The lungs regulate blood levels of carbon dioxide, a gas that combines with water to form carbonic acid. Increased levels of carbonic acid decrease pH.
○ Chemoreceptors in the medulla of the brain sense pH changes and vary the rate and depth of breathing to compensate.

▲ **ALERT** *Breathing faster or deeper eliminates more carbon dioxide from the lungs, which decreases the amount of carbonic acid made. As a result, pH rises. The body normalizes such a pH change by breathing slower or less deeply, reducing carbon dioxide excretion.*

- To assess the effectiveness of ventilation, look at the partial pressure of carbon dioxide in arterial blood ($Paco_2$). Normally, $Paco_2$ is 35 to 45 mm Hg. $Paco_2$ values reflect carbon dioxide levels in the blood. As those levels increase, so does $Paco_2$.
- As a buffer, the respiratory system can maintain acid-base balance twice as effectively as can chemical buffers because it can handle twice the amount of acids and bases.

AGE AWARE The respiratory system of an older adult may be compromised and less able to regulate acid-base balance.

- Although the respiratory system responds to pH changes within minutes, it can restore normal pH only temporarily. The kidneys are responsible for long-term adjustments to pH.

ALERT If a lack of bicarbonate causes acidosis, the rate of breathing increases, which blows off carbon dioxide and helps to raise the pH to normal. If an excess of bicarbonate causes alkalosis, the rate of breathing decreases, which retains carbon dioxide and helps lower the pH.

Renal buffers

- The kidneys maintain acid-base balance by reabsorbing acids and bases or excreting them into urine.
- They can also produce bicarbonate to replenish lost supplies. Such adjustments to pH take the kidneys hours to days to complete.
- The kidneys also regulate the bicarbonate level, which reflects the metabolic component of acid-base balance.
  - The bicarbonate level typically is reported with arterial blood gas results.
  - A normal bicarbonate level is 22 to 26 mEq/L.
  - Bicarbonate is also reported with serum electrolyte levels as total serum carbon dioxide content.
- If the blood contains too much acid or not enough base, the pH drops and the kidneys reabsorb sodium bicarbonate.
- The kidneys also excrete hydrogen along with phosphate or ammonia. Although urine tends to be acidic because the body usually produces slightly more acids than bases, in such situations urine becomes more acidic than normal.

AGE AWARE Because ammonia production decreases with age, the kidneys of an older adult can't handle excess acid as well as the kidneys of a younger adult.

- The reabsorption of bicarbonate and the increased excretion of hydrogen causes more bicarbonate to be formed in the renal tubules and eventually retained in the body. The bicarbonate level in the blood then rises to a more normal level, increasing pH.

Normal pH

This illustration shows that the blood pH normally stays slightly alkaline, between 7.35 and 7.45, a point at which the amount of acid (H) is balanced with the amount of base (bicarbonate). Typically, pH is maintained in a ratio of 20 parts bicarbonate to 1 part carbonic acid. A pH below 7.35 is abnormally acidic; a pH above 7.45, abnormally alkaline. A pH below 6.8 or above 7.8 typically is fatal.

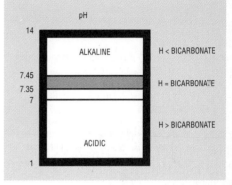

- If the blood contains more base and less acid, pH rises. The kidneys compensate by excreting bicarbonate and retaining more hydrogen ions. Urine becomes more alkaline, and the blood bicarbonate level drops. Conversely, if the blood contains less bicarbonate and more acid, the pH drops.

ALERT If the respiratory system disturbs the acid-base balance, the kidneys can compensate by altering levels of bicarbonate and hydrogen ions. When the $Paco_2$ is high (acidosis), the kidneys retain bicarbonate and excrete more acid to raise the pH. When the $Paco_2$ level is low (alkalosis), the kidneys excrete bicarbonate and hold on to more acid to lower the pH.

Fluid and electrolyte replacement

Isotonic solutions

○ Isotonic crystalloids
- These solutions contain about the same concentration of osmotically active particles as extracellular fluid.
- Fluid doesn't shift between the extracellular and intracellular areas.
○ Dextrose 5% in water (D_5W)
- D_5W has an osmolality (or concentration) of 275 to 295 mOsm/L.
- The dextrose metabolizes quickly, acting like a hypotonic solution and leaving water behind.
- Large amounts of D_5W may cause hyperglycemia.
○ Normal saline solution
- This solution contains only the electrolytes sodium and chloride.
○ Other isotonic fluids
- These fluids are more like extracellular fluid.
- Ringer's solution contains sodium, potassium, calcium, and chloride.
- Lactated Ringer's solution contains those electrolytes plus lactate, which the liver converts to bicarbonate.

Hypotonic fluids

○ Hypotonic crystalloids
- These solutions are less concentrated than extracellular fluid.

- They move from the bloodstream into the cell, causing the cell to swell.
○ Hypotonic fluids have an osmolality of less than 275 mOsm/L.
○ Examples of hypotonic fluids include half-normal saline solution, 0.33% sodium chloride solution, and dextrose 2.5% in water.
○ Hypotonic solutions should be given cautiously because fluid moves from the extracellular space into cells, causing them to swell and increasing the risk of cardiovascular collapse from vascular fluid depletion.
○ These solutions also can cause increased intracranial pressure (ICP) from fluid shifting into brain cells.
- They shouldn't be given to a patient at risk for increased ICP—for example, a patient who has had a cerebrovascular accident, head trauma, or neurosurgery.
- Signs of increased ICP include a change in the patient's level of consciousness; motor or sensory deficits; and changes in pupil size, shape, or response to light.
○ Hypotonic solutions also shouldn't be used for patients who have abnormal fluid shifts into the interstitial space or the body cavities—for example, as a result of liver disease, a burn, or trauma.

Hypertonic solutions

○ Hypertonic crystalloids
- These solutions are more highly concentrated than extracellular fluid.
- Fluid moves into the bloodstream from the cells, causing the cells to shrink. (See *Comparing fluid tonicity.*)

Comparing fluid tonicity

The illustrations below show the effects of different types of I.V. fluids on fluid movement and cell size.

Isotonic fluids
These fluids have a concentration of dissolved particles, or tonicity, equal to that of intracellular fluid. Osmotic pressure is therefore the same inside and outside the cells, so they neither shrink nor swell with fluid movement. Normal saline solution is an example of an isotonic solution.

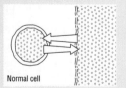

Normal cell

Hypertonic fluids
These fluids have a tonicity greater than that of intracellular fluid, so osmotic pressure is unequal inside and outside the cells. Dehydration or rapidly infused hypertonic fluids, such as 3% saline or 50% dextrose, draws water out of the cells into the more highly concentrated extracellular fluid.

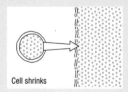

Cell shrinks

Hypotonic fluids
These fluids have a tonicity less than that of intracellular fluid. Osmotic pressure draws water into the cells from the extracellular fluid. Half-normal saline solution is an example of a hypotonic fluid. Severe electrolyte losses or inappropriate use of I.V. fluids can make body fluids hypotonic.

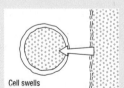

Cell swells

○ Hypertonic solutions have an osmolality greater than 295 mOsm/L.
○ Examples of hypertonic solutions include:
  – dextrose 5% in half-normal saline solution
  – dextrose 5% in normal saline solution
  – dextrose 5% in lactated Ringer's solution
  – dextrose 10% in water.
○ A hypertonic solution draws fluids from the intracellular space, causing cells to shrink and the extracellular space to expand.

▽ **ALERT** *Patients with cardiac or renal disease may be unable to tolerate extra fluid. Watch for fluid overload and pulmonary edema.*

○ Because hypertonic solutions draw fluids from cells, patients at risk for cellular dehydration (those with diabetic ketoacidosis, for example) shouldn't receive them.

Colloids

○ A colloid is a large molecule, such as albumin, that normally doesn't cross the capillary membrane. A crystalloid is a solute, such as sodium or glucose, that crosses the capillary membrane in solution.
○ The use of colloids over crystalloids is controversial. Still, a colloid — also known as a plasma expander — may be prescribed if your patient's blood volume doesn't improve with crystalloids.
○ Examples of colloids include:
  – albumin (available in 5% solutions, which are osmotically equal to plasma, and 25% solutions, which draw about four times their volume in interstitial fluid into the circulation within 15 minutes)
  – plasma protein fraction
  – dextran
  – hetastarch.
○ Colloids pull fluid into the bloodstream. The effects of colloids last several days if the lining of the capillaries is normal.
○ The patient needs to be closely monitored during a colloid infusion for increased blood pressure, dyspnea, and bounding pulse, which are all signs of hypervolemia.
○ If neither crystalloids nor colloids are effective in treating the imbalance, the patient may need a blood transfusion or other treatment.

Blood products and transfusions

Compatibility

○ Blood contains various antigens that affect whether one person's blood is compatible with another's.
○ Antigens include:
– ABO blood group
– rhesus (Rh) factor
– human leukocyte antigen (HLA) blood group.
○ These characteristics — especially Rh factor and ABO blood type — are crossmatched to ensure compatibility between donor and recipient before transfusion.

ABO group

○ The ABO method of typing blood identifies two antigens on red blood cells (RBCs).
– A person may have both A and B antigens (type AB blood).
– He may have only one antigen (either type A blood or type B blood).
– He may have neither antigen (type O blood).
○ In the United States, 85% of the population has either type A or type O blood (with type O being the most common), 10% has type B, and 5% has type AB.
○ A person with A antigens has anti-B antibodies in his plasma. If he has B antigens, he has anti-A antibodies in his plasma. Receiving a blood type for which he has antibodies may cause a transfusion reaction.
○ People with type AB blood are called universal recipients. They have no antibodies and, therefore, can receive blood of any type without a reaction.
○ People with type O blood are universal donors. Their blood may be transfused into a person with any blood type. However, because type O blood contains both anti-A and anti-B antibodies, people with this blood type may receive only type O blood safely.
○ If a patient's blood type is available, he should receive blood that's compatible with his own blood type to keep transfusion reactions to a minimum. (See Identifying compatible blood types.)
○ In an emergency, when waiting for a crossmatch would be dangerous, blood from a universal donor or plasma volume expanders may be given. Perfluorocarbons — milky, white emulsions that act like plasma but carry oxygen like RBCs — may provide an alternative in some hospitals.

Rh factor

○ About 85% of the U.S. population is Rh-positive, which means their blood contains the Rh antigen on the membranes of RBCs.
○ No natural antibodies to Rh exist. However, Rh-negative people may develop an Rh antibody if exposed to Rh-positive blood. The first exposure usually causes sensitization, but the second exposure may result in a fatal hemolytic reaction. These reactions can occur during transfusions or pregnancy.

HLA group

○ HLA is located on the surface of circulating platelets, white blood cells (WBCs), and most tissue cells.
○ It causes febrile reactions in patients receiving a transfusion that contains platelets from several donors. The antigen-antibody reaction causes platelet destruction, making the patient less responsive to platelet transfusions.
○ Giving HLA-matched platelets greatly decreases the risk of such antigen-antibody reactions.
○ In general, HLA tests benefit patients who receive multiple transfusions over a long period or frequent transfusions during a short-term illness.

Blood products

Whole blood

○ Whole blood is available in 500-ml bags and may be used to treat hemorrhage, trauma, or major burns.
○ You'll rarely use it unless the patient has lost more than 25% of total blood volume.
○ ABO compatibility and Rh matching are required before administration.
○ Avoid whole blood if fluid overload is a concern.
○ Stored whole blood is high in potassium.
○ After 24 hours, the viability and function of RBCs decrease.

Packed red blood cells

○ Packed RBCs are prepared by removing about 90% of the plasma surrounding the cells and adding an anticoagulant preservative.
○ A 250-ml bag of packed RBCs can help restore or maintain the oxygen-carrying capacity of the blood in patients with anemia or can correct blood losses during or after surgery.
○ About 70% of the leukocytes in packed cells have been removed, which reduces the risk of febrile, nonhemolytic reactions.
○ ABO compatibility and Rh matching are still required for these transfusions.

White blood cells

○ Granulocyte, or WBC, transfusions are rarely indicated; however, they may be used to treat gram-negative sepsis or progressive soft-tissue infection unresponsive to antimicrobial drugs.
○ HLA compatibility tests are preferable, and Rh matching is required.

Fresh frozen plasma

○ Fresh frozen plasma is prepared by separating the plasma from the RBCs and freezing it within 6 hours of collection.

- The solution contains plasma proteins, water, fibrinogen, some clotting factors, electrolytes, glucose, vitamins, minerals, hormones, and antibodies.
- Fresh frozen plasma is used to treat hemorrhage, expand plasma volume, correct undetermined coagulation factor deficiencies, replace specific clotting factors, and correct factor deficiencies caused by liver disease.
- ABO compatibility testing isn't needed; Rh matching is preferred.
- Large-volume transfusions of fresh frozen plasma may require correction for hypocalcemia because citric acid in the transfusion binds with and depletes the patient's serum calcium level.

Cryoprecipitate

- Cryoprecipitate (also called factor VIII) is the insoluble portion of plasma recovered from fresh frozen plasma.
- It's used to treat von Willebrand's disease, hypofibrinogenemia, factor VIII deficiency (antihemophilic factor), hemophilia A, and disseminated intravascular coagulation.
- ABO compatibility testing isn't needed.

Albumin

- Albumin, which comes in an isotonic 5% solution and a hypertonic 25% solution, is extracted from plasma and contains globulin and other proteins.
- It's used for patients with acute liver failure, burns, or trauma; patients who have had surgery; and neonates with hemolytic disease when crystalloids prove ineffective.
- As a colloidal solution, albumin's large molecules increase plasma oncotic pressure, moving fluid from the interstitial space across capillary membranes and into the intravascular space.
- Albumin may actually do more harm than good in patients with shock by leaking through damaged capillary membranes and dragging intravascular fluid along to worsen interstitial edema.
- Albumin is also used to treat hypoproteinemia with or without edema.
- ABO matching isn't needed.

Platelets

- Platelets are given to patients with platelet dysfunction or thrombocytopenia and to those who have had multiple transfusions of stored blood, acute leukemia, or bone marrow abnormalities.
- Platelet transfusion may cause febrile or mild allergic reactions.
- Rh matching is preferred.

Transfusion reactions

- Endogenous transfusion reactions (those caused by antigen-antibody reactions) include:
  - allergic

Identifying compatible blood types

A transfusion most likely will be safe if the donor and recipient have compatible blood types. This illustration provides a key to blood-type compatibility.

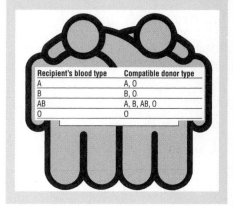

Recipient's blood type	Compatible donor type
A	A, O
B	B, O
AB	A, B, AB, O
O	O

- bacterial contamination
- febrile
- hemolytic
- plasma protein incompatibility.
- Exogenous transfusion reactions (those caused by external factors in administered blood) include:
  - bleeding tendencies
  - circulatory overload
  - hypocalcemia
  - hypothermia
  - potassium intoxication.
- With human immunodeficiency virus (HIV)–antibody testing being done on all donated blood and stringent criteria being used to exclude high-risk blood donors, studies now show that HIV transmission through infusion is rare.
- Testing for hepatitis B and hepatitis C viruses has become more specific, which has helped to make the blood supply safer.

Total parenteral nutrition

Solution components

○ Total parenteral nutrition (TPN) formulas provide nutritional supplementation tailored to the patient's specific needs.
○ Nutritional support teams consisting of nurses, doctors, pharmacists, and dietitians assess, prescribe for, and monitor patients receiving TPN.
○ TPN solutions may contain:
  – protein (amino acids in a 2.5% to 8.5% solution), with varying types available for patients with renal or liver failure
  – dextrose (15% to 50% solution)
  – fat emulsions (10% to 20% solution)
  – electrolytes
  – vitamins
  – trace element mixtures
  – drugs. (See *Understanding common TPN additives.*)

Understanding common TPN additives

Common components of total parenteral nutrition (TPN) solutions—such as dextrose 5% in water (D_5W), amino acids, and other additives—are used for specific purposes. For instance, D_5W provides calories for metabolism. Here's a list of other common additives and the purposes each serves. (Lipids may be infused separately.)

Electrolytes
● *Calcium* promotes development of bones and teeth and aids in blood clotting.
● *Chloride* regulates acid-base balance and maintains osmotic pressure.
● *Magnesium* helps the body absorb carbohydrates and protein.
● *Phosphorus* is essential for cellular energy and calcium balance.
● *Potassium* is needed for cellular activity and cardiac function.
● *Sodium* helps control water distribution and maintain normal fluid balance.

Vitamins
● *Folic acid* is needed for DNA formation and promotes growth and development.
● *Vitamin B* complex helps the final absorption of carbohydrates and protein.
● *Vitamin C* helps in wound healing.
● *Vitamin D* is essential for bone metabolism and maintenance of serum calcium levels.
● *Vitamin K* helps prevent bleeding disorders.

Other additives
● *Acetate* prevents metabolic acidosis.
● *Micronutrients* (such as zinc, cobalt, and manganese) help in wound healing and red blood cell synthesis.
● *Amino acids* provide the proteins needed for tissue repair.

Lipid emulsions

○ Lipid emulsions supply essential fatty acids and calories.
○ These thick solutions assist in wound healing, red blood cell production, and prostaglandin synthesis.
○ Although they're typically given with TPN, they may be given alone through a peripheral or central venous line, or they may be mixed with amino acids and dextrose in one container (providing a three-in-one-system) and infused over 24 hours.
○ Lipid emulsions should be given cautiously to patients with hepatic or pulmonary disease, anemia, or a coagulation disorder and to patients at risk for fat embolism.
○ These emulsions shouldn't be given to patients who have conditions that disrupt normal fat metabolism, such as pathologic hyperlipidemia, lipid nephrosis, and acute pancreatitis.

Adverse reactions

○ Signs and symptoms of electrolyte imbalances caused by TPN administration include:
  – abdominal cramps
  – lethargy
  – confusion
  – malaise
  – muscle weakness
  – tetany
  – seizures
  – cardiac arrhythmias.
○ Acid-base imbalances can also occur as a result of the patient's condition or the contents of the TPN.
○ Other complications may include:
  – heart failure or pulmonary edema from fluid and electrolyte administration, conditions that can lead to tachycardia, lethargy, confusion, weakness, and labored breathing
  – hyperglycemia from infusing dextrose too quickly, a condition that may require adjustment of the patient's insulin dosage
  – adverse reactions to drugs in the TPN solution— such as hypoglycemia from added insulin, which can cause confusion, restlessness, lethargy, pallor, and tachycardia
  – complications from I.V. cannulas and central venous catheters.
○ Immediate or early adverse reactions from lipid emulsions may include:
  – back and chest pain
  – cyanosis
  – diaphoresis or flushing
  – dyspnea
  – headache

- hypercoagulability
- irritation at the site
- lethargy or syncope
- nausea or vomiting
- slight pressure over the eyes
- thrombocytopenia.
○ Delayed complications from prolonged use of lipid emulsions may include:
- blood dyscrasias
- fatty liver syndrome
- hepatomegaly
- jaundice
- splenomegaly.

Hemodialysis basics

Overview

- Is performed to remove toxic wastes from the blood of patients in renal failure
- Removes blood from the body, circulates it through a purifying dialyzer, and then returns the blood to the body
- May be delivered through various types of access sites, although long-term treatment typically is delivered via an arteriovenous (AV) fistula (See *Hemodialysis access sites.*)
- Works on the principle of differential diffusion across a semipermeable membrane, which extracts byproducts of protein metabolism, such as urea and uric acid, as well as creatinine and excess water
- Restores or maintains balance of the body's buffer system and electrolyte level, promoting rapid return to normal serum values and preventing complications of uremia
- Provides temporary support for patients with acute reversible renal failure
- Is used for regular long-term treatment of patients with chronic end-stage renal disease
- Is performed less commonly for acute poisoning, such as barbiturate or analgesic overdose
- Depends on patient's condition (rate of creatinine accumulation and weight gain) for number and duration of treatments
- Is usually performed in hemodialysis unit by specially trained staff
- May be done at bedside in intensive care unit if patient is acutely ill and unstable
- May be available for use at home (special hemodialysis units)

Contraindications

- Hemodynamic instability

Special considerations

- Obtain blood samples from the patient, as ordered, usually before hemodialysis starts.

  ▶ **ALERT** *To avoid pyrogenic reactions and bacteremia with septicemia resulting from contamination, use strict sterile technique when preparing the dialysis machine.*

- Immediately report any machine malfunction or equipment defect.
- Avoid unnecessary handling of hemodialysis tubing.
- Assess the catheter insertion site for signs of infection, such as purulent drainage, inflammation, and tenderness.

  ▶ **ALERT** *Make sure you complete each step in the dialysis procedure correctly to avoid unnecessary blood loss or inefficient treatment from*

Hemodialysis access sites

Hemodialysis requires vascular access. The site and type of access may vary with the expected duration of dialysis, the surgeon's preference, and the patient's condition.

Subclavian vein catheterization
Using the Seldinger technique, a doctor or surgeon inserts an introducer needle into the subclavian vein, inserts a guidewire through the introducer needle, and removes the needle. Using the guidewire, he then threads a 5" to 12" (12.5- to 30.5-cm) plastic or Teflon catheter (with a Y hub) into the patient's vein.

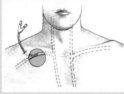

Native arteriovenous fistula
To create a native arteriovenous (AV) fistula, the surgeon makes an incision into the patient's wrist or lower forearm, a small incision in the side of an artery, and another small incision in the side of a vein. He sutures the edges of the incisions together to make a common opening 3 to 7 mm long.

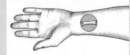

Femoral vein catheterization
Using the Seldinger technique, a doctor or surgeon inserts an introducer needle into the left or right femoral vein, inserts a guidewire through the introducer needle, and removes the needle. Using the guidewire, he then threads a 5" to 12" plastic or Teflon catheter into the vein with a Y hub or two catheters, one for inflow and another placed about 1/2" (1.3 cm) distal to the first for outflow.

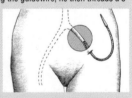

Prosthetic arteriovenous fistula
To create an AV fistula with synthetic material, the surgeon makes an incision in the patient's forearm, upper arm, or thigh. He then tunnels a synthetic graft under the skin and sutures the distal end to an artery and the proximal end to a vein.

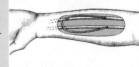

poor clearances or inadequate fluid removal. For example, allowing a saline solution bag to run dry while priming and soaking the dialyzer can cause air to enter the patient portion of the dialysate system. Ultimately, failure to perform accurate hemodialysis therapy can lead to patient injury and even death.

○ If bleeding continues after you remove an AV fistula needle, apply just enough pressure with a sterile, absorbable gelatin sponge or topical thrombin solution to stop the bleeding.
○ Monitor the patient's vital signs throughout hemodialysis at least hourly or as often as every 15 minutes, if needed.
○ After dialysis is complete, assess the patient's weight, vital signs, and mental status, and compare the findings with your predialysis assessment.
○ Perform periodic tests of clotting time on the patient's blood samples and samples from the dialyzer.
○ If the patient receives meals during treatment, make sure they're light.
○ Continue needed drug therapy during dialysis unless the drug would be removed in the dialysate; if so, give the drug after dialysis.
○ Provide emotional support.

Complications

○ Air embolism
○ Angina
○ Cardiac arrhythmias
○ Dialysis disequilibrium syndrome
○ Exsanguination
○ Fever
○ Hemolysis
○ Hyperglycemia
○ Hypernatremia
○ Hyperosmolarity
○ Hyperthermia
○ Hypotension
○ Hypovolemia
○ Stenosis of AV fistula
○ Thrombosis of AV fistula

Patient teaching

Be sure to cover:
○ how to care for the vascular access site at home
○ how to perform hemodialysis at home if possible — usually a complex process requiring 2 to 3 months to feel comfortable and be competent
○ the telephone number of the dialysis center.

Documentation

○ Time treatment began
○ Any problems with treatment
○ Vital signs and weight before and during treatment
○ Time blood specimens were taken for testing, the test results, and treatment for complications
○ Time the treatment was completed
○ Patient's response to treatment
○ Condition of vascular access site and site care

Managing hemodialysis

Hemodialysis of all types

Equipment

○ Hemodialysis machine with appropriate dialyzer
○ I.V. solution
○ Administration sets, lines, and related equipment
○ Dialysate
○ Optional: heparin, 3-ml syringe with needle, medication label
○ Hemostats

Equipment preparation

○ Prepare the hemodialysis equipment according to manufacturer's instructions and hospital protocol.
○ Test the dialyzer and dialysis machine for residual disinfectant after rinsing, and test all the alarms.

Essential steps

○ Wash your hands thoroughly before all procedures.
○ If the patient is having hemodialysis for the first time, explain the procedure in detail.
○ Maintain sterile technique to prevent pathogens from entering the patient's bloodstream during dialysis.
○ Wear appropriate personal protective equipment, as needed, during all procedures.
○ Weigh the patient and compare it to his weight after the last dialysis and his target weight to determine ultrafiltration needs.
○ Record baseline vital signs, taking blood pressure while the patient's sitting and standing; auscultate the heart for rate, rhythm, and abnormalities; assess the patient for edema; observe respiratory rate, rhythm, and quality; and check the patient's mental status.
○ Assess the condition and patency of the access site.
○ Check for problems since the last dialysis session, and evaluate previous laboratory data.
○ Help the patient into a comfortable position (supine or sitting in a reclining chair with feet elevated).
○ Support the access site and rest it on a clean drape.

Hemodialysis with a double-lumen catheter

Equipment

Starting hemodialysis
○ Povidone-iodine pads
○ Two sterile 4″ × 4″ gauze pads
○ Two 3-ml and two 5-ml syringes
○ Tape
○ Heparin bolus syringe
○ Clean gloves
Stopping hemodialysis
○ Sterile gauze pads
○ Povidone-iodine pads
○ Clean gloves
○ Sterile gloves
○ Normal saline solution
○ Alcohol pads
○ Heparin flush solution
○ Luer-lock injection caps
○ Transparent occlusive dressing

Essential steps

Starting hemodialysis
○ If extension tubing isn't already clamped, clamp it to prevent air from entering the catheter.
○ Clean each catheter extension tube, clamp, and Luer-lock injection cap with povidone-iodine pads to remove contaminants.
○ Place a sterile 4″ × 4″ gauze pad under the extension tubing, and place two 5-ml syringes and two sterile gauze pads on the drape.
○ Prepare the anticoagulant regimen as ordered.
○ Identify arterial and venous blood lines, and place them near the drape.
○ To remove clots and ensure catheter patency, remove catheter caps, attach syringes to each catheter port, open the clamp, aspirate 1.5 to 3 ml of blood, close the clamp, and flush each port with 5 ml of heparin flush solution.
○ To gain patient access, remove the syringe from the arterial port, attach the line to the arterial port, and give the heparin according to protocol to prevent clotting in the extracorporeal circuit.
○ Grasp the venous blood line and attach it to the venous port, open the clamps on the extension tubing, and secure the tubing to the patient's limb with tape to reduce tension on the tube and minimize trauma to the insertion site.
○ Begin hemodialysis according to your facility's protocol.

Stopping hemodialysis
○ Clamp the extension tubing to prevent air from entering the catheter.
○ Clean all connection points on the catheter and blood lines as well as the clamps to reduce the risk of systemic or local infections.
○ Place a clean drape under the catheter, and place two sterile 4″ × 4″ gauze pads on the drape beneath the catheter lines.
○ Soak the pads with povidone-iodine solution.
○ Prepare the catheter flush solution with normal saline or heparin flush solution, as ordered.
○ Put on clean gloves.
○ Grasp each blood line with a gauze pad and disconnect each line from the catheter.
○ Flush each port with saline solution to clean the extension tubing and catheter of blood.
○ Give additional heparin flush solution as ordered to ensure catheter patency. Then attach Luer-lock injection caps to prevent entry of air or loss of blood.
○ Clamp the extension tubing.
○ Re-dress the catheter insertion site; also re-dress it if it's occluded, soiled, or wet.

- During the dressing change, position the patient in a supine position with his face turned away from the insertion site so that he doesn't contaminate the site by breathing on it.
- Change gloves after washing your hands, and remove the outer occlusive dressing.
- Put on sterile gloves, remove the old inner dressing, and discard the gloves and the inner dressing.
- Set up a sterile field, and observe the site for drainage, obtaining a drainage sample for culture if needed.
- Notify the doctor if the suture seems to be missing.
- Put on sterile gloves and clean the insertion site with an alcohol pad to remove skin oils.
- Clean the site with a povidone-iodine pad and allow it to air dry.
- Place a precut gauze dressing under the catheter, and place another gauze dressing over the catheter.
- Apply a skin barrier preparation to the skin surrounding the gauze dressing and cover the gauze and catheter with a transparent occlusive dressing.
- Apply a 4″ to 5″ (10- to 12.5-cm) piece of 2″ tape over the cut edge of the dressing to reinforce the lower edge.

Hemodialysis with an AV fistula

Equipment

Starting hemodialysis
- Two winged fistula needles (each attached to a 10-ml syringe filled with heparin flush solution)
- Linen-saver pad
- Povidone-iodine pads
- Sterile 4″ × 4″ gauze pads
- Tourniquet
- Clean gloves
- Adhesive tape
- Hemostats

Stopping hemodialysis
- Clean gloves
- Hemostats
- Sterile gauze pads
- Two adhesive bandages

Essential steps

Starting hemodialysis
- Flush the fistula needles using attached syringes with heparinized saline solution, and set them aside.
- Place a linen-saver pad under the patient's arm.
- Using sterile technique, clean a 3″ × 10″ (8 × 25 cm) area of skin over the fistula with povidone-iodine pads. If the patient is sensitive to iodine, use chlorhexidine gluconate or alcohol instead.
- Discard each pad after one wipe.
- Apply a tourniquet above the fistula to distend the veins and facilitate venipuncture, making sure you don't occlude the fistula.

- Put on clean gloves.
- Remove the fistula needle guard and squeeze the wing tips firmly together.
- Insert the arterial needle at least 1″ (2.5 cm) above the anastomosis, being careful not to puncture the fistula.
- Release the tourniquet and flush the needle with heparin flush solution to prevent clotting.
- Clamp the arterial needle tubing with a hemostat, and secure the wing tips of the needle to the skin with adhesive tape to prevent it from dislodging inside the vein.
- Perform another venipuncture with the venous needle a few inches above the arterial needle.
- Flush the venous needle with heparin flush solution.
- Clamp the venous needle tubing, and secure the wing tips of the venous needle as you did with the arterial needle.
- Remove the syringe from the end of the arterial tubing, uncap the arterial line from the hemodialysis machine, and connect the two lines.
- Tape the connection securely to prevent it from separating during the procedure.
- Remove the syringe from the end of the venous tubing, uncap the venous line from the hemodialysis machine, and connect the two lines.
- Tape the connection securely to prevent it from separating during the procedure.
- Release the hemostats and start hemodialysis.

Stopping hemodialysis
- Turn the blood pump on the hemodialysis machine to 50 to 100 ml/minute.
- Put on clean gloves and remove the tape from the connection site of the arterial lines.
- Clamp the needle tubing with the hemostat and disconnect the lines. The blood in the machine's arterial line will continue to flow toward the dialyzer, followed by a column of air. Just before the blood reaches the point where the saline solution enters the line, clamp the blood line with another hemostat.
- Unclamp the saline solution to allow a small amount to flow through the line.
- Unclamp the hemostat on the machine line to allow all blood to flow into the dialyzer where it passes through the filter and back to the patient through the venous line.
- After the blood is retransfused, clamp the venous needle tubing and the machine's venous line with hemostats and turn off the blood pump.
- Remove the tape from the connection site of the venous lines and disconnect the lines.
- Remove the venipuncture needle and apply pressure to the site with a folded 4″ × 4″ gauze pad until all bleeding stops, usually within 10 minutes.
- Apply an adhesive bandage.
- Repeat the procedure on the arterial line.
- Disinfect and rinse the delivery system according to the manufacturer's instructions.

Peritoneal dialysis

Overview

- Is indicated for patients with chronic renal failure who can't tolerate hemodialysis
- Also is indicated for patients who prefer it or who refuse hemodialysis
- May be indicated for patients who prefer home dialysis but have no one trained for home hemodialysis
- Is performed by instilling dialysate into the peritoneal cavity by catheter (inserted surgically) to draw waste products, excess fluid, and electrolytes from the blood across the peritoneal membrane
- Requires dialysate to be drained from the peritoneal cavity after prescribed period, removing impurities with it
- Is repeated with new dialysate each time until waste removal is complete and fluid, electrolyte, and acid-base balance is restored

Contraindications and cautions

- Peritonitis
- Documented loss of peritoneal function or extensive abdominal adhesions that limit dialysate flow
- Uncorrectable mechanical defects
- Fresh intra-abdominal foreign bodies
- Peritoneal leaks
- Intolerance to volumes needed to reach an adequate peritoneal dialysis dose
- Inflammatory or ischemic bowel disease
- Abdominal wall or skin infection
- Morbid obesity
- Severe malnutrition
- Frequent episodes of diverticulitis

Equipment

- Must be sterile
- Commercially packaged dialysis kits or trays
- Prescribed dialysate (in 1- or 2-L bottles or bags)
- Warmer, heating pad, or water bath
- Face masks
- Dialysis administration set with drainage bag
- Two pairs of sterile gloves
- I.V. pole
- Fenestrated sterile drape

Equipment preparation

- Wash your hands thoroughly before all procedures.
- Bring all equipment to the patient's bedside.
- Make sure the dialysate is at body temperature to reduce discomfort and reduce vasoconstriction of the peritoneal capillaries.
- Place the container in a warmer or a water bath, or wrap it in a heating pad set at 98.6° F (37° C) for 30 to 60 minutes to warm the solution.

Essential steps

- Explain all procedures to the patient.
- Maintain asepsis throughout all procedures.
- Wash your hands and close the door to the room.
- Wear appropriate personal protective equipment during all procedures.
- Assess and record vital signs, weight, and abdominal girth to establish baseline levels.
- Place the patient in a supine position if tolerated and have him put on a sterile face mask.

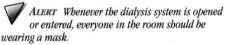 **ALERT** *Whenever the dialysis system is opened or entered, everyone in the room should be wearing a mask.*

- Inspect the warmed dialysate, which should appear clear and colorless.
- Put on a sterile face mask.
- Add prescribed drugs to the dialysate, using strict sterile technique, immediately before the solution is hung and used.
- Disinfect multiple-dose vials by soaking them in povidone-iodine solution for 5 minutes.
- Prepare the dialysis administration set. (See *Setup for peritoneal dialysis*.)
- Close the clamps on all lines.
- Place the drainage bag below the patient to facilitate gravity drainage and connect the drainage line to it.
- Connect the dialysate infusion lines to the bottles or bags of dialysate.
- Hang the bottles or bags on the I.V. pole at the patient's bedside.
- Open the infusion lines and let the solution flow until all lines are primed; then close all clamps.
- Connect the catheter to the administration set.
- Unclamp the lines to the patient and instill the prescribed amount of dialysate into the peritoneal cavity to test the catheter's patency.
- Clamp the lines to the patient.
- As soon as the dialysate container empties, clamp the lines to the patient immediately to prevent air from entering the tubing.
- Let the solution dwell in the peritoneal cavity for the prescribed time.
- Warm the solution for the next infusion.
- At the end of the prescribed dwell time, unclamp the line to the drainage bag and let solution drain from the peritoneal cavity (usually 20 to 30 minutes).
- Repeat the infuse-dwell-drain cycle as prescribed (usually 4 to 5 times daily).

ALERT *To reduce the risk of peritonitis, use strict sterile technique during catheter insertion, dialysis, and dressing changes.*

- Change the dressing at least every 24 hours or whenever it becomes wet or soiled.
- To prevent respiratory distress, position the patient for maximal lung expansion, turn the patient often, and encourage deep-breathing exercises.

ALERT *If the patient develops severe respiratory distress during the dwell phase of dialysis, drain the peritoneal cavity and notify the doctor.*

Special considerations

○ To prevent protein depletion, the doctor may order a high-protein diet or a protein supplement and monitoring of serum albumin levels.

○ Dialysate is available in three concentrations: 4.25% dextrose, 2.5% dextrose, and 1.5% dextrose. If your patient receives the 4.25% dextrose solution, watch for excess fluid loss and hyperglycemia.

○ Patients with low serum potassium levels may need potassium in the dialysate to prevent further losses.

○ To help prevent fluid imbalance, monitor fluid volume balance, blood pressure, and pulse and notify the doctor if the patient retains 500 ml or more of fluid for three consecutive cycles or loses at least 1 L of fluid for three consecutive cycles.

○ Weigh the patient at the same time each day to assess how much fluid is being removed during dialysis.

○ If inflow and outflow are slow or absent, check the tubing for kinks, raise the I.V. pole, reposition the patient, or apply manual pressure to the lateral aspects of the patient's abdomen. If these maneuvers fail, notify the doctor.

○ Normally, outflow fluid (effluent) is clear or pale yellow, but pink-tinged effluent may appear during the first three or four cycles.

○ If the effluent is pink-tinged or grossly bloody, suspect bleeding into the peritoneal cavity and notify the doctor.

○ If the outflow contains feces, which suggests bowel perforation, or if it's cloudy, which suggests peritonitis, notify the doctor and obtain a sample for culture and Gram's stain.

○ If the patient has pain during the procedure, determine when it occurs, its quality and duration, and whether it radiates, and notify the doctor.

ALERT *Pain during infusion usually results from dialysate that's too cool or acidic. It also may result from rapid inflow; slowing the inflow rate may reduce the pain. Severe, diffuse pain with rebound tenderness and cloudy effluent may indicate peritoneal infection. Pain that radiates to the shoulder commonly results from air accumulation under the diaphragm. Severe, persistent perineal or rectal pain can result from improper catheter placement.*

○ To minimize the patient's discomfort, perform daily care during the drain phase of the cycle, when the patient's abdomen is less distended.

Complications

○ Abdominal or pericatheter infection
○ Amyloidosis
○ Bladder perforation
○ Bowel perforation

Setup for peritoneal dialysis

The proper setup for peritoneal dialysis is shown below.

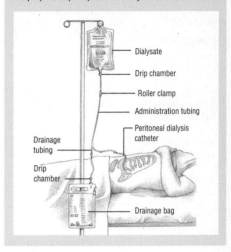

- Dialysate
- Drip chamber
- Roller clamp
- Administration tubing
- Peritoneal dialysis catheter
- Drainage tubing
- Drip chamber
- Drainage bag

○ Electrolyte imbalances
○ Hyperglycemia
○ Hypotension and shock
○ Peritonitis and sclerosing encapsulating peritonitis
○ Protein depletion
○ Respiratory distress
○ Tunnel abscess (in continuous ambulatory peritoneal dialysis)

Patient teaching

Be sure to cover:
○ performing the procedure using sterile technique
○ dressing changes and skin care
○ signs and symptoms of peritonitis and other complications to report
○ the need to record weight and blood pressure daily
○ the importance of keeping accurate intake records
○ name and telephone number of a person to call for assistance and questions.

Documentation

○ Date and time of dialysis
○ Exchange number
○ Volume of dialysate infused and drained
○ Infusion, dwell, and drain times
○ Drugs added to the solution
○ Color and character of effluent
○ Complications and treatment
○ Daily weight
○ Vital signs before, during, and after dialysis
○ Patient teaching
○ Total fluid balance after each exchange
○ Pericatheter skin assessment

Continuous renal replacement therapy

Overview

Description

○ Is used to manage fluid and electrolyte imbalance in hemodynamically unstable patients.
○ Removes toxins from the blood
○ Doesn't cause dramatic changes in blood pressure, as hemodialysis may, because fluid exits slowly
○ Is performed by a specially trained nurse in a critical care setting
○ Requires special equipment, supplies, and staff training

Types of continuous renal replacement therapy

○ Continuous arteriovenous hemofiltration (CAVH)

Following the circuit of continuous renal replacement therapy

In continuous renal replacement therapy (CRRT), a dual-lumen venous catheter provides access to the patient's blood. A pulsatile pump propels the blood through the tubing circuit.

This illustration shows the standard setup for one type of CRRT called continuous venovenous hemofiltration. The patient's blood enters the hemofilter from a line connected to one lumen of the venous catheter, flows through the hemofilter, and returns to the patient through the second lumen of the catheter.

At the first pump, an anticoagulant may be added to the blood. A second pump moves dialysate through the hemofilter. A third pump adds replacement fluid if needed. The ultrafiltrate (plasma water and toxins) removed from the blood drains into a collection bag.

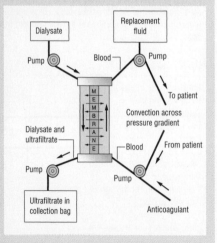

- Simple technology using a semipermeable membrane and an extracorporeal circuit
- Uses arterial pressure to move blood through the extracorporeal circuit and semipermeable membrane
- High risk for blood loss from clotting in the circuit
- High risk for bleeding from arterial cannulation
○ Continuous arteriovenous hemodiafiltration
- Same procedure as CAVH
- Uses dialysate to promote waste removal
○ Continuous venovenous hemofiltration (CVVH)
- Blood flow through a semipermeable fiber filter and an extracorporeal circuit
- Uses a pump to propel blood through the circuit and semipermeable membrane
- Decreased risk of clotting because pump rotates to move the blood
- Decreased risk of blood loss from a double-lumen, large-bore venous catheter to gain access to the patient's blood
- Alarms on the equipment to signal machine or patient problem
○ Continuous venovenous hemodialysis (CVVHD)
- Same procedure as CVVH
- Uses dialysate to increase solute removal
○ Continuous venovenous hemofiltration
- Same procedure as CVVHD
- Uses a replacement solution to maximize uremic toxin removal through convective clearance (See *Following the circuit of continuous renal replacement therapy.*)

Contraindications

○ Coagulopathy
○ Liver disease
○ Life-threatening hyperkalemia

Cautions

○ The patient needs to be in an intensive care unit.
○ Access must be secure and functional.
○ The nurse performing CRRT must have specialized knowledge of the machine and the procedure.
○ The patient has limited mobility during treatment.

Equipment

○ Dialysis machine at the patient's bedside
○ Access, such as a femoral catheter, internal arteriovenous (AV) graft, or AV shunt
○ Hemofilter for the dialysis machine, made up of about 5,000 hollow fiber capillaries, which filters the blood at about 250 ml/minute
○ Dialysate solution
○ Flush solution
○ Heparin, if ordered
○ Collection bag

Equipment preparation

○ May be prepared by dialysis nurse, based on facility policy

Essential steps

○ Consult with the nephrologist.
○ Establish access for dialysis.
○ Set up equipment for the appropriate type of CRRT.
○ Monitor the patient's response to therapy.

Special considerations

○ Requires one-to-one nursing care
○ Requires continuous monitoring of vital signs, cardiac rhythm, fluid status, electrolyte balance, mental status, and signs of bleeding
○ Requires certification of nurse performing CRRT
○ Requires meticulous documentation of intake and output

Complications

○ Bradycardia
○ Dyspnea
○ Electrolyte and acid-base imbalance
○ Fluid volume overload
○ Hypotension
○ Hypothermia
○ Hypovolemia
○ Removal of drugs across the semipermeable membrane (may need to increase doses of cardiac drugs and antibiotics)
○ Uncontrolled bleeding

Patient teaching

Be sure to cover:
○ the need for CRRT
○ equipment needed for procedure
○ how the procedure is performed
○ precautions needed during the procedure
○ length of treatment (days to weeks).

Documentation

○ Use specialized flowsheets for accurate documentation of intake and output.
○ Document vital signs, hemodynamic parameters, and laboratory values according to facility policy.
○ Note the patient's response to the procedure.

Part two

Disorders related to fluid and electrolyte imbalance

Acute poststreptococcal glomerulonephritis

Overview

Description

○ Renal disease in which the glomeruli become inflamed
○ Relatively common
○ Usually occurs after an infection, commonly a streptococcal infection of the respiratory tract or, less commonly, a skin infection such as impetigo
○ Full recovery in up to 95% of children and 70% of adults
○ May lead to chronic renal failure within months in geriatric patients
○ Also called acute glomerulonephritis

Pathophysiology

○ Antigen-antibody complexes are produced in response to group A beta-hemolytic *Streptococcus* infection.
○ Antigen-antibody complexes are trapped and collect in the glomerular capillary membranes.
○ Inflammatory damage results, impeding glomerular function.
○ Immune complement may further damage the glomerular membrane.
○ Damaged and inflamed glomeruli lose the ability to be selectively permeable.
○ Red blood cells (RBCs) and proteins filter through as glomerular filtration rate decreases.
○ Uremic poisoning may result.

Risk factors

○ Group A beta-hemolytic *Streptococcus* infection of the respiratory tract
○ Impetigo

Causes

○ Immune system reaction to untreated group A beta-hemolytic *Streptococcus* infection, especially of the respiratory tract

Prevalence

○ Most common in boys ages 4 to 6
○ May occur at any age
○ Actual prevalence unknown

Complications

○ Anemia
○ Hypertension
○ Progressive deterioration of renal function

Assessment

History

○ Decreased urination
○ Dyspnea
○ Fatigue
○ Malaise
○ Orthopnea
○ Smoky or coffee-colored urine
○ Untreated respiratory streptococcal infection within previous 1 to 3 weeks

Physical assessment

○ Bibasilar crackles (with heart failure)
○ Generalized edema
○ Hematuria
○ Mild to moderate periorbital edema
○ Mild to severe hypertension
○ Oliguria

Test results

Laboratory
○ Electrolyte imbalances
○ Elevated blood urea nitrogen (BUN) and creatinine levels
○ Decreased serum protein levels
○ RBCs, white blood cells, mixed cell casts, and protein in urine (indicate renal failure)
○ High levels of fibrin-degradation products and C3 protein

✳ *AGE AWARE* *If the patient is elderly, expect the proteinuria to be less pronounced than it would be in a younger patient.*

○ Decreased serum complement levels and increased antistreptolysin-O (80% of patients), streptozyme, and anti-DNase B titers, which verify recent streptococcal infection
○ Group A beta-hemolytic streptococci in throat culture
Imaging
○ Kidney-ureter-bladder X-rays show bilateral kidney enlargement.
○ Chest X-rays may show central venous congestion in a hilar pattern.
Diagnostic procedures
○ Renal biopsy or assessment of renal tissue shows inflammatory changes, which confirm the diagnosis.

Nursing diagnoses

○ Acute pain
○ Decreased cardiac output
○ Fatigue
○ Risk for imbalanced fluid volume
○ Risk for infection
○ Risk for injury

Key outcomes

The patient will:
- maintain fluid balance
- report increased comfort
- identify risk factors that worsen the condition and modify lifestyle accordingly
- maintain hemodynamic stability.

Interventions

General

- Correction of electrolyte imbalances (possibly with dialysis)
- Fluid restriction
- High-calorie, low-protein, low-sodium, low-potassium diet
- Bed rest

Nursing

- Give prescribed drugs.
- Encourage the patient to talk.
- Provide support.

Drug therapy

- Antibiotics if appropriate
- Antihypertensives
- Loop diuretics, such as metolazone or furosemide

Monitoring

- Creatinine clearance
- Daily weight
- Electrolyte values
- Intake and output
- Serum creatinine and BUN levels
- Vital signs

Patient teaching

Be sure to cover:
- the disorder, diagnosis, and treatment
- the importance of follow-up examinations to monitor renal function
- drug regimen, dosages, and possible adverse effects.

Discharge planning

- Refer the patient to appropriate resources for information and support.

Acute pyelonephritis

Overview

Description

- Inflammation of the kidney
- Affects mainly interstitial tissue and renal pelvis, occasionally renal tubules
- May affect one or both kidneys
- Rarely causes extensive permanent damage
- Good prognosis
- Also called acute infective tubulointerstitial nephritis

Pathophysiology

- Infection spreads from bladder to ureters to kidneys, commonly through vesicoureteral reflux.
- Vesicoureteral reflux may result from congenital weakness at the junction of the ureter and bladder.
- Bacteria refluxed to intrarenal tissues may create colonies of infection in 24 to 48 hours.

Risk factors

- Female sex
- Genitourinary obstruction
- Hematogenic infection, such as septicemia
- Neurogenic bladder
- Pregnancy in women
- Renal disease
- Renal procedures that involve instrumentation, such as cystoscopy
- Sexual activity in women

Causes

- Bacterial infection of the kidneys

Prevalence

- Community-acquired form: 15 cases per 100,000 people per year
- Hospital-acquired form: 7 cases per 10,000 people per year
- More common in women than men because of difference in anatomy

Complications

- Chronic pyelonephritis
- Multisystem infection
- Renal abscess
- Renal calculi
- Renal failure
- Septic shock

Assessment

History

- Anorexia
- Burning during urination
- Diarrhea
- Dysuria
- Fatigue
- Hematuria
- Nocturia
- Pain over one or both kidneys
- Symptoms that develop rapidly over a few hours or a few days
- Urinary frequency
- Urinary urgency
- Vomiting

Physical assessment

- Ammonia-like or fishy odor to urine
- Cloudy urine
- Fever of 102° F (38.9° C) or higher
- Pain with flank palpation
- Shaking chills

Test results

Laboratory

- Pyuria
- Significant bacteriuria
- Low urine specific gravity and osmolality
- Slightly alkaline urine pH
- Elevated white blood cell count
- Elevated neutrophil count
- Elevated erythrocyte sedimentation rate
- Proteinuria, glycosuria, and ketonuria (less common)

Imaging

- Kidney-ureter-bladder X-rays show calculi, tumors, or cysts in the kidneys or urinary tract.
- Excretory urography shows asymmetrical kidneys, which may indicate frequent infection.

Nursing diagnoses

- Acute pain
- Decreased cardiac output
- Fatigue
- Risk for imbalanced fluid volume
- Risk for infection
- Risk for injury

Key outcomes

The patient will:
- maintain fluid balance
- report increased comfort
- identify risk factors that worsen the condition, and modify lifestyle accordingly
- maintain hemodynamic stability.

Interventions

General

- Identification and correction of predisposing factors to infection, such as obstruction or calculi

- Short courses of therapy for uncomplicated infection
- Increased fluid intake

Nursing
- Give prescribed drugs.

Drug therapy
- Antibiotics
- Urinary analgesics, such as phenazopyridine

Monitoring
- Characteristics of urine
- Daily weight
- Intake and output
- Pattern of urination
- Renal function studies
- Vital signs

Patient teaching

Be sure to cover:
- the disorder, diagnosis, and treatment
- hygienic toileting practices that reduce the risk of bacterial contamination, such as wiping the perineum from front to back after bowel movements for women
- proper technique for collecting a clean-catch urine specimen
- drug regimen, dosages, and possible adverse effects
- routine checkups if the patient has a history of urinary tract infections
- signs and symptoms of recurrent infection.

Discharge planning

- Refer the patient to a nephrologist for recurring infections, as needed.

Acute respiratory distress syndrome

Overview

Description

- Severe form of alveolar injury or acute lung injury
- A form of pulmonary edema
- May be difficult to recognize
- Hypoxemia despite increased supplemental oxygen (hallmark sign)
- Occurs in four stages that may rapidly progress to fatal hypoxemia
- Little or no permanent lung damage in patients who recover
- May coexist with disseminated intravascular coagulation (DIC)
- Also known as adult respiratory distress syndrome and shock, stiff lung, white lung, wet lung, or Da Nang lung

Pathophysiology

- Increased permeability of the alveolocapillary membranes allows fluid to accumulate in the lung interstitium, alveolar spaces, and small airways, causing the lungs to stiffen.
- Impaired ventilation reduces oxygenation of pulmonary capillary blood.
- Elevated capillary pressure increases interstitial and alveolar edema.
- Alveolar closing pressure exceeds pulmonary pressures.
- Alveoli collapse.

Risk factors

- Chronic disease
- Old age

Causes

- Acute miliary tuberculosis
- Anaphylaxis
- Aspiration of gastric contents
- Coronary artery bypass grafting
- Diffuse pneumonia (especially viral)
- Drug overdose
- Hemodialysis
- Idiosyncratic drug reaction
- Indirect or direct lung trauma (most common)
- Inhalation of noxious gases
- Leukemia
- Near-drowning
- Oxygen toxicity
- Pancreatitis
- Thrombotic thrombocytopenic purpura
- Uremia
- Venous air embolism

Prevalence

- 85% probability in people who have three of the causes listed

Complications

- Cardiac arrest
- Metabolic acidosis
- Multiple organ dysfunction syndrome
- Respiratory acidosis

Assessment

History

- Causative factor (one or more)
- Dyspnea, especially on exertion

Physical assessment

Stage I
- Dyspnea, especially on exertion
- Normal to increased respiratory and pulse rates
- Reduced breath sounds

Stage II
- Anxiety
- Basilar crackles
- Bloody, sticky secretions
- Cool, clammy skin
- Dry cough with thick, frothy sputum
- Increased blood pressure
- Pallor
- Respiratory distress
- Restlessness
- Tachycardia
- Tachypnea
- Use of accessory muscles for respiration

Stage III
- Labile blood pressure
- Pale, cyanotic skin
- Possible crackles and rhonchi
- Productive cough
- Respiratory rate exceeding 30 breaths/minute
- Tachycardia with arrhythmias

Stage IV
- Acute respiratory failure with severe hypoxia
- Bradycardia with arrhythmias
- Deteriorating mental status (possible coma)
- Hypotension
- Lack of spontaneous respirations
- Metabolic and respiratory acidosis
- Pale, cyanotic skin

Test results

Laboratory
- Initial arterial blood gas (ABG) analysis: partial pressure of arterial oxygen (Pao_2) below 60 mm Hg and partial pressure of arterial carbon dioxide ($Paco_2$) below 35 mm Hg
- Later ABG analysis: Pao_2 decreased despite oxygen therapy, $Paco_2$ above 45 mm Hg, and bicarbonate levels below 22 mEq/L

- Infectious organism seen with Gram's stain, sputum culture and sensitivity testing, or blood cultures
- Drug overdose revealed by toxicology tests
- Increased serum amylase in pancreatitis

Imaging
- Early chest X-rays may show bilateral infiltrates.
- Later chest X-rays show a ground-glass appearance and, eventually, "whiteouts" of both lung fields.

Diagnostic procedures
- Pulmonary artery catheterization may find a pulmonary artery wedge pressure of 12 to 18 mm Hg.

Nursing diagnoses

- Anxiety
- Deficient fluid volume
- Impaired gas exchange
- Ineffective tissue perfusion: cardiopulmonary
- Risk for impaired skin integrity

Key outcomes

The patient will:
- maintain adequate ventilation
- maintain a patent airway
- maintain fluid volume balance
- use effective coping strategies
- maintain skin integrity
- report feelings of increased comfort.

Interventions

General

- Correction of electrolyte and acid-base imbalances
- Possible tracheotomy
- Treatment of the underlying cause

For mechanical ventilation
- Bed rest
- Fluid restriction
- Low tidal volumes
- Plateau pressures less than or equal to 40 cm H_2O
- Positive end-expiratory pressure (PEEP) as needed
- Tube feedings or parenteral nutrition
- Use of increased respiratory rates

Nursing

- Give prescribed drugs.
- Maintain a patent airway.
- Perform tracheal suctioning, as needed.
- Ensure adequate humidification.
- Reposition the patient often.
- Consider prone positioning for alveolar recruitment.
- Give tube feedings or parenteral nutrition, as ordered.
- Allow periods of uninterrupted sleep.
- Perform passive range-of-motion exercises.
- Provide meticulous skin care.
- Reposition the endotracheal tube according to facility policy.
- Provide emotional support.

- Provide alternative nonverbal means of communication.

Drug therapy

- Bronchodilators
- Diuretics
- Humidified oxygen

For mechanical ventilation
- Antimicrobials if the patient has nonviral infection
- Fluids and vasopressors if the patient is hypotensive
- Neuromuscular blocking drugs
- Opioids
- Sedatives
- Short course of high-dose corticosteroids if the patient has fatty emboli or chemical injury
- Sodium bicarbonate if the patient has severe metabolic acidosis

Monitoring

- Complications, such as cardiac arrhythmias, DIC, gastrointestinal (GI) bleeding, infection, malnutrition, or pneumothorax
- Daily weight
- Hemodynamics
- Intake and output
- Laboratory studies
- Level of consciousness
- Mechanical ventilator settings
- Nutritional status
- Respiratory status (breath sounds, ABG results)
- Response to treatment
- Sputum characteristics
- Vital signs and pulse oximetry

> **ALERT** Because PEEP may lower cardiac output, check for hypotension, tachycardia, and decreased urine output. To maintain PEEP, suction only as needed.

For mechanical ventilation
- Complications of mechanical ventilation
- Cuff pressure
- Endotracheal tube position and patency
- Signs and symptoms of stress ulcer
- Ventilator settings

Patient teaching

Be sure to cover:
- the disorder, diagnosis, and treatment
- drug regimen and possible adverse reactions
- when to contact a doctor
- complications, such as GI bleeding, infection, and malnutrition
- recovery time.

Discharge planning

- Refer the patient to a pulmonary rehabilitation program, if needed.

Acute respiratory failure

Overview

Description
○ Inadequate ventilation resulting from the inability of the lungs to maintain arterial oxygenation or eliminate carbon dioxide

Pathophysiology
○ If respiratory failure is mainly hypercapnic, it results from inadequate alveolar ventilation.
○ If respiratory failure is mainly hypoxemic, it results from inadequate oxygen exchange between the alveoli and capillaries.
○ Many people with respiratory failure have combined hypercapnic and hypoxemic failure.

Risk factors
○ Any condition that increases the work of breathing and decreases the respiratory drive of patients with chronic obstructive pulmonary disease

Causes
○ Accumulated secretions from cough suppression
○ Airway irritants
○ Bronchospasm
○ Central nervous system depression
○ Gas exchange failure
○ Endocrine or metabolic disorders
○ Heart failure
○ Myocardial infarction (MI)
○ Pulmonary emboli
○ Respiratory tract infection
○ Thoracic abnormalities
○ Ventilatory failure

Prevalence
○ Occurs in patients with hypercapnia and hypoxemia
○ Occurs in patients who have an acute deterioration in arterial blood gas (ABG) values

Complications
○ Chronic respiratory acidosis
○ Metabolic alkalosis
○ Respiratory and cardiac arrest
○ Tissue hypoxia

Assessment

History
○ Cough suppression and resulting accumulated pulmonary secretions
○ Exposure to irritants (smoke or fumes)
○ Heart failure
○ Infection
○ Metabolic acidosis
○ MI
○ Myxedema
○ Precipitating event
○ Pulmonary emboli
○ Trauma

Physical assessment
○ Ashen skin
○ Asymmetrical chest movement
○ Cold, clammy skin
○ Crackles (in pulmonary edema)
○ Cyanosis of the oral mucosa, lips, and nail beds
○ Decreased tactile fremitus over an obstructed bronchus or pleural effusion
○ Hyperresonance
○ Increased tactile fremitus over consolidated lung tissue
○ Nasal flaring
○ Pursed-lip breathing
○ Rapid breathing
○ Reduced or absent breath sounds
○ Rhonchi (in bronchitis)
○ Wheezes (in asthma)
○ Yawning and use of accessory muscles

Test results
Laboratory
○ Hypercapnia and hypoxemia in ABG analysis
○ Increased serum white blood cell count if the patient has a bacterial infection
○ Decreased oxygen-carrying capacity as revealed by serum hemoglobin level and hematocrit
○ Hypokalemia
○ Hypochloremia
○ Pathogen present in blood cultures, Gram's stain, or sputum culture
Imaging
○ Chest X-rays may show underlying pulmonary disorders, such as emphysema, atelectasis, lesions, pneumothorax, infiltrates, or effusion.
Diagnostic procedures
○ Electrocardiography may show arrhythmias, cor pulmonale, or myocardial ischemia.
○ Pulse oximetry may show decreased arterial oxygen saturation.
○ Pulmonary artery catheterization may show pulmonary or cardiovascular changes that could cause acute respiratory failure.

Nursing diagnoses

○ Anxiety
○ Impaired gas exchange
○ Ineffective coping
○ Ineffective tissue perfusion: cardiopulmonary
○ Risk for imbalanced fluid volume
○ Risk for impaired skin integrity

Key outcomes

The patient will:
- maintain a patent airway
- maintain adequate ventilation
- use a support system to assist with coping
- maintain skin integrity
- express feelings of increased comfort
- modify lifestyle to minimize the risk of decreased tissue perfusion
- maintain fluid volume balance.

Interventions

General

- Activity as tolerated
- Fluid restriction if the patient has heart failure
- High-frequency ventilation if the patient doesn't respond to conventional mechanical ventilation
- Mechanical ventilation with an endotracheal or a tracheostomy tube
- Possible tracheostomy

Nursing

- Give prescribed drugs.
- Orient the patient often.
- Give oxygen.
- Maintain a patent airway.
- Encourage pursed-lip breathing.
- Encourage the use of an incentive spirometer.
- Reposition the patient every 1 to 2 hours.
- Help clear the patient's secretions with postural drainage and chest physiotherapy.
- Assist with or perform oral hygiene.
- Position the patient for comfort and optimal gas exchange.
- Maintain normothermia.
- Schedule care to provide frequent rest periods.

For mechanical ventilation
- Obtain blood samples for ABG analysis, as ordered.
- Suction the trachea after hyperoxygenation, as needed.
- Provide humidification.
- Secure the endotracheal (ET) tube according to facility policy.
- Prevent infection.
- Prevent tracheal erosion.
- Maintain skin integrity.
- Provide alternative nonverbal means of communication.
- Provide sedation, as needed.

Drug therapy

- Antacids
- Antibiotics
- Bronchodilators
- Cautious oxygen therapy to increase partial pressure of arterial oxygen
- Corticosteroids
- Diuretics
- Histamine-receptor antagonists
- Positive inotropic drugs
- Vasopressors

Monitoring

- Cardiac rate and rhythm
- Chest X-rays
- Complications
- Daily weight
- Intake and output
- Laboratory studies
- Respiratory status (breath sounds and ABG results)
- Signs and symptoms of infection
- Sputum quality, consistency, and color
- Vital signs and pulse oximetry

For mechanical ventilation
- Complications of mechanical ventilation
- Cuff pressures
- ET tube position and patency
- Signs and symptoms of stress ulcers
- Ventilator settings

Patient teaching

Be sure to cover:
- the disorder, diagnosis, and treatment
- drug regimen and possible adverse reactions
- when to contact a doctor
- smoking cessation, if appropriate
- communication techniques, if intubated
- signs and symptoms of respiratory infection.

Discharge planning

- Refer the patient to a smoking-cessation program, if applicable.

Acute tubular necrosis

Overview

Description
- Injury to the tubular segment of the nephron resulting from ischemic or nephrotoxic injury
- Causes renal failure and uremic syndrome
- Also known as acute tubulointerstitial nephritis

Pathophysiology
- Ischemic injury—as from circulatory collapse, severe hypotension, traumatic injury, hemorrhage, dehydration, cardiogenic or septic shock, surgery, anesthetics, or a transfusion reaction—may disrupt blood flow to the kidneys.
- Nephrotoxic injury may result from a hypersensitivity reaction in the kidneys, or it may follow ingestion of certain chemicals, such as contrast medium or an antibiotic.

Risk factors
- Diabetic nephropathy
- Liver disease

Causes
- Diseased tubular epithelium
- Ischemic injury to glomerular epithelial cells or vascular endothelium
- Obstructed urine flow

Prevalence
- Accounts for about 3 in 4 cases of acute renal failure
- The most common cause of acute renal failure in critically ill patients

Complications
- Anemia
- Anorexia
- Heart failure
- Intractable vomiting
- Poor wound healing from debilitation
- Pulmonary edema
- Uremic lung
- Uremic pericarditis

> ◢ ALERT *Fever and chills may signal the onset of an infection, the leading cause of death in patients with acute tubular necrosis.*

Assessment

- Diagnosis is usually delayed until the condition has progressed to an advanced stage.

History
- Fever and chills
- Ischemic or nephrotoxic injury

- Low urine output (less than 400 ml in 24 hours)

Physical assessment
- Cardiac arrhythmia, if the patient is hyperkalemic
- Dry mucous membranes
- Dry, pruritic skin
- Evidence of bleeding abnormalities, such as petechiae and ecchymosis
- Muscle weakness
- Uremic breath

Test results
Laboratory
- Red blood cells (RBCs) and casts in urine sediment
- Decreased urine specific gravity
- Decreased urine osmolality (less than 400 mOsm/kg)
- Increased urine sodium level (40 to 60 mEq/L)
- Increased blood urea nitrogen and serum creatinine levels
- Anemia
- Defects in platelet adherence
- Metabolic acidosis
- Hyperkalemia

Diagnostic procedures
- Electrocardiography may show arrhythmias and, with hyperkalemia, a widening QRS complex, disappearing P waves, and tall, peaked T waves.

Nursing diagnoses

- Acute pain
- Decreased cardiac output
- Fatigue
- Risk for imbalanced fluid volume
- Risk for infection
- Risk for injury

Key outcomes
The patient will:
- maintain fluid balance
- report increased comfort
- identify risk factors that worsen the condition and modify lifestyle accordingly
- maintain hemodynamic stability.

Interventions

General
Acute phase
- Vigorous supportive measures until normal kidney function resumes

Long-term management
- Daily replacement of projected fluid loss (including insensible loss)
- Peritoneal dialysis or hemodialysis if the patient is catabolic or if hyperkalemia and fluid volume overload aren't controlled by other measures

- Fluid restriction
- Low-sodium, low-potassium diet
- Rest periods when fatigued

Nursing

- Give prescribed drugs and blood products.
- Restrict high-sodium and high-potassium foods.
- Use aseptic technique, particularly when handling catheters.
- Perform passive range-of-motion exercises.
- Provide good skin care.

Drug therapy

- Antibiotics
- Diuretics
- Emergency I.V. administration of 50% glucose, regular insulin, and sodium bicarbonate (with hyperkalemia)
- Epoetin alfa
- Sodium polystyrene sulfonate with sorbitol by mouth or enema (with hyperkalemia)
- Transfusion of packed RBCs

Monitoring

- Complications
- Intake and output
- Laboratory studies
- Vital signs

Patient teaching

Be sure to cover:
- the disorder, diagnosis, and treatment
- signs of infection and when to report them to a doctor
- dietary restrictions
- how to set goals that are realistic for the patient's prognosis.

Discharge planning

- Refer the patient to appropriate supportive services or social service.

Adrenal hypofunction

Overview

Description

Primary hypofunction
- Originates in the adrenal gland
- Characterized by decreased secretion of mineralo-corticoids, glucocorticoids, and androgens
- Also known as Addison's disease

Secondary hypofunction
- Originates in a process outside the adrenal gland, such as impaired pituitary secretion of corticotropin
- Characterized by decreased glucocorticoid secretion

Adrenal crisis
- A critical deficiency of mineralocorticoids and gluco-corticoids
- Typically follows acute stress, sepsis, traumatic injury, surgery, or the omission of corticosteroid therapy in a patient with chronic adrenal insufficiency
- A medical emergency that needs immediate, vigorous treatment
- Also known as addisonian crisis

Pathophysiology
- Adrenal hypofunction results from partial or complete destruction of the adrenal cortex.
- Levels of corticotropin and corticotropin-releasing hormone increase with destruction of the adrenal cortex.
- Addison's disease involves all zones of the cortex and causes deficient secretion of adrenocortical hormones, glucocorticoids, androgens, and mineralo-corticoids.
- Symptoms reflect deficient production of the adreno-cortical hormones cortisol, aldosterone, and androgen.
- Cortisol deficiency decreases liver gluconeogenesis (formation of glucose from noncarbohydrate molecules); as a result, blood glucose levels may become dangerously low in patients who take insulin routinely.
- Aldosterone deficiency increases renal sodium loss and potassium reabsorption.
- Hypotension may result from sodium excretion.
- Production of angiotensin II increases because of low plasma volume and arteriolar pressure.
- Androgen deficiency may decrease hair growth in axillary and pubic areas (less noticeable in men) and on the limbs of women.

Risk factors
- Autoimmune disease
  - Graves' disease
  - Hypoparathyroidism
  - Hypopituitarism
  - Myasthenia gravis
  - Type 1 diabetes

Causes

Primary hypofunction
- Autoimmune process in which circulating antibodies react specifically to adrenal tissue
- Bilateral adrenalectomy
- Family history of autoimmune disease, which may predispose the patient to Addison's disease and other endocrinopathies
- Hemorrhage into the adrenal gland
- Infection, such as histoplasmosis and cytomegalo-virus
- Neoplasm
- Tuberculosis (once the chief cause, now responsible for less than 20% of adult cases)

Secondary hypofunction
- Abrupt withdrawal of long-term corticosteroid therapy
- Hypopituitarism
- Removal of a corticotropin-secreting tumor

Adrenal crisis
- Exhausted body stores of glucocorticoids in a patient with adrenal hypofunction after traumatic injury, surgery, or other physiologic stress

Prevalence

Primary hypofunction
- Relatively uncommon
- May occur at any age and in both sexes

Autoimmune Addison's disease
- Most common in white women, probably from genetic predisposition
- More common in patients with a familial predisposition to autoimmune endocrine diseases

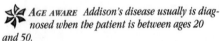 AGE AWARE *Addison's disease usually is diagnosed when the patient is between ages 20 and 50.*

Complications
- Hyperpyrexia
- Inadequate or excessive corticosteroid treatment
- Profound hypoglycemia
- Psychotic reactions
- Shock
- Ultimate vascular collapse, renal shutdown, coma, and death (if untreated)

Assessment

History
- Adrenal surgery
- Amenorrhea (in women)
- Craving for salty food
- Decreased tolerance for stress
- Dehydration
- Fatigue
- Gastrointestinal disturbances
- Impotence (in men)
- Muscle weakness

- Recent infection
- Use of synthetic steroids
- Weight loss

Physical assessment

- Areas of vitiligo
- Bronze coloration of the skin, darkening of scars
- Decreased axillary and pubic hair (in women)
- Hypotension
- Increased pigmentation of mucous membranes
- Poor coordination
- Weak, irregular pulse

Test results

Laboratory

- Increased corticotropin level in rapid corticotropin stimulation test (primary disorder)
- Decreased corticotropin level in rapid corticotropin stimulation test (secondary disorder)
- Decreased plasma cortisol level (less than 10 mcg/dl in the morning)
- Decreased serum sodium level
- Decreased fasting blood glucose level
- Increased serum potassium, calcium, and blood urea nitrogen levels
- Elevated hematocrit
- Increased lymphocyte and eosinophil counts

Imaging

- Chest X-ray shows a small heart.
- Computed tomography scan of the abdomen shows adrenal calcification if the cause is infectious.

Nursing diagnoses

- Decreased cardiac output
- Ineffective coping
- Risk for imbalance fluid volume
- Risk for infection

Key outcomes

The patient will:
- maintain stable vital signs
- maintain an adequate fluid balance
- remain free from signs and symptoms of infection
- develop adequate coping skills.

Interventions

General

- I.V. fluids
- Periods of rest
- Small, frequent, high-protein meals

Nursing

- Until onset of mineralocorticoid effect, encourage fluids to replace excessive fluid loss.

- Arrange for a diet that maintains sodium and potassium balances; if the patient is anorexic, suggest six small meals daily to increase calorie intake.
- Watch for cushingoid signs, such as fluid retention around the eyes and face.
- Check for petechiae.
- If the patient receives glucocorticoids alone, watch for orthostatic hypotension or electrolyte abnormalities.

Drug therapy

- Hydrocortisone
- I.V. saline and glucose solutions (for adrenal crisis)
- Lifelong corticosteroid replacement, usually with cortisone or hydrocortisone
- Oral fludrocortisone

Monitoring

- Blood glucose levels
- Cardiac rhythm
- Daily weight
- Hyperkalemia before treatment
- Hypokalemia after treatment
- Intake and output
- Signs of shock (decreased level of consciousness and urine output)
- Vital signs

Patient teaching

Be sure to cover:
- lifelong need for corticosteroid therapy
- symptoms of corticosteroid overdose (swelling, weight gain) and underdose (lethargy, weakness)
- possible need for increased dosage during times of stress or illness (when the patient has a cold, for example)
- risk of adrenal crisis during infection, injury, or profuse sweating in hot weather
- the importance of wearing or carrying medical identification showing that the patient takes a corticosteroid, including the drug name and dosage
- procedure for giving a hydrocortisone injection
- need to keep an emergency kit containing hydrocortisone in a prepared syringe available for use in times of stress
- stress management techniques.

Discharge planning

- Refer the patient to the National Adrenal Diseases Foundation for support and information.

Adrenogenital syndrome

Overview

Description

- A group of disorders resulting from hyperplasia of the adrenal cortex
- May be inherited, as in congenital adrenal hyperplasia (CAH)
- May be acquired, usually from an adrenal tumor (adrenal virilism)
- May cause fatal adrenal crisis in neonates (salt-losing CAH)

Pathophysiology

- Deficiencies occur in the enzymes needed for adrenocortical secretion of cortisol and possibly aldosterone.
- Compensatory corticotropin secretion produces varying degrees of adrenal hyperplasia.

Simple virilizing congenital adrenal hyperplasia
- Deficiency of the enzyme 21-hydroxylase results in underproduction of cortisol.
- Cortisol deficiency causes increased secretion of corticotropin, producing large amounts of cortisol precursors and androgens that don't require 21-hydroxylase for synthesis.

Salt-losing congenital adrenal hyperplasia
- 21-hydroxylase is almost completely absent.
- Corticotropin secretion increases, causing excessive production of cortisol precursors, including salt-wasting compounds.
- Plasma cortisol and aldosterone levels — both dependent on 21-hydroxylase — fall precipitously and, combined with excessive production of salt-wasting compounds, precipitate acute adrenal crisis.
- Corticotropin hypersecretion stimulates adrenal androgens and produces masculinization.

Causes

- Transmitted as an autosomal recessive trait

Prevalence

- Rare (acquired adrenal virilism)
- Affects twice as many female as male children

✳ *AGE AWARE CAH is the most prevalent adrenal disorder in infants and children; simple virilizing CAH and salt-losing CAH are the most common forms.*

Complications

- Adrenal crisis
- Adrenal tumor

- Altered growth, external genitalia, and sexual maturity
- Hyperkalemic infertility
- Hypertension

Salt-losing congenital adrenal hyperplasia
- Cardiac arrest
- Cardiovascular collapse

Assessment

History

Simple virilizing congenital adrenal hyperplasia
- Failure to start menstruation (girls)
- Frequent erections at an early age (boys)

Salt-losing congenital adrenal hyperplasia
- Apathy, failure to eat, and diarrhea (infants)
- Symptoms of adrenal crisis in the first week after birth (vomiting, dehydration from hyponatremia, hyperkalemia)

Physical assessment

- Pseudohermaphroditism in girls
- Precocious puberty in either sex

Salt-losing congenital adrenal hyperplasia
- May be taller than other children of the same age
- Progressive virilization at an early age: early appearance of pubic and axillary hair, deep voice, acne, facial hair
- Small testes

Test results

Laboratory
- Elevated levels of plasma 17-ketosteroids (17-KS), which can be suppressed with oral dexamethasone
- Elevated urinary levels of hormone metabolites, particularly pregnanetriol
- Elevated plasma 17-hydroxyprogesterone level
- Normal or decreased urinary levels of 17-hydroxycorticosteroids

✳ *AGE AWARE Adrenal hypofunction or adrenal crisis in the first week after birth suggests salt-losing CAH. Hyperkalemia, hyponatremia, and hypochloremia with excessive urinary 17-KS and pregnanetriol and decreased urinary aldosterone levels confirm it.*

Diagnostic procedures
- Gonadal biopsy and chromosomal studies confirm hermaphroditism.
- Sex chromatin and karyotype studies determine the genetic sex of patients with ambiguous genitalia.

Nursing diagnoses

- Decreased cardiac output
- Deficient knowledge: adrenal hypofunction
- Risk for imbalanced fluid volume

Key outcomes

The patient will:
○ maintain stable vital signs
○ maintain adequate fluid balance
○ have normal laboratory test results
○ express understanding of the disorder and treatment, as will his family.

Interventions

General

○ No activity restriction
○ Reconstructive surgery based on the determined sex and external genitalia
○ Well-balanced diet

Nursing

○ Maintain I.V. access, infuse fluids, and give corticosteroids, as ordered.
○ Watch for cyanosis, hypotension, tachycardia, tachypnea, and signs of shock.
○ Minimize external stressors.
○ If a child is receiving maintenance therapy with corticosteroid injections, rotate I.M. injection sites to prevent atrophy, and tell the parents to do the same.

Drug therapy

Simple virilizing congenital adrenal hyperplasia
○ Cortisone or hydrocortisone given daily
Salt-losing congenital adrenal hyperplasia with adrenal crisis
○ Desoxycorticosterone I.M.
○ Hydrocortisone I.V.
○ Immediate I.V. infusion of sodium chloride and glucose
○ Maintenance: mineralocorticoid replacement (desoxycorticosterone, fludrocortisone, or both) and glucocorticoid replacement (cortisone or hydrocortisone)

Monitoring

○ Blood pressure
○ Body weight
○ Edema, weakness, and hypertension if the patient receives desoxycorticosterone or fludrocortisone
○ Serum electrolyte levels

Patient teaching

Be sure to cover:
○ possible adverse effects (cushingoid symptoms) of long-term therapy
○ need for lifelong maintenance therapy with hydrocortisone, cortisone, or the mineralocorticoid fludrocortisone

○ the importance of not stopping drugs suddenly because life-threatening adrenal hypofunction will result
○ need to report stress and infection, which warrant increased corticosteroid dosages
○ the importance of wearing or carrying medical identification showing that the patient takes a corticosteroid, including the drug name and dosage.

Discharge planning

○ Refer the patient for psychological counseling to help accept this disorder.

Alport's syndrome

Overview

Description
○ Hereditary nephritis
○ Characterized by recurrent gross or microscopic hematuria
○ Accompanied by deafness, albuminuria, and variably progressive azotemia

Pathophysiology
○ Genetic mutations lead to abnormalities in the basement membrane of the glomerulus.
○ Abnormalities lead to hematuria and glomerulosclerosis.

Risk factors
○ Genetic predisposition

Causes
○ Genetic transmission as an X-linked, autosomal trait

Prevalence
○ Usually arises during childhood
○ Affects males more often and more severely than females

✴ *AGE AWARE Many men with hematuria and proteinuria from Alport's syndrome develop end-stage renal disease in their 30s or 40s.*

◥ *ALERT Respiratory infection commonly causes recurrent bouts of hematuria in those with Alport's syndrome.*

Assessment

History
○ Deafness (especially to high-frequency sounds)
○ Family history of recurrent hematuria and renal failure (especially in men)
○ Flank pain
○ Recurrent hematuria, which typically appears during early childhood

Physical assessment
○ Deafness
○ Flank pain
○ Hematuria
○ Hypertension (commonly related to progressive renal failure)
○ Ocular changes, possibly including cataracts and, less commonly, keratoconus, myopia, retinitis pigmentosa, and nystagmus

Test results

Laboratory
○ Immunoglobulins and complement components in blood studies
○ Proteinuria
○ Pyuria
○ Red cell casts in urine

Diagnostic procedures
○ Audiology reveals hearing loss.
○ Electron microscopy reveals characteristic changes in basement membrane and confirms diagnosis.
○ Renal biopsy confirms the diagnosis when electron microscopy shows basement membrane changes.

✴ *AGE AWARE Symptoms of Alport's syndrome in children almost always include hearing loss and such ocular defects as lenticonus, posterior polymorphous corneal dystrophy, and retinal flecks.*

Nursing diagnoses

○ Deficient knowledge: Alport's syndrome
○ Impaired urinary elimination
○ Ineffective coping

Key outcomes
The patient will:
○ express understanding of the disorder, diagnostic testing, and treatment
○ show appropriate coping mechanisms
○ use available support systems
○ regain or maintain adequate renal function.

Interventions

General
○ Dialysis
○ Eyeglasses or contact lenses
○ Hearing aid
○ Kidney transplantation
○ Supportive and symptomatic care

Nursing
○ Provide emotional support.
○ Pursue an effective communication system.

Drug therapy
○ Antibiotics
○ Antihypertensives

Monitoring
○ Blood pressure
○ Laboratory values
○ Urine color
○ Urine output

Patient teaching

Be sure to cover:
- the diagnosis, testing, and treatment
- the need to monitor urine function
- when to contact a doctor.

Discharge planning

- Refer the patient and family for genetic counseling as appropriate.

Amyloidosis

Overview

Description

- A rare, chronic disease characterized by accumulation of an abnormal fibrillar scleroprotein (amyloid) that infiltrates organs and soft tissues
- May be primary or secondary
- May affect the inner coats of blood vessels (perireticular type)
- May affect the outer coats of blood vessels and the parenchyma (pericollagen type)
- Variable prognosis based on type and on site and extent of involvement
- Sometimes causes permanent — possibly life-threatening — organ damage
- Sometimes linked to a Mediterranean ethnic origin (familial Mediterranean fever [FMF]), although only 50% of those with FMF have a family history of the disorder
- Sometimes diagnosed as multiple myeloma

Pathophysiology

- Accumulation and infiltration of amyloid causes pressure on and atrophy of nearby cells.
- Some types of amyloidosis cause reticuloendothelial cell dysfunction and abnormal immunoglobulin synthesis.

Risk factors

- Age older than 50
- Chronic infection or inflammatory disease
- Increased protein in diet
- Multiple myeloma

Causes

- Primary amyloidosis: no apparent cause
- Secondary amyloidosis: disorders that cause chronic inflammation, such as tuberculosis, Crohn's disease, rheumatoid arthritis, Hodgkin's disease, and syphilis
- May accompany Alzheimer's disease
- Linked to type 2 diabetes mellitus
- Ethnic origin in the Mediterranean area (hereditary form)

Prevalence

- In the United States, evidence of amyloidosis in 0.5% of autopsies
- Difficult to determine actual occurrence

Complications

- Heart failure
- Nephrotic syndrome
- Renal failure

Assessment

History

- Usually asymptomatic until organs are affected
- Constipation or diarrhea

Physical assessment

- Variable signs and symptoms based on system affected

Renal system
- Edema
- Low urine output

Cardiac system
- Faint heart sounds
- Irregular heartbeat
- Shortness of breath

Gastrointestinal (GI) system
- Abdominal pain
- Clay-colored stools
- GI bleeding
- Signs of malnutrition
- Stiffness and enlargement of the tongue

Skin
- Papules
- Purpura

Respiratory system
- Trouble breathing
- Wheezing

Neurologic system
- Carpal tunnel symptoms
- Muscle weakness
- Numbness and tingling

Test results

Laboratory
- Proteinuria
- Histologic confirmation, via polarizing or electron microscope, of aspirated tissue from rectal mucosa and abdominal fat pad (less hazardous than kidney or liver biopsy) or possibly from gingiva, skin, or nerves

Imaging
- A chest X-ray may show an enlarged heart and congestive heart failure.

Diagnostic procedures
- Electrocardiography may show low-voltage and conduction or rhythm abnormalities resembling those of a myocardial infarction.

Nursing diagnoses

- Deficient knowledge: amyloidosis
- Ineffective airway clearance
- Ineffective coping
- Risk for impaired skin integrity

Key outcomes

The patient will:
○ show effective coping mechanisms
○ use available support systems
○ express understanding of the disorder and its treatment
○ maintain a patent airway
○ avoid a break in skin integrity.

Interventions

General

○ Elimination of the underlying cause
○ Supportive care based on symptoms
○ Total parenteral nutrition
○ Transplantation of affected organ, although this action doesn't halt the disorder

Nursing

○ Offer emotional support.
○ Provide care as needed based on symptoms.
○ Supply meticulous mouth care if the tongue is involved.
○ Establish an alternate nonverbal means of communication if the patient can't talk.
○ Regularly assess airway patency if the patient's tongue is involved, and prevent respiratory tract compromise with gentle and adequate suctioning, if needed. Keep a tracheostomy tray at bedside.

Drug therapy

○ Analgesics
○ Antibiotics
○ Colchicine
○ Laxatives

Monitoring

○ Complications
○ Intake and output
○ Laboratory values
○ Nutritional status

Patient teaching

Be sure to cover:
○ the disorder, diagnostic tests, and treatment
○ when to contact a doctor
○ drug regimen, dosages, and adverse effects.

Discharge planning

○ Refer the patient for speech therapy, if needed.

Anaphylaxis

Overview

Description
- Dramatic, acute atopic reaction to an allergen
- Marked by sudden onset of rapidly progressive urticaria and respiratory distress
- Severity greater as time between exposure to the antigen and appearance of signs and symptoms decreases
- May include vascular collapse, systemic shock, and possibly death if reaction is severe

Pathophysiology
- After initial exposure to an antigen, the immune system produces immunoglobulin (Ig) antibodies in the lymph nodes. Helper T cells enhance the process.
- IgE antibodies bind to membrane receptors on mast cells and basophils.
- When the antigen reappears, the IgE antibodies, or cross-linked IgE receptors, recognize the antigen as foreign, activating the release of powerful chemical mediators that produce signs and symptoms of an allergic reaction.
- IgG or IgM antibodies take part in the reaction and activate the release of complement factors.

Risk factors
- History of allergies
- History of asthma
- Previous anaphylactic reaction

Causes
- Systemic exposure to sensitizing drugs, foods, insect venom, or other specific antigens

Prevalence
- Most common anaphylaxis-causing antigen: penicillin, which causes a reaction in 1 to 4 of every 10,000 patients treated

Complications
- Respiratory obstruction
- Systemic vascular collapse
- Death

Assessment

History
- Complaints of shortness of breath and chest tightness
- Complaints of sweating and weakness
- Immediately after exposure, complaints of a feeling of impending doom or fright
- Reports of sneezing and nasal itching
- Reports of a lump in the throat (angioedema)

Physical assessment
- Angioedema
- Apprehension, restlessness
- Cool and clammy skin
- Cyanosis
- Diarrhea
- Dizziness, drowsiness
- Edema
- Erythema
- Headache
- Hoarseness or stridor
- Hypotension, shock
- Nausea
- Seizures
- Severe abdominal cramps
- Tachypnea
- Urinary urgency and incontinence
- Urticaria
- Wheezing
- Angina and cardiac arrhythmias (less common)

Test results
- Not needed, although skin testing may help identify a particular allergen
- Diagnosis established by signs, symptoms, and history

Nursing diagnoses
- Acute pain
- Decreased cardiac output
- Impaired gas exchange
- Ineffective airway clearance
- Ineffective tissue perfusion (renal)
- Risk for injury

Key outcomes
The patient will:
- maintain a patent airway
- maintain adequate ventilation
- express feelings of increased comfort and decreased pain
- maintain normal cardiac output and normal heart rate
- identify causative allergen
- maintain fluid balance.

Interventions

General
- Airway establishment and maintenance
- Bed rest until stable
- Cardiopulmonary resuscitation if needed
- Nothing by mouth until stable

Nursing
- Provide supplemental oxygen and prepare to assist with insertion of an endotracheal tube, if needed.

○ Insert a peripheral I.V. line.
○ Continually reassure the patient, and explain all tests and treatments.
○ If the patient has skin or scratch testing, watch for signs of a serious allergic response. Keep emergency resuscitation equipment readily available.

▼ *ALERT If a patient must receive a drug to which he's allergic, prevent a severe reaction by making sure he either receives corticosteroids before the allergenic drug or he undergoes careful desensitization with gradually increasing doses of the antigen. Monitor the patient closely, and keep resuscitation equipment and epinephrine readily available.*

Drug therapy
○ Aminophylline I.V.
○ Antihistamines
○ Corticosteroids
○ Diphenhydramine I.V.
○ Dopamine
○ Immediate injection of epinephrine 1:1,000 aqueous solution, 0.1 to 0.5 ml S.C. or I.V.
○ Norepinephrine
○ Vasopressors
○ Volume expander infusions, as needed

Monitoring
○ Adverse reactions to radiographic contrast media
○ Complications
○ Degree of edema
○ Neurologic status
○ Respiratory status
○ Response to treatment
○ Serious allergic response after skin or scratch testing
○ Vital signs

Patient teaching

Be sure to cover:
○ the risk of delayed symptoms and the importance of reporting them immediately
○ the need to avoid exposure to known allergens
○ the importance of carrying and knowing how to use an anaphylaxis kit
○ the need to wear medical identification jewelry to identify the allergy.

Discharge planning

○ Refer the patient to an allergist or pulmonary specialist as indicated.

Aneurysm, abdominal aortic

Overview

Description

○ Abnormal dilation in the arterial wall of the aorta, commonly between the renal arteries and iliac branches
○ May be fusiform (spindle-shaped), saccular (pouch-like), or dissecting

Pathophysiology

○ Degenerative changes develop into a focal weakness in the tunica media layer of the aorta, which allows the tunica intima and tunica adventitia layers to stretch outward.
○ Pressure from blood in the aorta progressively weakens vessel walls and enlarges the aneurysm.

Risk factors

○ Age older than 50
○ Atherosclerosis
○ Caucasian
○ Diabetes
○ Family history of abdominal aortic aneurysm
○ History of smoking
○ Hypertension
○ Increased cholesterol level
○ Male sex

Causes

○ Arteriosclerosis or atherosclerosis (95%)
○ Infection
○ Syphilis
○ Traumatic injury

Prevalence

○ Seven times more common in hypertensive men than in women
○ Most common in whites ages 50 to 80

Complications

○ Dissection
○ Hemorrhage
○ Shock

Assessment

History

○ Asymptomatic until the aneurysm enlarges and compresses surrounding tissue
○ Syncope when aneurysm ruptures
○ Possible resolution of symptoms when a clot forms and bleeding stops

○ Possible abdominal pain from bleeding into the peritoneum

Physical assessment

Intact aneurysm

○ Gnawing, generalized, steady abdominal pain
○ Lower back pain unaffected by movement
○ Gastric or abdominal fullness
○ Sudden onset of severe abdominal pain or lumbar pain with radiation to flank and groin
○ Possible pulsating mass in the periumbilical area

 ALERT *If the patient has a pulsating mass in the periumbilical area, don't palpate it.*

Ruptured aneurysm

○ Absent distal peripheral pulses
○ Decreased level of consciousness
○ Diaphoresis
○ Distended abdomen
○ Ecchymosis or hematoma in the abdominal, flank, or groin area
○ Gastrointestinal bleeding with massive hematemesis and melena with rupture into the duodenum
○ Hypotension
○ Mottled skin from poor distal perfusion
○ Oliguria
○ Paraplegia if rupture reduces blood flow to the spine
○ Severe, persistent abdominal and back pain with rupture in to the peritoneal cavity
○ Systolic bruit over the aorta
○ Tachycardia
○ Tenderness over the affected area

Test results

Imaging

○ Anteroposterior and lateral abdominal X-rays can detect aortic calcification, which outlines the mass at least 75% of the time.
○ Computed tomography scan may be used to determine the effect of the aneurysm on nearby organs.

Diagnostic procedures

○ Abdominal ultrasonography or echocardiography may determine the size, shape, and location of the aneurysm.
○ Aortography shows the condition of vessels proximal and distal to the aneurysm and the extent of the aneurysm.

 ALERT *Aortography may underestimate the diameter of an aneurysm because it shows only the flow channel and not the surrounding clot.*

Nursing diagnoses

○ Acute pain
○ Anxiety
○ Decreased cardiac output
○ Deficient fluid volume
○ Deficient knowledge: abdominal aortic aneurysm

○ Ineffective tissue perfusion: cardiopulmonary

Key outcomes

The patient will:
○ maintain adequate cardiac output
○ maintain hemodynamic stability
○ maintain palpable pulses distal to the aneurysm site
○ maintain adequate urine output (equivalent to intake)
○ express feelings of increased comfort and decreased pain
○ relate an understanding of the disease process and treatment.

Interventions

General

Small, asymptomatic aneurysm
○ Activity, as tolerated
○ Careful control of hypertension
○ Fluid and blood replacement
○ Low-fat diet
○ Weight reduction, if appropriate

Large or symptomatic aneurysm
○ Bypass if perfusion distal to aneurysm is poor
○ Endovascular grafting
○ Repair and graft replacement for a ruptured aneurysm
○ Surgical resection

Nursing

In a nonacute situation
○ Let the patient express his fears and concerns.
○ Identify effective coping strategies.
○ Offer the patient and his family psychological support.
○ Before elective surgery, weigh the patient, insert an indwelling urinary catheter and an I.V. line, and assist with insertion of the arterial line and pulmonary artery catheter to monitor hemodynamic balance.
○ Give prescribed preventive antibiotics.

In an acute situation
○ Insert an I.V. line with at least a 14G needle to facilitate blood replacement.
○ Obtain blood samples for laboratory tests, as ordered.
○ Give prescribed drugs.

 ALERT *Watch carefully for signs of rupture, which may be immediately fatal. If an aneurysm ruptures, the patient will need surgery immediately. Medical antishock trousers may be used during transport.*

After surgery
○ Assess peripheral pulses for graft failure or occlusion.
○ Watch for signs of retroperitoneal bleeding from the graft site.

○ Maintain the patient's blood pressure in the prescribed range using fluids and drugs.

 ALERT *Assess the patient for severe back pain, which may indicate that the graft is tearing.*

○ Have the patient cough, or suction the endotracheal tube, as needed.
○ Turn the patient often, and assist with ambulation as soon as the patient is able.

Drug therapy

○ Analgesics
○ Antibiotics
○ Antihypertensives
○ Beta blockers

Monitoring

○ Abdominal dressings
○ Arterial blood gas values, as ordered
○ Cardiac rhythm and hemodynamics
○ Daily weight
○ Fluid status
○ Intake and output hourly
○ Laboratory studies
○ Nasogastric intubation for patency, amount, and type of drainage
○ Neurologic status
○ Pulse oximetry
○ Respirations and breath sounds at least every hour
○ Vital signs
○ Wound site for infection

Patient teaching

Be sure to cover:
○ surgical procedure and expected postoperative care
○ importance of taking all prescribed drugs and carrying a list of these drugs at all times, in case of an emergency
○ physical activity restrictions until the patient is cleared by the doctor
○ the need for regular examinations and ultrasound checks to monitor progression of the aneurysm if the patient didn't have surgery.

Discharge planning

○ Refer the patient for follow-up visits with a cardiologist as appropriate.

Aneurysm, thoracic aortic

Overview

Description
○ Abnormal widening of the ascending, transverse, or descending part of the aorta
○ May be saccular (outpouching), fusiform (spindle-shaped), or dissecting
○ Usually an emergency with a poor prognosis

Pathophysiology
○ Circumferential or transverse tear of the aortic wall intima, usually in the medial layer

Risk factors
○ Hypertension
○ Cigarette smoking

Causes
○ Atherosclerosis
○ Bacterial infections, usually at an atherosclerotic plaque
○ Blunt chest trauma
○ Coarctation of the aorta
○ Marfan syndrome
○ Rheumatic vasculitis
○ Syphilis

Prevalence
○ Ascending thoracic aorta the most common site
○ Occurs mainly in hypertensive men younger than age 60
○ Descending thoracic aortic aneurysms most common in younger people who have had chest trauma

Complications
○ Cardiac tamponade
○ Dissection
○ Death

Assessment

History
○ No signs and symptoms until aneurysm expands and begins to dissect
○ Sudden pain and possibly syncope

Physical assessment
○ Abrupt loss of radial and femoral pulses and right and left carotid pulses
○ Abrupt onset of intermittent neurologic deficits
○ Cyanosis
○ Diaphoresis
○ Dyspnea
○ Increasing area of flatness over the heart, suggesting cardiac tamponade and hemopericardium
○ Pallor
○ Transient paralysis
○ Weak legs

Dissecting ascending aneurysm
○ Boring, tearing, or ripping pain in the thorax or the right anterior chest that may extend to the neck, shoulders, lower back, and abdomen
○ Diastolic murmur of aortic insufficiency
○ Normal or significantly increased blood pressure, with a large difference in systolic blood pressure between the right and left arms
○ Pain most intense at onset
○ Pericardial friction rub if the patient has hemopericardium

Dissecting descending aneurysm
○ Carotid and radial pulses present and equal bilaterally
○ Possible bilateral crackles and rhonchi if the patient has pulmonary edema
○ Sharp, tearing pain between the shoulder blades that usually radiates to the chest
○ Systolic blood pressure that's equal bilaterally

Dissecting transverse aneurysm
○ Dry cough
○ Dysphagia
○ Dyspnea
○ Hoarseness
○ Sharp, boring, tearing pain that radiates to the shoulders
○ Throat pain

Test results

Laboratory
○ Possible decreased hemoglobin level from blood loss through a leaking aneurysm

Imaging
○ Posteroanterior and oblique chest X-rays may show widening of the aorta and mediastinum.
○ Magnetic resonance imaging and computed tomography may be used to confirm and locate a dissection.

Diagnostic procedures
○ Electrocardiography will show no evidence of a myocardial infarction.
○ Aortography may be used to determine the lumen, size, and location of the aneurysm.
○ Echocardiography may be used to identify a dissecting aneurysm of the aortic root.
○ Transesophageal echocardiography may be used to measure an aneurysm in the ascending and descending aorta.

Nursing diagnoses

○ Acute pain
○ Decreased cardiac output
○ Deficient fluid volume

- Ineffective gas exchange
- Risk for infection

Key outcomes

The patient will:
- maintain adequate cardiac output and hemodynamic stability
- maintain adequate ventilation
- express feelings of increased comfort and decreased pain
- show no signs or symptoms of infection
- maintain adequate fluid volume.

Interventions

General

- I.V. fluids and whole blood transfusions, if needed
- Low-fat diet
- No activity restrictions unless the patient has surgery
- Surgical resection with a Dacron or Teflon graft
- Weight reduction, if appropriate

Nursing

- In a nonemergency situation, give the patient time to express his fears and concerns and to identify and use effective coping strategies.
- Offer the patient and his family psychological support.
- Give prescribed analgesics to relieve pain.

After repair of a thoracic aneurysm
- Maintain blood pressure in the prescribed range using fluids and drugs.
- Give prescribed analgesics.
- After stabilization of vital signs, encourage and assist the patient in turning, coughing, and deep breathing.
- Help the patient walk as soon as he's able.
- Assist the patient with range-of-motion leg exercises.

Drug therapy

- Analgesics
- Antibiotics
- Antihypertensives
- Beta blockers
- Negative inotropic drugs

Monitoring

- Chest tube drainage
- Distal pulses
- Heart and lung sounds
- I.V. therapy and intake and output
- Laboratory results
- Level of consciousness and pain
- Signs of infection
- Vital signs and hemodynamics

▼ **ALERT** *After surgical repair, watch for signs and symptoms similar to those of the initial dissecting aneurysm; they suggest a tear at the graft site.*

Patient teaching

Be sure to cover:
- diagnosis
- procedure and expected postoperative care, if surgery is scheduled
- compliance with antihypertensive therapy, including the need for drugs and their expected adverse effects
- monitoring of blood pressure
- the need to call a doctor if the patient has any sharp pain in the chest or back of the neck.

Discharge planning

- Refer the patient to a smoking-cessation program, if indicated.

Aneurysm, ventricular

Overview

Description

- An outpouching of a ventricle, almost always the left, that produces ventricular wall dysfunction
- May develop days to weeks after myocardial infarction (MI) or may be delayed for years

Pathophysiology

- When an MI destroys a large section of muscle in the left ventricle, necrosis reduces the ventricular wall to a thin sheath of fibrous tissue.
- Under intracardiac pressure, the thin sheath stretches and forms a separate noncontractile sac.
- The affected ventricular wall moves abnormally.
- During systolic ejection, abnormal muscle wall movements cause the remaining normal myocardial fibers to contract more forcefully to maintain stroke volume and cardiac output.
- At the same time, a portion of the stroke volume is lost to passive distention of the noncontractile sac.

Risk factors

- History of MI

Causes

- MI

Prevalence

- Occurs in about 20% of patients who have an MI

Complications

- Cerebral embolization
- Heart failure
- Ventricular arrhythmias

Assessment

History

- Dyspnea
- Fatigue
- Previous MI

Physical assessment

- Arrhythmias, such as premature ventricular contractions
- Crackles and rhonchi
- Distended jugular veins, if heart failure is present
- Double, diffuse, or displaced apical impulse
- Edema
- Gallop rhythm
- Irregular peripheral pulse rhythm
- Pulsus alternans
- Visible or palpable systolic precordial bulge

Test results

Imaging

- If the aneurysm is large, a chest X-ray may show an abnormal bulge that distorts the heart's contour (may be normal if the aneurysm is small).

Diagnostic procedures

- Electrocardiography may show persistent ST–T wave elevations.
- Two-dimensional echocardiography shows abnormal motion in the left ventricular wall.
- Left ventriculography may be used to show left ventricular enlargement with an area of akinesia or dyskinesia (during cineangiography) and diminished cardiac function.
- Noninvasive nuclear cardiology may indicate the site of infarction and the area of aneurysm.

Nursing diagnoses

- Acute pain
- Anxiety
- Decreased cardiac output
- Deficient fluid volume
- Fatigue

Key outcomes

The patient will:
- maintain adequate cardiac output
- maintain hemodynamic stability
- maintain adequate fluid balance
- express feelings of increased energy and decreased fatigue
- express feelings of decreased anxiety.

Interventions

General

- Depends on the size of the aneurysm and the presence of complications
- Aneurysmectomy with myocardial revascularization
- Embolectomy
- Low-fat diet
- May warrant only routine medical examination to follow the patient's condition
- May warrant aggressive measures, such as cardioversion, defibrillation, and endotracheal intubation
- No activity restrictions unless the patient undergoes surgery
- Weight reduction, if appropriate

Nursing

- Give prescribed drugs.
- Prepare the patient for surgery, if indicated.
- Provide psychological support for the patient and his family.

  ▶ **ALERT** *Stay alert for sudden changes in sensorium, which may indicate cerebral embolization, and for signs that suggest renal failure or an MI.*

Drug therapy

○ Analgesics
○ Antiarrhythmics
○ Anticoagulants
○ Antihypertensives
○ Cardiac glycosides
○ Diuretics
○ Fluid and electrolyte replacement
○ Nitrates

Monitoring

Heart failure

○ Cardiac rhythm, especially for ventricular arrhythmias
○ Blood urea nitrogen and serum creatinine levels
○ Fluid and electrolyte balance
○ Intake and output
○ Vital signs and heart sounds

After surgery

○ Pulmonary artery catheter pressures
○ Signs and symptoms of infection
○ Type and amount of chest tube drainage

Patient teaching

Be sure to cover:
○ the disorder, diagnosis, and treatment
○ prescribed drugs and their potential adverse reactions
○ when to contact a doctor
○ expected postoperative care, if the patient is scheduled to undergo resection
○ how to monitor pulse irregularity and rate changes.

Discharge planning

○ Refer the patient (or his family) to a community-based cardiopulmonary resuscitation training program.
○ Refer the patient to a weight-reduction program, if needed.
○ Refer the patient to a smoking-cessation program, if needed.

Anorexia nervosa

Overview

Description
- A psychological disorder of self-imposed starvation
- Results from a distorted body image and an intense and irrational fear of gaining weight
- Loss of appetite (rare)
- May occur with bulimia nervosa

Pathophysiology
- Decreased calorie intake depletes body fat and protein stores.
- Lack of lipid substrate for synthesis causes estrogen deficiency and amenorrhea in women.
- Testosterone levels fluctuate in men, decreasing erectile function and sperm count.
- Increased use of fat as energy leads to ketoacidosis.

Risk factors
- Compulsive personality
- High achievement goals
- Feeling of pressure to achieve
- Issues with dependence and independence
- Low self-esteem
- Sexual abuse
- Social attitudes that equate slimness with beauty
- Stress caused by multiple responsibilities

Causes
- Exact cause unknown
- Subconscious need to exert personal control over life or to protect oneself from dealing with issues surrounding sexuality, dependence, achievement

Prevalence
- Affects 5% to 10% of the American population
- Affects females in more than 90% of cases

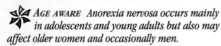 **AGE AWARE** *Anorexia nervosa occurs mainly in adolescents and young adults but also may affect older women and occasionally men.*

Complications
- Amenorrhea
- Anemia
- Decreased cardiac output
- Decreased left ventricular muscle mass and chamber size
- Dehydration
- Electrocardiogram changes
- Electrolyte imbalances
- Esophageal erosion, ulcers, tears, and bleeding
- Heart failure
- Hypotension
- Increased susceptibility to infection
- Malnutrition
- Suicide attempts
- Tooth and gum erosion and dental caries
- Death

Assessment

History
- Amenorrhea
- Angry disposition
- Compulsion to be thin
- Constipation or diarrhea
- Fatigue
- Infertility
- Intolerance to cold
- Loss of libido
- Loss of 15% or more of body weight for no known reason
- Morbid fear of being fat (See *Criteria for diagnosing anorexia nervosa.*)
- Ritualistic personality
- Sleep alterations
- Tendency to minimize weight loss

Physical assessment
- Atrophy of breast tissue
- Blotchy or sallow skin
- Bradycardia
- Dryness or loss of scalp hair
- Emaciated appearance
- Hypotension
- Lanugo on the face and body
- Loss of fatty tissue
- Skeletal muscle atrophy

With bulimia
- Abrasions or scars on the dorsum of the hand
- Bowel distention
- Calluses of the knuckles
- Dental caries
- Oral or pharyngeal abrasions
- Painless salivary gland enlargement
- Slowed reflexes

Test results
Laboratory
- Decreased hemoglobin level, platelet count, and white blood cell count
- Prolonged bleeding time
- Decreased erythrocyte sedimentation rate
- Decreased levels of serum creatinine, blood urea nitrogen, uric acid, cholesterol, total protein, albumin, sodium, potassium, chloride, calcium, and fasting blood glucose
- Elevated levels of alanine aminotransferase and aspartate aminotransferase in severe starvation states
- Elevated serum amylase levels
- In women, decreased levels of serum luteinizing hormone and follicle-stimulating hormone
- Decreased triiodothyronine levels
- Dilute urine

Diagnostic procedures
○ Electrocardiography may show nonspecific changes in ST interval and T wave, a prolonged PR interval, and possible ventricular arrhythmias.

Nursing diagnoses

○ Chronic low self-esteem
○ Deficient fluid volume
○ Delayed growth and development
○ Disturbed body image
○ Imbalanced nutrition: less than body requirements

Key outcomes
The patient will:
○ acknowledge a change in body image
○ express positive feelings about self
○ achieve and maintain an expected body weight
○ achieve an expected state of wellness
○ maintain fluid volume balance.

Interventions

General
○ Balanced diet with a normal eating pattern
○ Behavior modification
○ Curtailed activity if needed for cardiac arrhythmias
○ Gradual increase in physical activity with weight gain and stabilization
○ Group, family, or individual psychotherapy
○ Parenteral nutrition, if needed

Nursing
○ Support the patient's efforts to achieve a target weight.
○ Negotiate an adequate food intake with the patient.
○ Supervise the patient one-on-one during meals and for 1 hour afterward.

Drug therapy
○ Vitamin and mineral supplements

Monitoring
○ Activity for compulsive exercise
○ Electrolyte levels and complete blood count
○ Intake and output
○ Vital signs
○ Weight on a regular schedule

 ALERT *Monitor the patient for 1 hour after meals to rule out self-induced vomiting.*

Patient teaching

Be sure to cover:
○ nutrition
○ the importance of keeping a food journal

Criteria for diagnosing anorexia nervosa

According to the *Diagnostic and Statistical Manual of Mental Disorders,* 4th edition (text revision), these criteria must be documented before a patient can be diagnosed with anorexia nervosa:
● Refusal to maintain or achieve normal weight for age and height
● Intense fear of gaining weight or becoming fat, even though underweight
● Disturbed perception of body weight, size, or shape
● In women, the absence of at least three consecutive menstrual cycles when otherwise expected to occur.

○ the need for the patient to avoid discussions about food with her family.

Discharge planning

○ Refer the patient to support services.

Aortic insufficiency

Overview

Description

- A heart condition in which blood flows back into the left ventricle, causing excess fluid volume
- Also called aortic regurgitation

Pathophysiology

- Blood flows backward into the left ventricle during diastole, increasing left ventricular diastolic pressure.
- This process causes volume overload, dilation, and, eventually, hypertrophy of the left ventricle.
- Excess fluid volume also eventually increases left atrial pressure and pulmonary vascular pressure.

Risk factors

- History of any condition that weakens the aortic valve

Causes

- Aortic aneurysm
- Aortic dissection
- Connective tissue diseases
- Hypertension
- Idiopathic valve calcification
- Infective endocarditis
- Primary disease of the aortic valve leaflets, the wall or the aortic root, or both
- Rheumatic fever
- Traumatic injury

Prevalence

- Occurs most commonly among males
- When accompanied by mitral valve disease, more common among females

Complications

- Left-sided heart failure
- Myocardial ischemia
- Pulmonary edema

Assessment

History

- Angina, especially nocturnal
- Exertional dyspnea, orthopnea, paroxysmal nocturnal dyspnea
- Fatigue
- Palpitations, head pounding
- Sensation of a forceful heartbeat, especially when supine
- Symptoms of heart failure (late stages)

Physical assessment

- Austin Flint murmur

- Bisferious pulse
- Corrigan's pulse
- Diffuse, hyperdynamic apical impulse, displaced laterally and inferiorly
- Head bobbing with each heartbeat
- High frequency, blowing, early-peaking, diastolic decrescendo murmur best heard with the patient sitting down, leaning forward, and in deep fixed expiration (See *Identifying the murmur of aortic insufficiency.*)
- Pulsating nail beds and Quincke's sign
- S_3 gallop with increased left ventricular end-diastolic pressure
- Systolic thrill at base or suprasternal notch
- Tachycardia, peripheral vasoconstriction, and pulmonary edema if severe
- Water-hammer pulse
- Wide pulse pressure

Test results

Imaging

- Chest X-rays may show left ventricular enlargement and pulmonary vein congestion.

Diagnostic procedures

- Echocardiography may show left ventricular enlargement, increased motion of the septum and posterior wall, thickening of valve cusps, prolapse of the valve, flail leaflet, vegetations, or dilation of the aortic root.
- In severe disease, electrocardiography shows sinus tachycardia, left axis deviation, left ventricular hypertrophy, and left atrial hypertrophy.
- Cardiac catheterization shows the presence and degree of aortic insufficiency, left ventricular dilation and function, and coexisting coronary artery disease.

Nursing diagnoses

- Activity intolerance
- Decreased cardiac output
- Ineffective tissue perfusion: cardiopulmonary
- Excess fluid balance
- Impaired gas exchange
- Ineffective coping

Key outcomes

The patient will:

- carry out activities of daily living without excess fatigue or decreased energy
- maintain cardiac output, hemodynamic stability, and absence of arrhythmias
- maintain adequate fluid balance
- maintain adequate ventilation
- use available support systems.

Interventions

General

- Low-sodium diet

- Medical control of hypertension
- Periodic noninvasive monitoring of aortic insufficiency and left ventricular function with echocardiogram
- Planned rest periods to avoid fatigue
- Valve replacement

Nursing

- Give prescribed drugs.
- If the patient needs bed rest, stress its importance, and provide a bedside commode.
- Alternate periods of activity and rest.
- Allow the patient to express his concerns about the effects of activity restrictions on his responsibilities and routines.
- Keep the patient's legs elevated while he sits in a chair.
- Place the patient in an upright position, if needed, and give oxygen.
- Keep the patient on a low-sodium diet in consultation with a dietitian.
- After surgery, watch for hypotension, arrhythmias, and thrombus formation.

Drug therapy

- Antiarrhythmics
- Antihypertensives
- Cardiac glycosides
- Diuretics
- Infective endocarditis prophylaxis
- Vasodilators

▶ **ALERT** *Avoid using beta blockers in patients with aortic insufficiency because these drugs have negative inotropic effects.*

Monitoring

- Adverse reactions to drug therapy
- Complications
- Pulmonary edema
- Signs and symptoms of heart failure

After surgery
- Arterial blood gas levels
- Blood chemistry studies, prothrombin time, and International Normalized Ratio values
- Chest tube drainage
- Chest X-ray results
- Daily weight
- Heart sounds
- Intake and output
- Neurologic status
- Pulmonary artery pressures
- Vital signs and cardiac rhythm

Patient teaching

Be sure to cover:
- the disorder, diagnosis, and treatment
- prescribed drugs and their potential adverse reactions

Identifying the murmur of aortic insufficiency

Aortic insufficiency is characterized by a high-pitched, blowing decrescendo murmur that radiates from the aortic valve area to the left sternal as shown here.

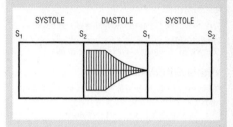

- when to contact a doctor
- the need for periodic rest periods in the patient's daily routine
- the need to elevate the legs whenever the patient sits
- diet restrictions
- signs and symptoms of heart failure
- the importance of consistent follow-up care
- how to monitor pulse rate and rhythm
- blood pressure control.

Discharge planning

- Refer the patient to an outpatient cardiac rehabilitation program, if indicated.
- Refer the patient to a smoking-cessation program, if needed.
- Refer the patient to a weight-reduction program, if needed.

Aortic stenosis

Overview

Description
- Narrowing of the aortic valve that affects blood flow in the heart
- Classified as either acquired or rheumatic

Pathophysiology
- Stenosis of the aortic valve impedes forward blood flow.
- The left ventricle must exert greater pressure to open the aortic valve.
- The increased workload increases myocardial oxygen demand.
- Reduced cardiac output reduces coronary artery blood flow.
- Left ventricular hypertrophy and failure result.

Risk factors
- Diabetes mellitus
- Hypercholesterolemia

Causes
- Atherosclerosis
- Congenital aortic bicuspid valve
- Idiopathic fibrosis and calcification
- Rheumatic fever

Prevalence
- May be asymptomatic until age 50 to 70, even though stenosis has been present since childhood
- Affects men in about 80% of cases

Complications
- Cardiac arrhythmias, especially atrial fibrillation
- Infective endocarditis
- Left-sided heart failure
- Left ventricular hypertrophy
- Right-sided heart failure
- Sudden death

Assessment

History
- Angina
- Dyspnea on exertion
- Exertional syncope
- Fatigue
- May be asymptomatic
- Palpitations
- Paroxysmal nocturnal dyspnea

Physical assessment
- Apex of the heart may be displaced inferiorly and laterally
- Diminished carotid pulses with delayed upstroke
- Distinct lag between carotid artery pulse and apical pulse
- Harsh, rasping, mid- to late-peaking systolic murmur best heard at the base that may radiate to carotids and apex (See *Identifying the murmur of aortic stenosis.*)
- Orthopnea
- Peripheral edema
- Prominent jugular vein A waves
- Prominent S_4
- Small, sustained arterial pulses that rise slowly
- Split S_2 as stenosis becomes more severe
- Suprasternal thrill

AGE AWARE An early systolic ejection murmur may be present in children and adolescents who have noncalcified valves. The murmur is low-pitched, rough, and rasping and is loudest at the base in the second intercostal space.

Test results

Imaging
- Chest X-rays show valvular calcification, left ventricular enlargement, pulmonary vein congestion and, in later stages, left atrial, pulmonary arterial, right atrial, and right ventricular enlargement.

Diagnostic procedures
- Echocardiography shows a decreased valve area, increased gradient, and increased thickness of the left ventricular wall.
- Electrocardiography may show left ventricular hypertrophy, atrial fibrillation, or another arrhythmia.
- Cardiac catheterization shows an increased pressure gradient across the aortic valve, increased left ventricular pressures, and the presence of coronary artery disease.

Nursing diagnoses

- Activity intolerance
- Decreased cardiac output
- Excess fluid volume
- Impaired physical mobility
- Ineffective coping
- Ineffective tissue perfusion: cardiopulmonary

Key outcomes
The patient will:
- perform activities of daily living without excess fatigue or exhaustion
- avoid complications
- maintain cardiac output
- show hemodynamic stability
- keep a balanced fluid status
- maintain joint mobility and range of motion
- develop and use adequate coping skills.

Interventions

General

- In adults, valve replacement after symptoms begin and hemodynamic evidence suggests severe obstruction
- In children without calcified valves, simple commissurotomy under direct visualization
- Lifelong treatment and management of congenital aortic stenosis
- Low-sodium, low-fat, low-cholesterol diet
- Percutaneous balloon aortic valvuloplasty
- Periodic noninvasive evaluation of the severity of valve narrowing
- Planned rest periods
- Ross procedure in patients younger than age 5

Nursing

- Give prescribed drugs.
- Maintain a low-sodium diet in consultation with a dietitian.
- If the patient needs bed rest, stress its importance; provide a bedside commode.
- Alternate periods of activity and rest.
- Keep the patient's legs elevated while he sits in a chair.
- Place the patient in an upright position and give oxygen, as needed.
- Allow the patient to express his fears and concerns.

Drug therapy

- Antibiotics to prevent infective endocarditis
- Cardiac glycosides

> ◥ **ALERT** *The use of diuretics and vasodilators in patients with aortic stenosis may lead to hypotension and an inadequate stroke volume.*

Monitoring

- Arrhythmias
- Daily weight
- Intake and output
- Respiratory status
- Signs and symptoms of heart failure
- Signs and symptoms of progressive aortic stenosis
- Vital signs

After surgery
- Arterial blood gas results
- Blood chemistry results
- Chest X-rays
- Hemodynamics
- Signs and symptoms of thrombus formation

Patient teaching

Be sure to cover:
- the disorder, diagnosis, and treatment

Identifying the murmur of aortic stenosis

Aortic stenosis is characterized by a low-pitched, harsh, crescendo-decrescendo murmur that radiates from the aortic valve area to the carotid artery as shown here.

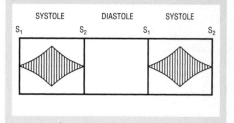

- prescribed drugs and their potential adverse reactions
- when to contact a doctor
- the need for rest periods in the patient's daily routine
- the need to elevate the legs when the patient sits
- diet and fluid restrictions
- the importance of consistent follow-up care
- signs and symptoms of heart failure
- prevention of infective endocarditis
- pulse rate and rhythm
- monitoring methods for atrial fibrillation and other arrhythmias

Discharge planning

- Refer the patient to a weight-reduction program, if needed.
- Refer the patient to a smoking-cessation program, if needed.

Asbestosis

Overview

Description
- Lung disease characterized by diffuse interstitial pulmonary fibrosis
- Results from prolonged exposure to airborne asbestos particles
- May develop 15 to 20 years after regular exposure to asbestos ceases
- Causes pleural plaques and mesotheliomas of the pleura and the peritoneum
- A form of pneumoconiosis
- Also known as mesothelioma

Pathophysiology
- Inhaled asbestos fibers travel down the airway and penetrate respiratory bronchioles and alveolar walls.
- Goblet cells and mucus production are stimulated to protect the airway and aid in expectoration.
- Fibers become encased in a brown, iron-rich, proteinlike sheath and are called asbestosis bodies.
- Chronic irritation by the fibers continues, causing edema of the airways.
- Fibrosis develops in response to the chronic irritation.

Risk factors
- Asbestos exposure
- Cigarette smoking

Causes
- Prolonged inhalation of asbestos fibers from such industries as mining and milling, construction, fireproofing, and textiles
- Production of paints, plastics, and brake and clutch linings
- Exposure to fibrous dust shaken off workers' clothing
- Exposure to fibrous dust or waste piles from nearby asbestos plants

Prevalence
- Commonly becomes symptomatic between ages 40 and 75
- Affects males more commonly than females

Complications
- Cor pulmonale
- Pulmonary fibrosis
- Pulmonary hypertension
- Respiratory failure

Assessment

History
- Chest pain
- Cough
- Exertional or resting dyspnea
- Exposure to asbestos fibers
- Recurrent respiratory tract infections

Physical assessment
- Characteristic dry crackles in the lung bases
- Clubbing of the fingers
- Tachypnea

Test results
Laboratory
- Decreased partial pressures of arterial oxygen and carbon dioxide in arterial blood gas analysis
Imaging
- Chest X-rays may show fine, irregular, and linear diffuse infiltrates; a honeycomb or ground-glass appearance in the lungs; and pleural thickening, pleural calcification, bilateral obliteration of costophrenic angles, and an enlarged heart with a "shaggy" border.
Diagnostic procedures
- Pulmonary function tests may show decreased vital capacity, forced vital capacity (FVC), and total lung capacity; decreased or normal forced expiratory volume in 1 second (FEV_1); a normal ratio of FEV_1 to FVC; and a reduced diffusing capacity for carbon monoxide.

Nursing diagnoses

- Deficient knowledge: asbestosis
- Fatigue
- Imbalanced nutrition: less than body requirements
- Impaired gas exchange
- Risk of imbalanced fluid volume

Key outcomes
The patient will:
- maintain adequate ventilation
- maintain adequate calorie intake
- express understanding of the illness
- identify measures to prevent or reduce fatigue
- maintain fluid volume balance.

Interventions

General
- Activity, as tolerated
- At least 3 qt (3 L) of fluids daily
- Controlled coughing and postural drainage with chest percussion and vibration
- High-calorie, high-protein, low-sodium diet

○ Lung transplantation in severe disease

Nursing
○ Give prescribed drugs.
○ Provide supportive care.
○ Provide chest physiotherapy.
○ Provide high-calorie, high-protein, low-sodium foods in small, frequent meals.
○ Encourage oral fluid intake.
○ Provide frequent rest periods.

Drug therapy
○ Antibiotics
○ Cardiac glycosides
○ Diuretics
○ Inhaled mucolytics
○ Supplemental oxygen

Monitoring
○ Complications
○ Daily weight
○ Intake and output
○ Mentation
○ Respiratory status (breath sounds, arterial blood gas results)
○ Sputum production
○ Vital signs

Patient teaching

Be sure to cover:
○ the disorder, diagnosis, and treatment
○ prescribed drugs and their potential adverse reactions
○ transtracheal catheter care, if applicable
○ prevention of infection
○ signs and symptoms of infection
○ the need for influenza and pneumococcus immunizations
○ home oxygen therapy, if needed
○ the importance of follow-up care
○ the need for chest physiotherapy
○ the need for a high-calorie, high-protein, low-sodium diet
○ the need for adequate oral fluid intake
○ energy conservation techniques.

Discharge planning

○ Refer the patient to a smoking-cessation program, if needed.

Asphyxia

Overview

Description

- A condition of insufficient oxygen and accumulating carbon dioxide in the blood and tissues
- Without prompt treatment, leads to cardiopulmonary arrest and death

Pathophysiology

- Asphyxia is an interference with respiration that causes an insufficient oxygen intake.
- Carbon dioxide accumulates as a result.
- Hypoxemia arises.
- Tissue perfusion is inadequate.

Risk factors

- Opioid abuse
- Spinal cord injury

Causes

- Opioid abuse
- Airway obstruction
- Aspiration
- Carbon monoxide poisoning
- Near drowning
- Pulmonary edema
- Respiratory muscle paralysis
- Smoke inhalation
- Strangulation
- Trauma to airway
- Tumor

Prevalence

- Can occur at any age

Complications

- Neurologic damage
- Death

Assessment

History

- Possibly an obvious cause
- Variable causes of signs and symptoms

Physical assessment

- Altered respiratory rate
- Anxiety or agitation
- Cherry-red mucous membranes (carbon monoxide poisoning)
- Confusion
- Cyanosis in mucous membranes, lips, and nail beds
- Decreased or absent breath sounds
- Dyspnea
- Erythema and petechiae on the upper chest (from trauma)
- Intercostal rib retractions
- Little or no air movement
- Pale skin
- Prominent neck muscles
- Wheezing and stridor

Test results

Laboratory
- Decreased partial pressure of arterial oxygen (less than 60 mm Hg) and increased partial pressure of arterial carbon dioxide (more than 50 mm Hg) on arterial blood gas (ABG) analysis
- Toxicology tests showing drugs, chemicals, or an abnormal hemoglobin level

Imaging
- Chest X-rays may detect a foreign body, pulmonary edema, or atelectasis.

Diagnostic procedures
- Pulmonary function tests may indicate respiratory muscle weakness.
- Bronchoscopy can be used to locate a foreign body.

Nursing diagnoses

- Decreased cardiac output
- Impaired gas exchange
- Ineffective airway clearance
- Risk for aspiration
- Risk for deficient fluid volume
- Risk for suffocation

Key outcomes

The patient will:
- maintain a patent airway
- maintain adequate ventilation
- maintain an acceptable cardiac output
- demonstrate knowledge of safety measures to prevent suffocation
- maintain fluid volume balance.

Interventions

General

- Activity based on outcome of interventions
- Established airway and ventilation
- Nothing by mouth until airway is protected
- Treatment for the underlying cause
- Tumor removal

Nursing

- Perform abdominal thrust maneuver if the patient has an airway obstruction.
- Maintain a patent airway.
- Begin cardiopulmonary resuscitation, if needed.
- Insert a nasogastric tube or an Ewald tube for lavage (for opioid abuse).

○ Give prescribed drugs.
○ Reassure the patient and his family.
○ Ensure I.V. access.

Drug therapy

○ Narcan (if caused by opioid abuse)
○ Oxygen

Monitoring

○ ABG levels, pulse oximetry
○ Cardiac status
○ Neurologic status
○ Respiratory status
○ Vital signs

Patient teaching

Be sure to cover:
○ the cause of asphyxia
○ ways to prevent recurrence (with patient and family members) if appropriate
○ safety measures if the patient is a child.

Discharge planning

○ Refer the patient to the proper authorities, if criminal intent was involved.
○ Refer the patient to resource and support services, if appropriate.

Asthma

Overview

Description

- A chronic reactive airway disorder involving episodic, reversible airway obstruction caused by bronchospasm, increased mucus secretion, and mucosal edema
- Signs and symptoms that range from mild wheezing and dyspnea to life-threatening respiratory failure
- Possibly persistent signs and symptoms of bronchial airway obstruction between acute episodes

Pathophysiology

- Tracheal and bronchial linings overreact to various stimuli, causing episodic smooth-muscle spasms that severely constrict the airways.
- Mucosal edema and thick secretions further block the airways.
- Immunoglobulin E (IgE) antibodies, attached to histamine-containing mast cells and receptors on cell membranes, initiate intrinsic asthma attacks.
- When exposed to an antigen such as pollen, the IgE antibodies combine with the antigen. With later exposure to that antigen, mast cells degranulate and release mediators.
- The mediators cause the bronchoconstriction and edema of an asthma attack.
- During an asthma attack, expiratory airflow decreases, trapping gas in the airways and causing alveolar hyperinflation.
- Atelectasis may develop in some lung regions.
- The increased airway resistance leads to labored breathing.

Risk factors

- Air pollution
- Occupational exposure to irritants
- Second-hand tobacco smoke

Causes

- Sensitivity to specific external allergens or internal, nonallergenic factors

Extrinsic asthma (atopic asthma)
- Animal dander
- Food additives containing sulfites and any other sensitizing substance
- House dust or mold
- Kapok or feather pillows
- Pollen

Intrinsic asthma (nonatopic asthma)
- Emotional stress
- Genetic factors

Bronchoconstriction
- Cold air
- Drugs, such as aspirin, beta blockers, and nonsteroidal anti-inflammatory drugs

- Exercise
- Hereditary predisposition
- Psychological stress
- Sensitivity to allergens or irritants such as pollutants
- Tartrazine
- Viral infections

Prevalence

- Can occur at any age
- Affects children younger than age 10 in about 50% of cases
- Affects twice as many boys as girls
- Onset between ages 10 and 30 in about one-third of patients
- Also occurs in at least one immediate family member about one-third of the time
- Occurs as both intrinsic and extrinsic asthma in many people

Complications

- Respiratory failure
- Status asthmaticus
- Death

Assessment

History

- Exposure to a particular allergen followed by a sudden onset of dyspnea, wheezing, chest tightness, and cough with thick, clear, or yellow sputum
- Irritants, emotional stress, fatigue, endocrine changes, temperature and humidity variations, and exposure to noxious fumes
- Possibly dramatic simultaneous onset of severe, multiple symptoms, or possibly a gradual increase in respiratory distress
- Previous severe respiratory tract infection (intrinsic asthma), especially in adults

Physical assessment

- Ability to speak only a few words before pausing for breath
- Cyanosis, confusion, and lethargy (at onset of life-threatening status asthmaticus and respiratory failure)
- Diaphoresis
- Diminished breath sounds
- Hyperresonance
- Increased anteroposterior thoracic diameter
- Inspiratory and expiratory wheezes
- Mild systolic hypertension
- Prolonged expiratory phase of respiration
- Tachycardia
- Tachypnea
- Use of accessory respiratory muscles
- Visible dyspnea

Test results

Laboratory
○ Hypoxemia on arterial blood gas (ABG) analysis
○ Increased serum IgE levels from an allergic reaction
○ Increased eosinophil count on complete blood count with differential

Imaging
○ Chest X-rays may show hyperinflation with areas of focal atelectasis.

Diagnostic procedures
○ Pulmonary function studies may show decreased peak flows and forced expiratory volume in 1 second, low-normal or decreased vital capacity, and increased total lung and residual capacities.
○ Skin testing may identify specific allergens.
○ Bronchial challenge testing shows the practical significance of allergens identified by skin testing.
○ Pulse oximetry may show decreased oxygen saturation.

Nursing diagnoses

○ Fear
○ Impaired gas exchange
○ Ineffective airway clearance
○ Ineffective breathing pattern
○ Ineffective coping
○ Risk for deficient fluid volume

Key outcomes
The patient will:
○ maintain adequate ventilation
○ maintain a patent airway
○ use effective coping strategies
○ report feelings of comfort
○ maintain fluid volume balance.

Interventions

General
○ Activity as tolerated
○ Desensitization to specific antigens
○ Establishment and maintenance of a patent airway
○ Fluid replacement
○ Identification and avoidance of precipitating factors

Nursing
○ Give prescribed drugs.
○ Place the patient in high Fowler's position.
○ Encourage pursed-lip and diaphragmatic breathing.
○ Give prescribed humidified oxygen.
○ Adjust the oxygen according to the patient's vital signs and ABG values.
○ Assist with intubation and mechanical ventilation, if needed.
○ Perform postural drainage and chest percussion, if tolerated.
○ Suction an intubated patient, as needed.

○ Treat the patient's dehydration with I.V. or oral fluids, as tolerated.
○ Anticipate bronchoscopy or bronchial lavage.
○ Keep the room temperature comfortable.
○ Use an air conditioner or a fan in hot, humid weather.

Drug therapy
○ Antibiotics
○ Anticholinergic bronchodilators
○ Bronchodilators
○ Corticosteroids
○ Heliox trial (before intubation)
○ Histamine antagonists
○ I.V. magnesium sulfate (controversial)
○ Leukotriene antagonists
○ Low-flow oxygen

▽ **ALERT** *The patient with increasingly severe asthma that doesn't respond to drug therapy is usually admitted for treatment with corticosteroids, epinephrine, and sympathomimetic aerosol sprays. The patient may need endotracheal intubation and mechanical ventilation.*

Monitoring
○ ABG results
○ Breath sounds
○ Complications of corticosteroids
○ Intake and output
○ Level of anxiety
○ Pulmonary function test results
○ Pulse oximetry
○ Response to treatment
○ Signs and symptoms of theophylline toxicity
○ Vital signs

Patient teaching

Be sure to cover:
○ the disorder, diagnosis, and treatment
○ prescribed drugs and their potential adverse reactions
○ when to contact a doctor
○ the need to avoid known allergens and irritants
○ how to use a metered-dose or dry powder inhaler
○ pursed-lip and diaphragmatic breathing
○ use of a peak flow meter
○ effective coughing techniques
○ maintaining adequate hydration.

Discharge planning

○ Refer the patient to a local asthma support group.

Atelectasis

Overview

Description

- Incomplete expansion of alveolar clusters or lung segments leading to partial or complete lung collapse
- May be chronic or acute
- Good prognosis with prompt removal of airway obstruction, relief of hypoxia, and reexpansion of the collapsed lung

Pathophysiology

- Incomplete expansion removes certain regions of the lung from gas exchange.
- Unoxygenated blood passes unchanged through these regions and produces hypoxia.
- Alveolar surfactant causes increased surface tension, permitting complete alveolar deflation.

Risk factors

- Anesthesia
- Lung disease
- Prolonged bed rest

Causes

- Bed rest in a supine position
- Bronchial occlusion
- Bronchiectasis
- Bronchogenic carcinoma
- Cystic fibrosis
- External compression
- General anesthesia
- Idiopathic respiratory distress syndrome of the neonate
- Inflammatory lung disease
- Oxygen toxicity
- Pleural effusion
- Pulmonary edema
- Pulmonary embolism
- Sarcoidosis

Prevalence

- Common after upper abdominal or thoracic surgery
- More common with prolonged immobility, mechanical ventilation, and central nervous system (CNS) depression
- Increased predisposition in patients who smoke and in those with chronic obstructive pulmonary disease (COPD)

Complications

- Acute respiratory failure
- Hypoxemia
- Pneumonia

Assessment

History

- CNS depression
- COPD
- Mechanical ventilation
- Prolonged immobility
- Recent abdominal surgery
- Rib fractures, tight chest dressings
- Smoking

Physical assessment

- Anxiety
- Cyanosis
- Decreased chest wall movement
- Decreased fremitus
- Decreased or absent breath sounds
- Diaphoresis
- Dullness or flatness over lung fields
- End-inspiration crackles
- Mediastinal shift to the affected side
- Substernal or intercostal retractions
- Tachycardia

Test results

Laboratory
- Hypoxia on arterial blood gas analysis

Imaging
- Chest X-rays show characteristic horizontal lines in the lower lung zones and characteristic dense shadows.

Diagnostic procedures
- Bronchoscopy may show an obstructing neoplasm, foreign body, or pneumonia.
- Pulse oximetry shows decreased oxygen saturation.

Nursing diagnoses

- Acute pain
- Impaired gas exchange
- Ineffective coping
- Ineffective airway clearance
- Risk for deficient fluid volume

Key outcomes

The patient will:
- maintain a patent airway
- maintain adequate ventilation
- report feelings of increased comfort
- use support systems to manage anxiety and fear
- maintain fluid volume balance.

Interventions

General

- Activity (not bed rest) as tolerated
- Bronchoscopy if other measures fail

- Chest percussion
- Diet based on patient's condition, as tolerated
- Frequent coughing and deep breathing
- Humidity
- Incentive spirometry
- Increased fluids
- Intermittent positive-pressure breathing therapy
- Possibly radiation for an obstructing neoplasm
- Postural drainage
- Surgery for an obstructing neoplasm

Nursing

- Give prescribed drugs.
- Encourage coughing and deep breathing.
- Reposition the patient often.
- Encourage and assist with ambulation as soon as possible.
- Help the patient use an incentive spirometer.
- Humidify inspired air.
- Encourage adequate fluid intake.
- Loosen secretions with postural drainage and chest percussion.
- Provide suctioning, as needed.
- Offer reassurance and emotional support.

Drug therapy

- Analgesics after surgery
- Bronchodilators

Monitoring

- Intake and output
- Pulse oximetry
- Respiratory status (breath sounds, arterial blood gas results)
- Vital signs

Patient teaching

Be sure to cover:
- use of an incentive spirometer
- postural drainage and percussion
- coughing and deep-breathing exercises
- the importance of splinting an incision
- energy conservation techniques
- stress reduction strategies
- the importance of mobilization.

Discharge planning

- Refer the patient to a smoking-cessation program, if needed.
- Refer the patient to a weight-reduction program, if needed.

Blood transfusion reaction

Overview

Description

○ A hemolytic reaction caused by transfusion of mismatched blood
○ Accompanies or follows I.V. delivery of blood components
○ Mediated by immune or nonimmune factors
○ Varies from mild to severe

Pathophysiology

○ Recipient's antibodies — immunoglobulin (Ig) G or IgM — bind to donor red blood cells (RBCs), leading to widespread clumping and destruction of the recipient's RBCs.
○ Transfusion with Rh-incompatible blood triggers a less serious reaction, known as Rh isoimmunization, within several days to 2 weeks. (See *Understanding the Rh system*.)
○ A febrile nonhemolytic reaction — the most common type — develops when cytotoxic or agglutinating antibodies in the recipient's plasma attack antigens on transfused lymphocytes, granulocytes, or plasma cells.

Causes

○ Transfusion of incompatible blood or blood products

Understanding the Rh system

The Rh system contains more than 30 antibodies and antigens. About 85% of people are Rh-positive, which means that their red blood cells carry the D or Rh antigen. Everyone else is Rh-negative; they don't have this antigen.

Effects of sensitization
When an Rh-negative person receives Rh-positive blood for the first time, he becomes sensitized to the D antigen but shows no immediate reaction to it. If he receives Rh-positive blood a second time, he'll have a massive hemolytic reaction.

For example, an Rh-negative mother who delivers an Rh-positive baby is sensitized by the baby's Rh-positive blood. During her next Rh-positive pregnancy, her sensitized blood will cause a hemolytic reaction in the fetal circulation.

Preventing sensitization
To prevent the formation of antibodies against Rh-positive blood in her next pregnancy, an Rh-negative mother should receive Rho(D) immune globulin (human) (RhoGAM) I.M. within 72 hours after delivering an Rh-positive baby.

Prevalence

○ Mild reactions: 1% to 2% of transfusions

Complications

○ Acute tubular necrosis leading to acute renal failure
○ Anaphylactic shock
○ Bronchospasm
○ Disseminated intravascular coagulation
○ Vascular collapse

Assessment

History

○ Chest or back pain
○ Chest tightness
○ Chills
○ Nausea
○ Transfusion of blood or blood product
○ Vomiting

Physical assessment

○ Angioedema
○ Apprehension
○ Dyspnea
○ Fever
○ Hypotension
○ Tachycardia
○ Urticaria
○ Wheezing
○ In a surgical patient: blood oozing from mucous membranes or the incision site
○ In a hemolytic reaction:
  – Fever
  – Unexpected decrease in serum hemoglobin level
  – Frank blood in urine
  – Jaundice

Test results

Laboratory
○ Decreased serum hemoglobin level
○ Increased serum bilirubin level
○ Increased indirect bilirubin level
○ Hemoglobinuria in urinalysis
○ Serum anti-A or anti-B antibodies in indirect Coombs' test or serum antibody screen
○ Increased prothrombin time
○ Decreased fibrinogen level
○ Increased blood urea nitrogen level
○ Increased serum creatinine level

Nursing diagnoses

○ Acute pain
○ Decreased cardiac output
○ Impaired gas exchange
○ Impaired tissue integrity
○ Powerlessness
○ Risk for imbalanced body temperature
○ Risk for imbalanced fluid volume
○ Risk for injury

Key outcomes

The patient will:
○ maintain hemodynamic stability
○ show no signs of active bleeding
○ maintain adequate ventilation
○ express understanding of the reaction
○ maintain adequate fluid volume.

Interventions

General

○ Bed rest
○ Dialysis (may be needed if acute tubular necrosis develops)
○ Diet, as tolerated
○ Immediate halt of transfusion

Nursing

○ Stop the transfusion.
○ Maintain a patent I.V. line with normal saline solution.
○ Insert an indwelling urinary catheter.
○ Report early signs of complications.
○ Cover the patient with blankets to ease chills.
○ Give supplemental oxygen, as needed.
○ Document the transfusion reaction on the patient's chart, noting the duration of the transfusion and the amount of blood absorbed.
○ Follow your facility's blood transfusion policy and procedure.

Drug therapy

○ Antipyretics
○ Corticosteroids
○ Diphenhydramine
○ Epinephrine
○ I.V. normal saline solution
○ I.V. vasopressors
○ Osmotic or loop diuretics

Monitoring

○ Intake and output
○ Laboratory test results
○ Signs of shock
○ Vital signs

Patient teaching

Be sure to cover:
○ before the transfusion, the type of transfusion needed
○ signs and symptoms of a reaction
○ after recovery, the type of reaction that occurred.

Discharge planning

○ Urge the patient to inform other health care providers about the transfusion reaction.

Bronchitis, chronic

Overview

Description

- Inflammation of the lining of the bronchial tubes
- A form of chronic obstructive pulmonary disease
- Excessive production of tracheobronchial mucus
- A cough lasting 3 or more months each year for 2 consecutive years
- Severity linked to amount of cigarette smoke or other pollutants inhaled and duration of inhalation
- Respiratory tract infections that typically worsen the cough and related symptoms
- Significant airway obstruction in some patients

Pathophysiology

- Bronchial mucous glands undergo hypertrophy and hyperplasia.
- Goblet cells increase.
- Cilia are damaged.
- Columnar epithelium undergoes squamous metaplasia.
- Bronchial walls are chronically infiltrated by leukocytes and lymphocytes.
- Additional effects include widespread inflammation, narrowing of the airways, and mucus in the airways.
- All effects produce resistance in the small airways and, in turn, a severe ventilation-perfusion imbalance. (See *What happens in chronic bronchitis*.)

Causes

- Cigarette smoking
- Environmental pollution
- Organic or inorganic dust
- Exposure to noxious gas
- Possibly genetic predisposition

Prevalence

- About 20% of men
- More prevalent in women than men
- Diagnosed in more than 8.8 million Americans yearly
- Increased risk among children of parents who smoke

Complications

- Acute respiratory failure
- Cor pulmonale
- Pulmonary hypertension
- Right ventricular hypertrophy

Assessment

History

- Cough
  - Initially more common in winter
  - Gradually becoming year-round
- Exertional dyspnea
- Frequent upper respiratory tract infections
- Increasingly severe coughing episodes
- Longtime smoker
- Productive cough
- Worsening dyspnea

Physical assessment

- Accessory respiratory muscle use
- Cough that produces copious gray, white, or yellow sputum
- Cyanosis
- Neck vein distention
- Pedal edema
- Prolonged expiratory time
- Rhonchi
- Substantial weight gain
- Tachypnea
- Wheezing

Test results

Laboratory
- Decreased partial pressure of oxygen in arterial blood gas (ABG) analysis
- Normal or increased partial pressure of carbon dioxide in ABG analysis
- Microorganisms and neutrophils in sputum culture

Imaging
- Chest X-ray may show hyperinflation and increased bronchovascular markings.

Diagnostic procedures
- Electrocardiography may show abnormalities:
  - atrial arrhythmias
  - peaked P waves in leads II, III, and aVF
  - right ventricular hypertrophy.
- Pulmonary function tests show:
  - increased residual volume
  - decreased vital capacity
  - decreased forced expiratory flow
  - normal static compliance and diffusing capacity.

Nursing diagnoses

- Anxiety
- Deficient knowledge (chronic bronchitis)
- Fatigue
- Imbalanced nutrition: less than body requirements
- Impaired gas exchange
- Ineffective breathing patterns
- Risk for deficient fluid volume

In chronic bronchitis, irritants inhaled for a prolonged period inflame the tracheobronchial tree. The inflammation leads to increased mucus production and a narrowed or blocked airway.

As inflammation continues, the mucus-producing goblet cells hypertrophy, as do the ciliated epithelial cells that line the respiratory tract. Hypersecretion from the goblet cells blocks the free movement of cilia, which normally sweep irritants, dust, and mucus from the airways.

As a result, the airway stays blocked, and mucus and debris accumulate in the respiratory tract.

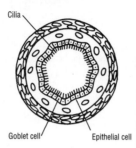

CROSS SECTION OF A NORMAL BRONCHIAL TREE

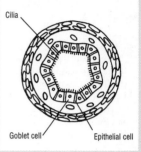

NARROWED BRONCHIAL TUBE IN CHRONIC BRONCHITIS

Key outcomes

The patient will:
- maintain adequate ventilation
- identify measures to prevent or reduce fatigue
- express understanding of the illness
- maintain a patent airway
- maintain fluid volume balance.

Interventions

General

- Activity as tolerated with frequent rest periods
- Adequate fluid intake
- Avoidance of air pollutants
- Chest physiotherapy
- High-calorie, protein-rich diet
- Smoking cessation
- Tracheostomy in advanced disease
- Ultrasonic or mechanical nebulizer treatments

Nursing

- Give prescribed drugs.
- Encourage expression of fears and concerns.
- Include the patient and his family in care decisions.
- Perform chest physiotherapy.
- Provide a high-calorie, protein-rich diet.
- Offer small, frequent meals.
- Encourage energy conservation techniques.
- Ensure adequate oral fluid intake.
- Perform frequent mouth care.
- Encourage daily activity.
- Provide diversional activities, as appropriate.
- Arrange frequent rest periods.

Drug therapy

- Antibiotics
- Bronchodilators
- Corticosteroids
- Diuretics
- Oxygen

Monitoring

- Breath sounds
- Daily weight
- Edema
- Intake and output
- Respiratory status
- Response to treatment
- Sputum production
- Vital signs

Patient teaching

Be sure to cover:
- the disorder, diagnosis, and treatment
- prescribed drugs and their possible adverse effects
- when to contact a doctor
- infection control practices
- influenza and pneumococcus immunizations
- home oxygen therapy, if needed
- postural drainage and chest percussion
- coughing and deep-breathing exercises
- use of an inhaler
- the need for high-calorie, protein-rich meals
- the need for adequate hydration
- avoidance of inhaled irritants
- prevention of bronchospasm.

Discharge planning

- Refer the patient to a smoking-cessation program, if needed.
- Refer the patient to the American Lung Association for information and support.

Bulimia nervosa

Overview

Description

- Behavioral disorder
- Binge eating
  - More food in a measured time (usually 2 hours) than an ordinary person would eat
  - Feeling of lack of control over eating
- Inappropriate behaviors to compensate for binges
  - Self-induced vomiting
  - Misuse of laxatives or enemas
  - Misuse of diuretics
  - Strict dieting or fasting
- Extreme concern about body image and weight

Pathophysiology

- Patient's behaviors and attitudes suggest that weight and body image are primary concerns.
- Patient eats large amounts of food without gaining weight.
- Patient creates complex schedules to hide binge-purge episodes.
- Patient visits the bathroom often, particularly after meals.
- Patient may withdraw from usual friends and activities.
- Bulimia commonly is accompanied by evidence of depression.

Causes

- Exact cause unknown
- Family disturbance or conflict
- Sexual abuse

Criteria for diagnosing bulimia nervosa

According to the *Diagnostic and Statistical Manual of Mental Disorders,* 4th edition (text revision), these criteria must be documented before a patient can be diagnosed with bulimia nervosa:

- Recurrent episodes of binge eating during which the person eats substantially more than most people would in the same period and during which the person feels a lack of control over what or how much is eaten
- Recurrent inappropriate compensatory behaviors to prevent weight gain, which may include self-induced vomiting; misuse of laxatives, diuretics, other drugs, or enemas; fasting; or excessive exercise
- Binges and compensatory behaviors that occur, on average, at least twice weekly for 3 months and not only during episodes of anorexia nervosa
- Undue concern over body image and weight.

Bulimia may be categorized as the purging type or the nonpurging type. In the former, the patient uses vomiting or misuses laxatives, diuretics, or enemas. In the latter, the patient uses mostly fasting or excessive exercise to compensate for binges.

- Maladaptive learned behavior
- Struggle for control or self-identity
- Cultural overemphasis on physical appearance
- Parental obesity

Prevalence

- Affects women about 80% of the time
- Affects 1% to 3% of adolescent and young women
- 5% to 15% of adolescent and young women have some symptoms of the disorder

 AGE AWARE   Bulimia typically starts in adolescence or early adulthood.

Complications

- Arrhythmia
- Cardiac failure
- Death
- Dehydration
- Dental caries
- Electrolyte imbalance
- Erosion of tooth enamel
- Esophageal tear
- Gastric rupture
- Gum infection
- Intestinal mucosal damage
- Parotitis
- Sudden death
- Suicide

Assessment

History

- Childhood trauma or abuse
- Continued eating until abdominal pain, sleep, or another person interrupts
- Depression
- Episodic binge eating
- Exaggerated sense of guilt
- Parental obesity
- Possible depression (Beck Depression Inventory)
- Preferred food usually sweet, soft, high-calorie, high-carbohydrate
- Unsatisfactory sexual relationships

Physical assessment

- Abdominal and epigastric pain
- Abnormal use of diuretics, laxatives, vomiting, and exercise (See *Criteria for diagnosing bulimia nervosa.*)
- Amenorrhea
- Calluses, abrasions, or scars on knuckles or back of the hand
- Eroded tooth enamel
- Hoarseness
- Normal weight or slightly overweight
- Painless swelling of salivary glands
- Throat irritation or lacerations
- Unusual swelling of cheeks or jaw area

Test results

Laboratory
- ○ Increased bicarbonate level
- ○ Decreased potassium level
- ○ Decreased sodium level

Nursing diagnoses

- ○ Chronic low self-esteem
- ○ Constipation
- ○ Disturbed body image
- ○ Disturbed sleeping pattern
- ○ Imbalanced nutrition: less than body requirements
- ○ Ineffective coping
- ○ Risk for deficient fluid volume

Key outcomes

The patient will:
- ○ acknowledge a change in body image
- ○ participate in decision-making about her care
- ○ express positive feelings about self
- ○ achieve an expected state of wellness
- ○ maintain fluid volume balance.

Interventions

General

- ○ Balanced diet
- ○ Drug rehabilitation
- ○ Inpatient or outpatient psychotherapy
- ○ Monitoring of activity
- ○ Monitoring of eating pattern
- ○ Self-help groups

Nursing

- ○ Supervise the patient during and for a specified period after meals, usually up to 1 hour.
- ○ Set a time limit for each meal.
- ○ Provide a pleasant, relaxed environment for eating.
- ○ Use behavior modification techniques.
- ○ Establish a food contract, specifying the amount and type of food to be eaten at each meal.
- ○ Encourage verbalization, and provide support.

Drug therapy

- ○ Antidepressants
- ○ Vitamin supplements

Monitoring

- ○ Activity
- ○ Complications
- ○ Eating patterns
- ○ Elimination patterns
- ○ Response to treatment
- ○ Suicide potential

Patient teaching

Be sure to cover:
- ○ the importance of keeping a food journal
- ○ risks of self-induced vomiting
- ○ risks of laxative and diuretic abuse
- ○ risks of fasting and excessive exercise
- ○ assertiveness training
- ○ prescribed drugs, dosages, and possible adverse effects.

Discharge planning

- ○ Refer the patient to support services or specialized inpatient care.
- ○ Refer the patient for psychological counseling.

Burns

Overview

Description
○ Heat or chemical injury to tissue
○ May be permanently disfiguring and incapacitating

Pathophysiology
First-degree burns
○ Superficial, partial thickness
○ Not life-threatening
Second-degree burns
○ Deep, partial thickness
○ Destruction of epidermis and some dermis
○ Thin-walled, fluid-filled blisters
○ Painful open nerve endings when blisters break
○ Lost barrier function of skin
Third- and fourth-degree burns
○ Painless; full thickness into subcutaneous tissue
○ Every body system and organ affected
○ Damage to muscle, bone, and interstitial tissues
○ Edema from interstitial fluids
○ Immediate immunologic response
○ Risk of wound sepsis

Causes
○ Fires
○ Traffic accidents
○ Improper use or storage of flammable materials
○ Malfunction of electrical devices
○ Contact with faulty electrical wiring
○ Chewing of electric cords
○ Contact with high-voltage power lines
○ Scalding accidents
○ Contact with or ingestion, inhalation, or injection of
  acids, alkali, or vesicants
○ Friction or abrasion
○ Sun exposure

Prevalence
○ Affects more than 2 million people each year
○ 70,000 hospitalizations, 20,000 in burn units

Complications
○ Anemia
○ Hypovolemic shock
○ Malnutrition
○ Multiple organ dysfunction syndrome
○ Respiratory complications
○ Sepsis

Assessment

History
○ Cause of the burn
○ Existing medical conditions

Physical assessment
○ Depth and size of the burn
○ Severity of the burn
  – Major burn: affects more than 10% of adult's or
    20% of child's body surface area (BSA)
  – Moderate burn: 3% to 10% of adult's or 10% to
    20% of child's BSA
  – Minor burn: less than 3% of adult's or less than
    10% of child's BSA
First-degree burns
○ Blanching
○ Chills
○ Erythema
○ Headache
○ Localized pain
○ Nausea and vomiting
Second-degree burns
○ Mild to moderate pain
○ Thin-walled, fluid-filled blisters
○ White, waxy appearance in damaged area
Third- and fourth-degree burns
○ No blisters
○ No pain
○ Pale, white, brown, or black leathery tissue
○ Visible thrombosed vessels
Electrical burns
○ Cardiac arrest
○ Hearing impairment
○ Muscle contractions
○ Numbness and tingling
○ Respiratory failure
○ Seizures
○ Silver colored, raised area at contact site
○ Unconsciousness
○ Weakness
Mucosal burns
○ Coughing, wheezing
○ Darkened sputum
○ Sores in mouth or nose
○ Voice changes

Test results
Laboratory
○ Evidence of smoke inhalation, decreased alveolar
  function, possible hypoxia in arterial blood gas tests
○ Decreased hemoglobin level and hematocrit in com-
  plete blood count if patient loses blood
○ Abnormal electrolyte levels from fluid loss and shifts
○ Increased blood urea nitrogen level with fluid loss
○ Decreased glucose level in children because of limit-
  ed glycogen storage
○ Myoglobinuria and hemoglobinuria in urinalysis
○ Increased carboxyhemoglobin level
Diagnostic procedures
○ Electrocardiography may show myocardial ischemia,
  injury, or arrhythmias, especially in electrical burns.
○ Fiber-optic bronchoscopy may show airway edema.

Nursing diagnoses

○ Acute pain
○ Anxiety
○ Deficient fluid volume
○ Deficient knowledge (burns)
○ Disturbed body image
○ Hypothermia
○ Imbalanced nutrition: less than body requirements
○ Impaired gas exchange
○ Impaired physical mobility
○ Impaired skin integrity
○ Ineffective coping
○ Ineffective protection
○ Ineffective tissue perfusion: all
○ Risk for infection

Key outcomes

The patient will:
○ report increased comfort and decreased pain
○ attain the highest degree of mobility possible
○ maintain fluid balance in an acceptable range
○ maintain a patent airway
○ use effective coping techniques.

Interventions

General

○ Stopping the burn source
○ Securing the airway
○ Preventing hypoxia
○ Giving I.V. fluids through a large-bore I.V. line (See *Fluid replacement after a burn.*)
  – Adult: urine output 30 to 50 ml/hour
  – Child less than 30 kg (66 lb): urine output 1 ml/kg/hour
○ Nasogastric tube and urinary catheter insertion
○ Wound care
○ Nothing by mouth until severity of burn is established; then high-protein, high-calorie diet
○ Increased hydration with high-calorie, high-protein drinks, not free water
○ Total parenteral nutrition if unable to eat
○ Activity limited based on extent and location of burn
○ Physical therapy
○ Loose tissue and blister debridement
○ Escharotomy
○ Skin grafting

Nursing

○ Apply immediate, aggressive burn treatment.
○ Use strict sterile technique.
○ Remove constricting items and smoldering clothes.
○ Perform appropriate wound care.
○ Provide adequate hydration.
○ Weigh the patient daily.
○ Encourage verbalization and provide support.

Fluid replacement after a burn

For a burned adult, use one of the following formulas:

First 24 hours

EVANS
● 1 ml × patient's weight in kg × % total body surface area (TBSA) burn (0.9% normal saline solution)
● 1 ml × patient's weight in kg × % TBSA burn (colloid solution)

BROOKE
● 1.5 ml × patient's weight in kg × % TBSA burn (lactated Ringer's solution)
● 0.5 ml × patient's weight in kg × % TBSA burn (colloid solution)

PARKLAND
● 4 ml × patient's weight in kg × % TBSA burn (lactated Ringer's solution). Give half of volume in first 8 minutes; then infuse remainder over 16 minutes.

Second 24 hours

EVANS
● 50% of first 24-hour replacement (0.9% normal saline solution)
● 2,000 ml (dextrose 5% in water [D_5W])

BROOKE
● 50% to 75% of first 24-hour replacement (lactated Ringer's solution)
● 2,000 ml (D_5W)

PARKLAND
● 30% to 60% of calculated plasma volume (25% albumin)
● Volume to maintain desired urine output (D_5W)

Drug therapy

○ Analgesics
○ Anxiolytics
○ Antibiotics
○ Booster of tetanus toxoid

Monitoring

○ Vital signs
○ Respiratory status
○ Signs of infection
○ Intake and output
○ Hydration and nutritional status

Patient teaching

Be sure to cover:
○ the injury, diagnosis, and treatment
○ appropriate wound care
○ prescribed drugs and possible adverse effects
○ developing a dietary plan
○ signs and symptoms of complications.

Discharge planning

○ Refer the patient to rehabilitation, if appropriate.
○ Refer the patient for psychological aid, if needed.
○ Refer the patient to resource and support services.

Cardiomyopathy, dilated

Overview

Description
○ Disease of the heart muscle fibers
○ Also called congestive cardiomyopathy

Pathophysiology
○ Extensively damaged myocardial muscle fibers reduce contractility in the left ventricle. (See *Understanding dilated cardiomyopathy.*)
○ As systolic function declines, cardiac output falls.
○ The sympathetic nervous system is stimulated to increase heart rate and contractility.
○ When compensatory mechanisms can no longer maintain cardiac output, the heart begins to fail.

Causes
○ Cardiotoxic effects of drugs or alcohol
○ Chemotherapy
○ Drug hypersensitivity
○ Hypertension
○ Ischemic heart disease
○ Peripartum syndrome related to toxemia
○ Valvular disease
○ Viral or bacterial infection

Prevalence
○ Most common among middle-age men but can occur in any age group

Complications
○ Arrhythmias
○ Emboli
○ Intractable heart failure

Understanding dilated cardiomyopathy

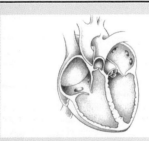

- Greatly increased chamber size
- Thinning of left ventricular muscle
- Increased atrial chamber size
- Increased myocardial mass
- Normal ventricular inflow resistance
- Decreased contractility

Assessment

History
○ Gradual onset of shortness of breath, orthopnea, dyspnea on exertion, paroxysmal nocturnal dyspnea, fatigue, dry cough at night, palpitations, and vague chest pain
○ Possible history of a disorder that can cause cardiomyopathy

Physical assessment
○ Ascites
○ Hepatomegaly
○ Irregular cardiac rhythms, diffuse apical impulses, pansystolic murmur
○ Jugular vein distention
○ Narrow pulse pressure
○ Peripheral cyanosis
○ Peripheral edema
○ Pulmonary crackles
○ Pulsus alternans in late stages
○ S_3 and S_4 gallop rhythms
○ Splenomegaly
○ Tachycardia even at rest

▼ **ALERT** *Dilated cardiomyopathy may need to be differentiated from other types of cardiomyopathy.* (*See* Assessment findings in cardiomyopathies.)

Test results
Imaging
○ Chest X-rays show moderate to marked cardiomegaly and possible pulmonary edema.
○ Echocardiography may show ventricular thrombi, global hypokinesis, and the degrees of left ventricular dilation and systolic dysfunction.
○ Gallium scans may identify patients with dilated cardiomyopathy and myocarditis.
Diagnostic procedures
○ Electrocardiography evaluates ischemic heart disease and identifies arrhythmias and intraventricular conduction defects.
○ Cardiac catheterization can show left ventricular dilation and dysfunction, elevated left (and often right) ventricular filling pressures, and diminished cardiac output.
○ Angiography rules out ischemic heart disease.
○ Transvenous endomyocardial biopsy may help determine the underlying disorder.

Nursing diagnoses

○ Activity intolerance
○ Anxiety
○ Decreased cardiac output
○ Deficient knowledge: dilated cardiomyopathy
○ Excess fluid volume
○ Fatigue

Assessment findings in cardiomyopathies

Type	Assessment findings
Dilated cardiomyopathy	• Generalized weakness, fatigue • Chest pain, palpitations • Syncope • Tachycardia • Narrow pulse pressure • Pulmonary congestion, pleural effusions • Jugular vein distention, peripheral edema • Paroxysmal nocturnal dyspnea, orthopnea, dyspnea on exertion
Hypertrophic cardiomyopathy	• Angina, palpitations • Syncope • Orthopnea, dyspnea with exertion • Pulmonary congestion • Loud systolic murmur • Life-threatening arrhythmias • Sudden cardiac arrest
Restrictive cardiomyopathy	• Generalized weakness, fatigue • Bradycardia • Dyspnea • Jugular vein distention, peripheral edema • Liver congestion, abdominal ascites

○ Hopelessness
○ Ineffective tissue perfusion: cardiopulmonary

Key outcomes

The patient will:
○ maintain adequate cardiac output and hemodynamic stability
○ maintain adequate ventilation
○ develop no complications of excess fluid volume
○ recognize and accept limitations of chronic illness
○ express feelings of increased energy and decreased fatigue.

Interventions

General

○ No ingestion of alcohol if cardiomyopathy results from alcoholism
○ Low-sodium diet with vitamin supplements
○ Rest periods
○ Heart transplantation
○ Possible cardiomyoplasty

�֍ AGE AWARE *A woman of childbearing age who has dilated cardiomyopathy should avoid pregnancy.*

Nursing

○ Alternate periods of rest with required activities of daily living.
○ Provide active or passive range-of-motion exercises.
○ Consult with a dietitian to provide a low-sodium diet.
○ Give oxygen, as needed.
○ Check serum potassium levels for hypokalemia, especially if therapy includes a cardiac glycoside.
○ Offer support, and let the patient express his feelings.

○ Let the patient and family express their fears and concerns, and help them identify effective coping strategies.

Drug therapy

○ Angiotensin-converting enzyme inhibitors
○ Antiarrhythmics
○ Anticoagulants
○ Beta blockers
○ Cardiac glycosides
○ Diuretics
○ Oxygen
○ Vasodilators

Monitoring

○ Daily weight
○ Evidence of progressive heart failure
○ Hemodynamics
○ Intake and output
○ Vital signs

Patient teaching

Be sure to cover:
○ the disorder, diagnosis, and treatment
○ prescribed drugs and potential adverse reactions
○ when to contact a doctor
○ sodium and fluid restrictions
○ evidence of worsening heart failure.

Discharge planning

○ Refer family members to community cardiopulmonary resuscitation classes.

Cardiomyopathy, hypertrophic

Overview

Description
○ Primary disease of cardiac muscle characterized by left ventricular hypertrophy
○ Also known as idiopathic hypertrophic subaortic stenosis, hypertrophic obstructive cardiomyopathy, and muscular aortic stenosis

Pathophysiology
○ The hypertrophied ventricle becomes stiff, noncompliant, and unable to relax during ventricular filling.
○ Tachycardia develops, reducing ventricular filling time.
○ Reduced ventricular filling time leads to low cardiac output. (See *Understanding hypertrophic cardiomyopathy.*)

Causes
○ Transmission by autosomal dominant trait (about half of all cases)
○ Associated with hypertension

Prevalence
○ More common in men than women
○ Affects 5 to 8 people per 100,000 in the United States
○ More common in Blacks than in other races

Understanding hypertrophic cardiomyopathy

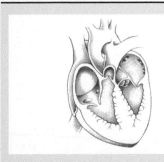

- Normal right and decreased left chamber size
- Left ventricular hypertrophy
- Thickened interventricular septum (hypertrophic obstructive cardiomyopathy)
- Atrial chamber size increased on left side
- Increased myocardial mass
- Increased ventricular inflow resistance
- Increased or decreased contractility

Complications
○ Heart failure
○ Pulmonary hypertension
○ Ventricular arrhythmias

Assessment

History
○ Usually, no discernible features until disease is well advanced
○ Blood flow to left ventricle abruptly reduced by atrial dilation and, sometimes, atrial fibrillation
○ Possible family history of hypertrophic cardiomyopathy
○ Orthopnea
○ Dyspnea on exertion
○ Angina
○ Fatigue
○ Syncope, even at rest

Physical assessment
○ Rapidly rising carotid arterial pulse possible
○ Pulsus biferiens
○ Double or triple apical impulse, possibly displaced laterally
○ Bibasilar crackles if the patient has heart failure
○ Harsh systolic murmur heard after S_1 at the apex near the left sternal border
○ Possible S_4

⚠ **ALERT** *Hypertrophic cardiomyopathy may need to be differentiated from other types of cardiomyopathy.*

Test results
Imaging
○ Chest X-rays may show mild to moderate increase in heart size.
○ Echocardiography shows left ventricular hypertrophy (a thick, asymmetrical intraventricular septum in the obstructive form or hypertrophy in various ventricular areas in the nonobstructive form).
○ Thallium scan usually reveals myocardial perfusion defects.
Diagnostic procedures
○ Electrocardiography usually shows left ventricular hypertrophy, ST-segment and T-wave abnormalities, left anterior hemiblock, left axis deviation, ventricular arrhythmias, atrial arrhythmias, and Q waves in leads II, III, aVF, and V4 to V6 (from hypertrophy, not infarction).
○ Cardiac catheterization reveals elevated left ventricular end-diastolic pressure and, possibly, mitral insufficiency.
○ Angiography reveals a dilated, diffusely hypokinetic left ventricle.

Nursing diagnoses

○ Activity intolerance
○ Anxiety
○ Decreased cardiac output
○ Deficient knowledge: hypertrophic cardiomyopathy
○ Excess fluid volume
○ Fatigue
○ Hopelessness
○ Ineffective tissue perfusion: cardiopulmonary

Key outcomes

The patient will:
○ maintain adequate cardiac output and hemodynamic stability
○ develop no complications of excess fluid volume
○ carry out activities of daily living without excess fatigue or decreased energy
○ express feelings of comfort and decreased pain
○ develop adequate coping mechanisms.

Interventions

General

○ Cardioversion for atrial fibrillation
○ Low-fat, low-salt diet
○ Fluid restrictions
○ Avoidance of alcohol
○ Activity limitations as needed
○ Bed rest, if needed
○ Ventricular myotomy alone or with mitral valve replacement
○ Heart transplantation

Nursing

○ Alternate periods of rest with required activities and treatments.
○ Provide personal care, as needed, to prevent fatigue.
○ Provide active or passive range-of-motion exercises.

▷ **ALERT** *If propranolol is being stopped, don't do so abruptly. Rebound effects could cause myocardial infarction or sudden death.*

○ Offer support, and let the patient express his feelings.
○ Let the patient and family express their fears and concerns and identify effective coping strategies.

Drug therapy

○ Amiodarone, unless the patient has atrioventricular block
○ Antibiotic prophylaxis
○ Beta blockers
○ Calcium channel blockers

▷ **ALERT** *Angiotensin-converting enzyme inhibitors, nitrates, and digoxin are contraindicated in hypertrophic cardiomyopathy.*

Monitoring

○ Hemodynamics
○ Intake and output
○ Vital signs

Patient teaching

Be sure to cover:
○ the possibility that propranolol can cause depression and the need to notify the doctor if symptoms occur
○ instructions to take drugs as ordered
○ the need to tell all doctors that the patient shouldn't receive nitroglycerin, digoxin, or diuretics because they can worsen obstruction
○ the need for antibiotic prophylaxis before dental work or surgery to prevent infective endocarditis
○ warnings against strenuous activity, which may cause syncope or sudden death
○ the need to avoid Valsalva's maneuver or sudden position changes.

Discharge planning

○ Refer family members to community cardiopulmonary resuscitation classes.

Cholera

Overview

Description
○ Acute enterotoxin-mediated gastrointestinal infection
○ Transmitted through food and water contaminated with the feces of carriers or people with active infections
○ Food poisoning caused by *Vibrio parahaemolyticus,* a similar bacterium
○ Also known as Asiatic cholera or epidemic cholera

Pathophysiology
○ Humans are the only hosts and victims of *Vibrio cholerae,* a motile, aerobic organism.

Risk factors
○ Deficiency or absence of hydrochloric acid

Causes
○ The gram-negative bacillus *V. cholerae*

Prevalence
○ Most common in Africa, Southern and Southeast Asia, and the Middle East, although outbreaks have occurred in Japan, Australia, and Europe
○ Occurs during warm months, usually among lower socioeconomic groups
○ Common among children ages 1 to 5 in India, but equally distributed among all age groups in other endemic areas

Complications
○ Dehydration
○ Hypovolemic shock
○ Metabolic acidosis
○ Uremia
○ Coma and death

Assessment

History
○ Profuse, watery diarrhea
○ Vomiting
○ Intense thirst
○ Weakness
○ Muscle cramps (especially in the limbs)

Physical assessment
○ Stools containing white flecks of mucus (rice-water stools)
○ Loss of skin turgor, wrinkled skin, sunken eyes
○ Pinched facial expression
○ Cyanosis
○ Tachycardia, tachypnea
○ Thready or absent peripheral pulses
○ Decreased blood pressure
○ Fever
○ Inaudible, hypoactive bowel sounds

Test results
Laboratory
○ A culture of *V. cholerae* from feces or vomitus
○ Rapidly moving bacilli (like shooting stars) with microscopic examination of fresh feces
○ Group- and type-specific antisera in agglutination testing

Nursing diagnoses
○ Diarrhea
○ Impaired urinary elimination
○ Risk for imbalanced fluid volume

Key outcomes
The patient will:
○ regain and maintain adequate fluid and electrolyte balance
○ have normal elimination patterns
○ have stable vital signs
○ produce adequate urine volume.

Interventions

General
○ Enteric precautions
○ Supportive care
○ Increased fluid intake

Nursing
○ Wear a gown and gloves when handling feces-contaminated articles.
○ Carefully observe neck veins.
○ Auscultate the lungs frequently.

Drug therapy
○ Rapid I.V. infusion of large amounts (50 to 100 ml/minute) of isotonic saline solution, alternating with isotonic sodium bicarbonate or sodium lactate
○ Tetracycline

Monitoring
○ Intake and output
○ I.V. infusion
○ Laboratory test results
○ Neck veins
○ Vital signs

Patient teaching

Be sure to cover:
○ administration of cholera vaccine to travelers in endemic areas
○ proper hand-washing technique
○ need for increased fluid intake.

Discharge planning

○ Explain the use of oral tetracycline to family members.
○ If the doctor orders a cholera vaccine, tell the patient that he'll need a booster 3 to 6 months later for continuing protection.

Chronic glomerulonephritis

Overview

Description
○ A slowly progressive disease characterized by inflammation of the glomeruli
○ Causes sclerosis, scarring, and eventual renal failure
○ Usually subclinical until the progressive phase begins, marked by proteinuria, cylindruria (presence of granular tube casts), and hematuria
○ Usually irreversible

Pathophysiology
○ Injury to the kidney reduces the size of the nephron.
○ The glomerular filtration rate decreases.
○ The remaining nephron develops hypertrophy and hyperfiltration.
○ Intraglomerular hypertension develops.
○ Glomerulosclerosis eventually occurs, along with further nephron loss, leading to renal failure.

Causes
○ Focal glomerulosclerosis
○ Goodpasture's syndrome
○ Hemolytic uremic syndrome
○ Lupus erythematosus
○ Membranoproliferative glomerulonephritis
○ Membranous glomerulopathy
○ Poststreptococcal glomerulonephritis
○ Primary renal disorders
○ Rapidly progressive glomerulonephritis

Prevalence
○ Third leading cause of end-stage renal disease in the United States

Complications
○ Cardiac hypertrophy
○ End-stage renal failure
○ Heart failure
○ Metabolic acidosis
○ Pericarditis
○ Pulmonary edema
○ Severe anemia
○ Severe hypertension

Assessment

History
○ Causative factor
○ Possibly no symptoms for many years
○ Leg cramps
○ Shortness of breath
○ Chest pain

○ Signs of uremia
  – Fatigue
  – Loss of appetite
  – Nausea
  – Peripheral neuropathy
  – Pruritus
  – Reversal of sleep pattern
  – Seizures
  – Vomiting
  – Weakness

Physical assessment
○ Hypertension
○ Jugular vein distension
○ Pulmonary crackles
○ Mild to severe edema

Test results
Laboratory
○ Proteinuria
○ Hematuria
○ Cylindruria
○ Red blood cell casts in urinalysis
○ Increased blood urea nitrogen level
○ Increased serum creatinine level
○ Increased potassium level
○ Anemia
Imaging
○ X-ray or ultrasound shows smaller kidneys.
Diagnostic procedures
○ Kidney biopsy identifies underlying disease.

Nursing diagnoses

○ Excess fluid volume
○ Fatigue
○ Imbalanced nutrition: less than body requirements
○ Impaired skin integrity
○ Ineffective tissue perfusion: renal
○ Risk for infection

Key outcomes
The patient will:
○ maintain fluid balance
○ report increased comfort
○ identify risks that worsen decreased tissue perfusion and modify lifestyle appropriately
○ maintain hemodynamic stability
○ avoid or minimize complications
○ have increased energy and decreased fatigue.

Interventions

General
○ Activity as tolerated
○ Correction of fluid and electrolyte imbalances through restrictions and replacement
○ Dialysis

- Kidney transplantation
- Sodium-restricted, low-protein diet
- Symptomatic care

Nursing

- Give drugs as prescribed.
- Watch for signs of fluid, electrolyte, and acid-base imbalances.
- Provide skin care (because of pruritus and edema) and oral hygiene.
- Provide emotional support.

Drug therapy

- Antibiotics for symptomatic urinary tract infection
- Antihypertensives
- Diuretics

Monitoring

- Daily weight
- Evidence of heart failure
- Intake and output
- Laboratory test results
- Vital signs

Patient teaching

Be sure to cover:
- disease process, diagnostic tests and procedures, and treatment plan
- the need for low-sodium, high-calorie meals with adequate protein.
- prescribed drugs, dosages, and possible adverse effects
- when to contact a doctor
- how to assess ankle edema
- signs of infection, particularly urinary tract infection, and the need to avoid contact with infected persons.

Discharge planning

- Encourage follow-up examinations to assess renal function.

Cirrhosis

Overview

Description
○ Chronic hepatic disease
○ Several types

Pathophysiology
○ Hepatic cells undergo diffuse destruction and fibrotic regeneration.
○ Necrotic tissue yields to fibrosis.
○ Liver structure and vasculature are altered.
○ Blood and lymph flow are impaired.
○ Hepatic insufficiency develops.

Causes
○ Alcoholism
○ Biliary obstruction
○ Hepatitis
○ Metabolic disorders
○ Toxins

Laënnec's or micronodular cirrhosis (alcoholic or portal cirrhosis)
○ Chronic alcoholism
○ Malnutrition

Postnecrotic or macronodular cirrhosis
○ Complication of viral hepatitis
○ Possible after exposure to such liver toxins as arsenic, carbon tetrachloride, and phosphorus

Biliary cirrhosis
○ Prolonged biliary tract obstruction or inflammation

Idiopathic cirrhosis (cryptogenic)
○ No known cause
○ Chronic inflammatory bowel disease
○ Sarcoidosis

Prevalence
○ Tenth most common cause of death in the United States
○ Most common among those ages 45 to 75
○ Occurs in twice as many men as women

Complications
○ Bleeding esophageal varices
○ Death
○ Hepatic encephalopathy
○ Hepatorenal syndrome
○ Portal hypertension

Assessment

History
○ Chronic alcoholism
○ Exposure to liver toxins such as arsenic and certain drugs
○ Malnutrition
○ Prolonged biliary tract obstruction or inflammation
○ Viral hepatitis

Early stage
○ Abdominal pain
○ Diarrhea, constipation
○ Fatigue
○ Muscle cramps
○ Nausea, vomiting
○ Vague signs and symptoms

Later stage
○ Bleeding tendency, such as frequent nosebleeds, easy bruising, and bleeding gums
○ Chronic dyspepsia
○ Constipation
○ Pruritus
○ Weight loss

Physical assessment
○ Anemia
○ Ascites
○ Asterixis
○ Clubbed fingers
○ Distended abdominal blood vessels
○ Ecchymosis
○ Enlarged spleen
○ Gynecomastia
○ Jaundice
○ Menstrual irregularities
○ Palmar erythema
○ Palpable, large, firm liver with a sharp edge (early finding)
○ Slurred speech, paranoia, hallucinations
○ Spider angiomas on the face, neck, arms, and trunk
○ Telangiectasis on the cheeks
○ Testicular atrophy
○ Thigh and leg edema
○ Umbilical hernia

Test results

Laboratory
○ Increased levels of liver enzymes, such as alanine aminotransferase, aspartate aminotransferase, total serum bilirubin, and indirect bilirubin
○ Decreased total serum albumin and protein levels
○ Prolonged prothrombin time
○ Decreased serum electrolyte levels, hemoglobin level, and hematocrit
○ Vitamins A, C, and K deficiency
○ Increased urine levels of bilirubin and urobilinogen
○ Decreased fecal urobilinogen levels

Imaging
○ Abdominal X-rays show liver and spleen size and cysts or gas in the biliary tract or liver; liver calcification; and massive ascites.
○ Computed tomography and liver scans determine liver size, identify liver masses, and reveal hepatic blood flow and obstruction.
○ Radioisotope liver scans show liver size, blood flow, and obstruction.

Diagnostic procedures

○ Liver biopsy is the definitive test for cirrhosis, revealing hepatic tissue destruction and fibrosis.
○ Esophagogastroduodenoscopy reveals bleeding esophageal varices, stomach irritation or ulceration, and duodenal bleeding and irritation.

Nursing diagnoses

○ Activity intolerance
○ Excess fluid volume
○ Hopelessness
○ Imbalanced nutrition: less than body requirements
○ Risk for impaired skin integrity
○ Risk for injury

Key outcomes

The patient will:
○ maintain caloric intake, as needed
○ maintain normal fluid volume
○ incur no injuries
○ have no bleeding
○ maintain intact skin.

Interventions

General

○ Blood transfusion
○ Esophageal balloon tamponade
○ Frequent rest periods, as needed
○ High-calorie diet
○ I.V. fluids
○ No alcohol intake
○ Paracentesis
○ Peritoneovenous shunt, if needed, to divert ascites into venous circulation
○ Portal-systemic shunt
○ Removal or alleviation of underlying cause
○ Restricted fluid intake
○ Restricted sodium consumption
○ Sclerotherapy

Nursing

○ Give prescribed I.V. fluids and blood products.
○ Give prescribed drugs.
○ Encourage verbalization and provide support.
○ Provide appropriate skin care.

Drug therapy

○ Ammonia detoxicant
○ Antacids
○ Antiemetics
○ Beta blockers
○ Potassium-sparing diuretics
○ Vasopressin
○ Vitamin and nutritional supplements

Monitoring

○ Abdominal girth
○ Ammonia level
○ Bleeding tendencies
○ Changes in mentation, behavior
○ Hydration and nutritional status
○ Laboratory test results
○ Skin integrity
○ Vital signs
○ Weight

Patient teaching

Be sure to cover:
○ the disorder, diagnosis, and treatment
○ over-the-counter medications that may increase bleeding tendencies
○ diet modifications
○ the need to avoid infections and abstain from alcohol
○ the need to avoid sedatives and acetaminophen (hepatotoxic)
○ the need for a high-calorie diet and small, frequent meals.

Discharge planning

○ Refer the patient to Alcoholics Anonymous, if appropriate.
○ Refer the patient for psychological counseling, if needed.

Crohn's disease

Overview

Description
- Inflammatory bowel disease that may affect any part of the gastrointestinal (GI) tract
- Commonly involves the terminal ileum
- Affects colon and small bowel in 50% of cases; terminal ileum in 33%; colon alone in 10% to 20%
- Extends through all layers of the intestinal wall
- May involve regional lymph nodes and mesentery

Pathophysiology
- Crohn's disease involves slow, progressive inflammation of the bowel.
- Enlarged lymph nodes cause lymphatic obstruction.
- Edema, mucosal ulceration, fissures, and abscesses develop.
- Elevated patches of closely packed lymph follicles (Peyer's patches) develop in the small intestinal lining.
- Fibrosis thickens the bowel wall and causes stenosis.
- Inflamed bowel loops adhere to other diseased or normal loops.
- The diseased bowel becomes thicker, shorter, and narrower.

Risk factors
- History of allergies
- Immune disorders
- Genetic predisposition
  - One or more affected relatives in 10% to 20% of patients with the disease
  - Sometimes occurs in monozygotic twins

Causes
- Exact cause unknown
- Lymphatic obstruction and infection among contributing factors

Prevalence
- Occurs equally in males and females
- More common in Jewish people
- Onset usually before age 30

Complications
- Anal fistula
- Fistulas of the bladder or vagina or to the skin in an old scar area
- Intestinal obstruction
- Nutritional deficiencies caused by malabsorption and maldigestion
- Perforation
- Perineal abscess

Assessment

History
- Diarrhea that may worsen after emotional upset or ingestion of poorly tolerated foods, such as milk, fatty foods, and spices
- Fatigue and weakness
- Fever, flatulence, nausea
- Gradual onset of signs and symptoms, marked by periods of remission and exacerbation
- Steady, colicky or cramping abdominal pain that usually occurs in the right lower abdominal quadrant
- Weight loss

Physical assessment
- Bloody diarrhea
- Hyperactive bowel sounds
- Perianal and rectal abscesses
- Possible abdominal mass, indicating adherent loops of bowel
- Possible soft or semiliquid stool, usually without gross blood
- Right lower abdominal quadrant tenderness or distention

Test results
Laboratory
- Occult blood in stools
- Decreased hemoglobin level and hematocrit
- Increased white blood cell count and erythrocyte sedimentation rate
- Decreased serum potassium, calcium, and magnesium levels
- Hypoglobulinemia from intestinal protein loss
- Vitamin B_{12} and folate deficiency

Imaging
- Small bowel X-rays may show irregular mucosa, ulceration, and stiffening.
- Barium enema reveals the string sign (segments of stricture separated by normal bowel) and may also show fissures and narrowing of the lumen.

Diagnostic procedures
- Sigmoidoscopy and colonoscopy show patchy areas of inflammation and may also reveal the characteristic coarse irregularity (cobblestone appearance) of the mucosal surface.
- Biopsy reveals granulomas in up to half of specimens.

Nursing diagnoses

- Chronic pain
- Deficient knowledge (Crohn's disease)
- Diarrhea
- Disturbed body image
- Imbalanced nutrition: less than body requirements
- Ineffective coping

- Ineffective tissue perfusion: GI
- Risk for deficient fluid volume
- Risk for impaired skin integrity

Key outcomes

The patient will:
- maintain adequate caloric intake
- maintain normal fluid volume
- regain normal bowel movements
- verbalize understanding of the disease process and treatment regimen
- use adequate coping mechanisms and seek appropriate sources of support
- express feelings of comfort.

Interventions

General

- Adequate caloric, protein, and vitamin intake
- Avoidance of foods that worsen diarrhea
- Avoidance of raw fruits and vegetables if blockage occurs
- Colectomy with ileostomy
- Parenteral nutrition, if needed
- Reduced physical activity
- Stress reduction

Nursing

- Provide emotional support to the patient and family.
- Provide meticulous skin care after each bowel movement.
- Schedule patient care to include rest periods throughout the day.
- Assist with diet modification.
- Give prescribed iron supplements and blood transfusions.
- Give prescribed analgesics.

Drug therapy

- Antibacterial and antiprotozoal drugs
- Antidiarrheals
- Anti-inflammatory drugs
- Antispasmodics
- Corticosteroids
- Immunosuppressants
- Opioids
- Sulfonamides
- Vitamin supplements

Monitoring

- Abdominal pain and distention
- Bleeding, especially with corticosteroid use
- Daily weight
- Intake and output, including amount of stool
- Serum electrolyte, glucose, and hemoglobin levels, and stools for occult blood
- Signs of infection or obstruction
- Vital signs

Patient teaching

Be sure to cover:
- information about the disease, symptoms, and complications
- ordered diagnostic tests and pretest guidelines
- the importance of adequate rest
- ways to identify and reduce sources of stress
- prescribed diet changes
- prescribed drugs, dosages, and possible adverse reactions.

Discharge planning

- Refer the patient to a smoking-cessation program, if appropriate.
- Refer the patient to an enterostomal therapist, if indicated.

Cushing's syndrome

Overview

Description

○ Evidence of glucocorticoid excess, particularly cortisol
○ May also reflect excess secretion of mineralocorticoids and androgens
○ Classified as primary, secondary, or iatrogenic, depending on etiology
○ Prognosis dependent on early diagnosis, identification of underlying cause, and effective treatment

Pathophysiology

○ Normal feedback inhibition by cortisol is lost.
○ Elevated cortisol levels don't suppress hypothalamic and anterior pituitary secretion of corticotropin releasing hormone and adrenocorticotropic hormone (ACTH).
○ The result is excessive levels of circulating cortisol.

Causes

○ Corticotropin-producing tumor in another organ
○ Cortisol-secreting adrenal tumor
○ Excess production of corticotropin
○ Long-term use of synthetic glucocorticoids or corticotropin
○ Pituitary microadenoma

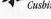 AGE AWARE *In neonates, the usual cause of Cushing's syndrome is adrenal carcinoma.*

Prevalence

○ More common in females than males
○ Can affect a person at any age

Complications

○ Diabetes mellitus
○ Dyslipidemia
○ Frequent infections
○ Heart failure
○ Hypertension
○ Impaired glucose tolerance
○ Ischemic heart disease
○ Menstrual disturbances
○ Osteoporosis and pathologic fractures
○ Peptic ulcer
○ Psychiatric problems ranging from mood swings to psychosis
○ Sexual dysfunction
○ Slow wound healing
○ Suppressed inflammatory response

Assessment

History

○ Amenorrhea
○ Decreased libido
○ Fatigue
○ Frequent infections
○ Headache
○ Impotence
○ Irritability; emotional instability
○ Muscle weakness
○ Polyuria
○ Sleep disturbances
○ Symptoms resembling those of hyperglycemia
○ Thirst
○ Use of synthetic corticosteroids
○ Water retention

Physical assessment

○ Acne
○ Buffalo hump
○ Central obesity
○ Delayed wound healing
○ Hirsutism
○ Hypertension
○ Moon-shaped face
○ Muscle wasting and weakness
○ Petechiae, ecchymoses, and purplish striae
○ Swollen ankles
○ Thin hair
○ Thin limbs

Test results

Laboratory
○ Increased salivary free cortisol level
○ Decreased ACTH level in adrenal disease; increased ACTH level with excessive pituitary or ectopic secretion
○ Hypernatremia
○ Hypokalemia
○ Hypocalcemia
○ Increased blood glucose level
○ Increased free cortisol level in urine
○ Increased serum cortisol level in the morning
○ Glycosuria
Imaging
○ Ultrasonography, computed tomography scan, and magnetic resonance imaging may show the location of a pituitary or adrenal tumor.
Diagnostic procedures
○ A low-dose dexamethasone suppression test shows that plasma cortisol levels aren't suppressed.

Nursing diagnoses

○ Activity intolerance
○ Deficient knowledge (Cushing's syndrome)

- Disturbed body image
- Excess fluid volume
- Impaired skin integrity
- Ineffective coping
- Risk for infection

Key outcomes

The patient will:
- maintain skin integrity
- remain free from infection
- perform activities of daily living as tolerated within the confines of the disorder
- express positive feelings about self
- express understanding of disorder.

Interventions

General

- Management to restore hormone balance and reverse Cushing's syndrome, including radiation, drug therapy, or surgery
- High-protein, high-potassium, low-calorie, low-sodium diet
- Activity, as tolerated
- Possible hypophysectomy or pituitary irradiation
- Bilateral adrenalectomy
- Excision of nonendocrine, corticotropin-producing tumor, followed by drug therapy

Nursing

- Give prescribed drugs.
- Consult a dietitian.
- Apply protective measures to reduce the patient's risk of infection.
- Use meticulous hand-washing technique.
- Schedule adequate rest periods.
- Institute safety precautions.
- Provide meticulous skin care.
- Encourage verbalization of feelings.
- Offer emotional support.
- Help the patient develop effective coping strategies.

After hypophysectomy with transsphenoidal approach
- Keep the head of the bed elevated at least 30 degrees.
- Maintain nasal packing.
- Provide frequent mouth care.
- Avoid activities that increase intracranial pressure (ICP).

Drug therapy

- Aminoglutethimide
- Antifungals
- Antihypertensives
- Antineoplastic antihormone drugs
- Diuretics
- Glucocorticoids
- Potassium supplements

◤ **ALERT** *Giving glucocorticoids on the morning of surgery can help prevent acute adrenal insufficiency during surgery. Cortisol therapy is essential during and after surgery to help the patient tolerate the physiologic stress caused by removal of the pituitary or adrenal glands.*

Monitoring

- Daily weights
- Intake and output
- Serum electrolyte results
- Vital signs

After bilateral adrenalectomy and hypophysectomy
- Adrenal hypofunction
- Bowel sounds
- Hemorrhage and shock
- Hypopituitarism
- Increased ICP
- Neurologic and behavioral status
- Severe nausea, vomiting, and diarrhea
- Transient diabetes insipidus

After hypophysectomy with transsphenoidal approach
- Cerebrospinal fluid leak

Patient teaching

Be sure to cover:
- the disorder, diagnosis, and treatment
- prescribed drugs, dosages, and potential adverse reactions
- when to contact a doctor
- lifelong corticosteroid replacement
- signs and symptoms of adrenal crisis
- the need for medical identification
- prevention of infection
- stress reduction strategies.

Discharge planning

- Refer the patient to a mental health professional for additional counseling, if needed.

Cystic fibrosis

Overview

Description

- Chronic, progressive, inherited, incurable disease affecting exocrine (mucus-secreting) glands
- Transmitted as an autosomal recessive trait
- Genetic mutation that involves chloride transport across epithelial membranes (more than 100 mutations of the gene identified)
- Characterized by major aberrations in sweat gland, respiratory, and gastrointestinal (GI) functions
- Accounts for almost all cases of pancreatic enzyme deficiency in children
- May be apparent soon after birth or take years to develop
- Death typically from pneumonia, emphysema, or atelectasis

Pathophysiology

- Viscosity of bronchial, pancreatic, and other mucous gland secretions increases, obstructing glandular ducts.
- Accumulation of tenacious secretions in bronchioles and alveoli causes respiratory changes and eventually severe atelectasis and emphysema.
- Disease also causes characteristic GI effects in the intestines, pancreas, and liver.
- Obstruction of pancreatic ducts causes trypsin, amylase, and lipase deficiency, which prevents conversion and absorption of fat and protein in the intestinal tract and interferes with the digestion of food and absorption of fat-soluble vitamins.
- In the pancreas, fibrotic tissue, multiple cysts, thick mucus, and fat replace the acini, producing signs of pancreatic insufficiency.

Causes

- Autosomal recessive mutation of gene on chromosome 7
- Causes of symptoms: increased viscosity of bronchial, pancreatic, and other mucous gland secretions and consequent destruction of glandular ducts

Prevalence

- Most common fatal genetic disease of white children
- Twenty-five percent chance of transmission with each pregnancy when both parents are carriers of the recessive gene
- Highest occurrence in people of northern European ancestry
- Less common in Blacks, Native Americans, and people of Asian ancestry
- Equally common in both sexes

Complications

- Arthritis
- Atelectasis
- Azoospermia in males
- Biliary disease
- Bronchiectasis
- Cardiac arrhythmias
- Clotting problems
- Cor pulmonale
- Death
- Dehydration
- Delayed sexual development
- Diabetes
- Distal intestinal obstructive syndrome
- Electrolyte imbalances
- Gastroesophageal reflux
- Hepatic disease
- Malnutrition
- Pneumonia
- Potentially fatal shock
- Retarded bone growth
- Secondary amenorrhea in females

Assessment

History

- Abdominal distention, vomiting, constipation
- Dry, nonproductive cough
- Frequent, bulky, foul-smelling, and pale stool with a high fat content
- Hematemesis
- Nasal polyps and sinusitis
- Poor growth
- Poor weight gain
- Ravenous appetite
- Recurring bronchitis and pneumonia
- Shortness of breath
- Wheezing

AGE AWARE Neonates may have meconium ileus and symptoms of intestinal obstruction: abdominal distention, vomiting, constipation, dehydration, and electrolyte imbalance.

Physical assessment

- Barrel chest
- Bibasilar crackles and hyperresonance
- Cyanosis
- Clubbing of fingers and toes
- Delayed sexual development
- Distended abdomen
- Dry, nonproductive, paroxysmal cough
- Dyspnea
- Failure to thrive
- Hepatomegaly
- Neonatal jaundice
- Rectal prolapse
- Sallow skin with poor turgor
- Tachypnea

- Thin limbs
- Wheezy respirations

Test results

Laboratory
- Absence of trypsin in stool specimen
- Delta F 508 deletion in deoxyribonucleic acid tests
- Possible hepatic insufficiency in liver enzyme tests
- Possible organisms — such as *Pseudomonas* and *Staphylococcus* — in sputum cultures
- Decreased serum albumin level
- Possible hypochloremia
- Possible hyponatremia
- Hypoxemia in arterial blood gas studies

Imaging
- Chest X-rays may show early signs of lung obstruction.
- High-resolution chest computed tomography scan shows bronchial wall thickening, cystic lesions, and bronchiectasis.

Diagnostic procedures
- Sweat tests using pilocarpine solution show positive results — increased sodium or chloride levels.
- Pulmonary function tests show decreased vital capacity, elevated residual volume, and decreased forced expiratory volume in 1 second.

Nursing diagnoses

- Anxiety
- Deficient knowledge (cystic fibrosis)
- Disabled family coping
- Imbalanced nutrition: less than body requirements
- Impaired gas exchange
- Ineffective airway clearance
- Ineffective breathing patterns
- Ineffective tissue perfusion: cardiopulmonary
- Risk for deficient fluid volume

Key outcomes

The patient will:
- maintain a patent airway and adequate ventilation
- consume adequate calories daily
- use a support system to assist with coping
- express an understanding of the illness
- maintain fluid balance.

Interventions

General
- Based on organ systems involved
- Chest physiotherapy, nebulization, and breathing exercises several times daily
- Postural drainage
- Gene therapy (experimental)
- Annual influenza vaccination
- Salt supplements
- High-fat, high-protein, high-calorie diet

- Activity, as tolerated
- Heart-lung transplantation

Nursing
- Give prescribed drugs.
- Give pancreatic enzymes with meals and snacks.
- Perform chest physiotherapy and postural drainage.
- Give oxygen therapy, as needed.
- Provide a well-balanced, high-calorie, high-protein diet; include adequate fats.
- Provide vitamin A, D, E, and K supplements, if indicated.
- Ensure adequate oral fluid intake.
- Provide exercise and activity periods.
- Encourage breathing exercises.
- Provide a young child with play periods.
- Enlist the help of physical and play therapists, if available.
- Provide emotional support.
- Include family members in all phases of the child's care.

Drug therapy
- Antibiotics
- Bronchodilators
- Dornase alfa, a pulmonary enzyme given by aerosol nebulizer
- Oral pancreatic enzymes
- Oxygen therapy, as needed
- Prednisone
- Vitamin A, D, E, and K supplements

Monitoring
- Daily weight
- Hydration
- Intake and output
- Pulse oximetry
- Respiratory status
- Vital signs

Patient teaching

Be sure to cover:
- the disorder, diagnosis, and treatment
- drugs and potential adverse reactions
- when to contact a doctor
- aerosol therapy
- chest physiotherapy
- evidence of infection
- complications.

Discharge planning

- Refer family members for genetic counseling, as appropriate.
- Refer patient and family to a local support group, such as the Cystic Fibrosis Foundation.

Cystinuria

Overview

Description

○ An autosomal recessive disorder
○ An inborn error of amino acid transport in the kidneys and intestine that allows excessive urinary excretion of cystine and other dibasic amino acids
○ Causes recurrent cystine renal calculi
○ The most common defect of amino acid transport
○ Good prognosis with proper treatment

Pathophysiology

○ Impaired renal tubular reabsorption of dibasic amino acids (cystine, lysine, arginine, and ornithine) results in excessive amino acid concentration and excretion in the urine.
○ Cystine concentration exceeds its solubility and precipitates and forms crystals, precursors of cystine calculi.

Causes

○ Inherited as an autosomal recessive defect

Prevalence

○ About 1 in 15,000 live births
○ More prevalent in persons of short stature, for unknown reasons
○ Affects both sexes
○ More severe in males

Complications

○ Obstruction and destruction of kidney and ureter tissue

Assessment

✳ AGE AWARE *The effects of cystinuria result from cystine or mixed cystine calculi, which typically develop between ages 10 and 30.*

History

○ Abdominal distention
○ Dull flank pain
○ Family history of renal disease or calculi
○ Nausea
○ Signs of secondary infection
  – Chills
  – Fever
  – Burning, itching, or pain on urination
  – Urinary frequency
  – Foul-smelling urine
○ Vomiting

Physical assessment

○ Hematuria
○ Tenderness in the costovertebral angle or over the kidneys

Test results

Laboratory
○ Cystine crystals in calculi
○ Hexagonal, flat cystine crystals in urine, visible by microscope
○ Cystine crystals that resemble benzene rings when glacial acetic acid is added to chilled urine
○ Increased serum white blood cell count
○ Increased clearance of cystine, lysine, arginine, and ornithine
○ Aminoaciduria with cystine, lysine, arginine, and ornithine
○ Usually a urine pH less than 5
○ Positive cyanide-nitroprusside test
Imaging
○ Kidney-ureter-bladder X-rays determine the size and location of calculi.
Diagnostic procedures
○ Excretory urography determines renal function.

Nursing diagnoses

○ Acute pain
○ Deficient knowledge (cystinuria)
○ Impaired urinary elimination
○ Risk for infection

Key outcomes

The patient will:
○ maintain urine specific gravity within designated limits
○ report increased comfort
○ identify risk factors that worsen decreased tissue perfusion, and modify lifestyle accordingly
○ avoid or minimize complications.

Interventions

General

○ Increasing fluid intake to maintain a minimum 24-hour urine volume of 4,000 ml (5,000 to 7,000 ml is optimal)
○ Alkaline-ash diet (high in vegetables and fruit, low in protein) to alkalinize urine, increasing cystine solubility, although this may increase the risk of calcium phosphate calculi
○ Surgical removal of calculi

Nursing

○ Give prescribed drugs.
○ Encourage increased oral fluid intake.
○ Provide emotional support.

Drug therapy

○ Antibiotics for secondary infection
○ Penicillamine (cautiously, because of toxic adverse effects and risk of allergic reaction)
○ Sodium bicarbonate

Monitoring

○ Intake and output
○ Serum bicarbonate level
○ Signs of infection
○ Urine pH

Patient teaching

Be sure to cover:
○ the disorder, diagnosis, and treatment
○ the need to maintain increased, evenly spaced fluid intake, even through the night
○ signs of renal calculi and urinary tract infection
○ prescribed drugs, dosages, and possible adverse effects.

Discharge planning

○ Refer the patient to a nephrologist for follow-up care.

Diabetes insipidus

Overview

Description

- Disorder of water balance regulation characterized by excessive fluid intake and hypotonic polyuria
- Failure of vasopressin secretion in response to normal physiologic stimuli
- Two types: primary and secondary
- May occur only during pregnancy, usually after the fifth or sixth month of gestation
- Good prognosis if uncomplicated
- Variable prognosis if complicated by underlying disorder, such as cancer
- Increased risk of complications with impaired or absent thirst mechanism

Pathophysiology

- Vasopressin (antidiuretic hormone) is synthesized in the hypothalamus and stored by the posterior pituitary gland.
- Once released into the general circulation, vasopressin acts on the distal and collecting tubules of the kidneys.
- Vasopressin increases permeability of the tubules to water and causes water reabsorption.
- Absence of vasopressin allows filtered water to be excreted in the urine instead of being reabsorbed.

Causes

- Certain drugs, such as lithium
- Congenital malformation of the central nervous system (CNS)
- Damage to hypothalamus or pituitary gland
- Failure of the kidneys to respond to vasopressin, called nephrogenic diabetes insipidus (DI)
- Familial
- Granulomatous disease
- Idiopathic
- Infection
- Neurosurgery, skull fracture, or head trauma
- Pregnancy (gestational DI)
- Psychogenic
- Trauma
- Tumors
- Vascular lesions

Prevalence

- Affects men and women equally
- Primary DI in 50% of patients

Complications

- Bladder distention
- Circulatory collapse
- CNS changes
- Hydronephrosis
- Hydroureter
- Hyperosmolality
- Hypovolemia
- Loss of consciousness

Assessment

History

- Abrupt onset of extreme polyuria
- Extreme thirst
- Extraordinarily large oral fluid intake
- Weight loss
- Dizziness, weakness, fatigue
- Constipation
- Nocturia

✳ *AGE AWARE In children, reports of enuresis, sleep disturbances, irritability, anorexia, thirst, and decreased weight gain and linear growth are common.*

Physical assessment

- Decreased muscle strength
- Dyspnea
- Fever
- Hypotension
- Pale, voluminous urine
- Poor skin turgor
- Signs of dehydration
- Tachycardia

Test results

Laboratory
- Colorless urine with low osmolality and specific gravity
- Increased serum sodium level
- Increased serum osmolality
- Decreased serum vasopressin level
- Decreased specific gravity and increased volume in 24-hour urine test
- Increased blood urea nitrogen (BUN) and creatinine levels

Diagnostic procedures
- Dehydration test or water deprivation test shows an increase in urine osmolality exceeding 9% after vasopressin administration.

Nursing diagnoses

- Deficient fluid volume
- Deficient knowledge (diabetes insipidus)
- Delayed growth and development
- Fear
- Impaired oral mucous membrane
- Impaired urinary elimination
- Ineffective coping

Key outcomes

The patient will:
○ demonstrate balanced fluid volume
○ display adaptive coping behaviors
○ avoid complications
○ have normal laboratory test results.

Interventions

General

○ Identification and treatment of underlying cause
○ Control of fluid balance
○ Dehydration prevention
○ Free access to oral fluids
○ With nephrogenic DI, low-sodium diet

Nursing

○ Give prescribed drugs.
○ Provide meticulous skin and mouth care.
○ Encourage verbalization of feelings.
○ Offer encouragement while providing a realistic assessment of the situation.
○ Help the patient develop effective coping strategies.

> ▼ **ALERT** *Use caution when giving vasopressin to a patient with coronary artery disease because it can cause coronary artery constriction.*

Drug therapy

○ I.V. fluids
  – Dextrose 5% in water if serum sodium level exceeds 150 mEq/L
  – Normal saline solution if serum sodium level is less than 150 mEq/L
○ Synthetic vasopressin analogue
○ Thiazide diuretics in nephrogenic DI
○ Vasopressin
○ Vasopressin stimulant

Monitoring

○ Cardiac rhythm
○ Daily weight
○ Evidence of hypovolemic shock
○ Intake and output
○ Mental or neurologic status
○ Serum electrolyte and BUN levels
○ Urine specific gravity
○ Vital signs

Patient teaching

Be sure to cover:
○ the disorder, diagnosis, and treatment
○ drugs, dosages, and possible adverse reactions
○ when to contact a doctor
○ evidence of dehydration
○ daily weight

○ intake and output
○ use of a hydrometer to measure urine specific gravity
○ need for medical identification
○ need for ongoing medical care.

Discharge planning

○ Refer the patient to a mental health professional for additional counseling as indicated.

Diabetes mellitus

Overview

Description

- Chronic disease of absolute or relative insulin deficiency or resistance
- Characterized by disturbances in carbohydrate, protein, and fat metabolism
- Two primary forms
  - Type 1, characterized by absolute insufficiency
  - Type 2, characterized by insulin resistance with varying degrees of insulin secretory defects

Pathophysiology

- The effects of diabetes mellitus result from insulin deficiency or resistance to endogenous insulin.
- Insulin allows glucose transport into the cells for use as energy or storage as glycogen.
- Insulin also stimulates protein synthesis and free fatty acid storage in adipose tissue.
- Insulin deficiency compromises the body's access to essential nutrients for fuel and storage.

Risk factors

- Certain drugs
  - Adrenal corticosteroids
  - Hormonal contraceptives
  - Thiazide diuretics
- Obesity (type 2)
- Physiologic or emotional stress
- Pregnancy
- Sedentary lifestyle (type 2)
- Viral infection (type 1)

Causes

- Autoimmune disease (type 1)
- Genetic factors

Prevalence

Type 1

- Usually occurs before age 30, although it may occur at any age
- More common in men

Type 2

- Occurrence increases with age
- Usually occurs in obese adults older than age 30, although it may occur in obese North American youths of African-American, Native American, or Hispanic descent
- Affects about 8% of the United States' population
- About one-third of patients undiagnosed

Complications

- Cardiovascular disease
- Cognitive dysfunction
- Diabetic dermopathy
- Hyperosmolar, hyperglycemic syndrome
- Impaired resistance to infection
- Ketoacidosis
- Nephropathy
- Peripheral vascular disease
- Retinopathy, blindness

AGE AWARE *If a diabetic mother's glucose levels aren't well controlled before and during pregnancy, her neonate has two to three times the risk of congenital malformations and fetal distress.*

Assessment

History

- Dehydration
- Dry, itchy skin
- Dry mucous membranes
- Frequent skin and urinary tract infections
- Nocturnal diarrhea
- Numbness or pain in hands or feet
- Polydipsia
- Polyuria, nocturia
- Poor skin turgor
- Postprandial feeling of nausea or fullness
- Sexual problems
- Weakness, fatigue
- Weight loss and hunger
- Vision changes

Type 1

- Rapidly developing symptoms

Type 2

- Family history of diabetes mellitus
- Other endocrine diseases
- Pregnancy
- Recent stress or trauma
- Severe viral infection
- Use of drugs that increase blood glucose levels
- Vague, long-standing symptoms that develop gradually

Physical assessment

- Characteristic "fruity" breath odor in ketoacidosis
- Cool skin temperature
- Decreased peripheral pulses
- Diminished deep tendon reflexes
- Dry mucous membranes
- Muscle wasting and loss of subcutaneous fat (type 1)
- Obesity, particularly in the abdominal area (type 2)
- Orthostatic hypotension
- Poor skin turgor
- Possible hypovolemia and shock in ketoacidosis and hyperosmolar hyperglycemic state
- Retinopathy or cataract formation
- Skin changes, especially on the legs and feet

Test results

Laboratory

- Fasting plasma glucose level greater than or equal to 126 mg/dl on at least two occasions

- Random blood glucose level greater than or equal to 200 mg/dl
- Two-hour postprandial blood glucose level greater than or equal to 200 mg/dl
- Increased glycosylated hemoglobin level
- Possible acetone or glucose in urine

Diagnostic procedures
- Ophthalmic examination may show diabetic retinopathy.

Nursing diagnoses

- Deficient fluid volume
- Imbalanced nutrition: less than body requirements
- Imbalanced nutrition: more than body requirements
- Impaired skin integrity
- Ineffective coping
- Ineffective tissue perfusion: renal, cardiovascular, peripheral
- Risk for infection
- Sexual dysfunction

Key outcomes

The patient will:
- maintain optimal body weight
- remain free from infection
- avoid complications
- verbalize understanding of the disorder and treatment
- demonstrate adaptive coping behaviors.

Interventions

General

- American Diabetes Association recommendations to reach target glucose, glycosylated hemoglobin, lipid, and blood pressure levels
- Exercise and diet control
- Modest calorie restriction for weight loss or maintenance
- Pancreas transplantation
- Regular aerobic exercise
- Tight glycemic control to prevent complications

Nursing

- Give prescribed drugs.
- Give rapidly absorbed carbohydrates for hypoglycemia or, if the patient is unconscious, glucagon or I.V. dextrose, as ordered.
- Give I.V. fluids and insulin replacement for hyperglycemic crisis, as ordered.
- Provide meticulous skin care, especially to the feet and legs.
- Treat all injuries, cuts, and blisters immediately.
- Avoid constricting hose, slippers, or bed linens.
- Encourage adequate fluid intake.
- Encourage verbalization of feelings.

- Offer emotional support.
- Help to develop effective coping strategies.

Drug therapy

- Exogenous insulin (type 1 or possibly type 2)
- Oral antihyperglycemics (type 2)

Monitoring

- Cardiovascular status
- Daily weight
- Intake and output
- Renal status
- Serum glucose
- Signs and symptoms of developing problems
  - Hypoglycemia
  - Hyperglycemia
  - Hyperosmolar coma
  - Urinary tract and vaginal infections
  - Diabetic neuropathy
- Urine acetone
- Vital signs

Patient teaching

Be sure to cover:
- the disorder, diagnosis, and treatment
- prescribed drugs, dosages, and possible adverse reactions
- methods of administering drugs
- when to contact a doctor
- prescribed meal plan
- prescribed exercise program
- signs and symptoms of problems
  - infection
  - hypoglycemia
  - hyperglycemia
  - diabetic neuropathy
- self-monitoring of blood glucose level
- complications of hyperglycemia
- foot care
- annual ophthalmologic examinations
- safety precautions
- management of diabetes during illness.

Discharge planning

- Refer the patient to a dietitian.
- Refer the patient to a podiatrist if needed.
- Refer the patient to an ophthalmologist.
- Refer an adult diabetic patient who is planning a family for preconception counseling.
- Refer the patient to the Juvenile Diabetes Research Foundation, the American Association of Diabetes Educators, and the American Diabetes Association to obtain additional information.

Diabetic ketoacidosis

Overview

Description
- Acute complication of diabetes mellitus
- Life-threatening
- Increased serum ketone and blood glucose levels
- Decreased serum pH (below 7.2)

Pathophysiology
- Absolute or relative insulin deficiency causes an increase in counter-regulatory hormones.
- Hepatic glyconeogenesis, glycogenolysis, and lipolysis occurs, causing hyperglycemia and an increase in serum free fatty acids.
- Ketonemia and ketonuria occur, resulting in metabolic acidosis and osmotic diuresis.
- Hypoglycemia may then occur.

Causes
- Uncontrolled type 1 diabetes mellitus
  - New diagnosis
  - Noncompliance
  - Concurrent illness
  - Medication
  - Stress (physical or psychological)
  - Idiopathic
- Occasionally uncontrolled type 2 diabetes mellitus

Prevalence
- Accounts for 50% of diabetes-related hospital admissions in young people
- Exact prevalence unknown
- More common among Whites, as is diabetes mellitus
- Affects women slightly more than men

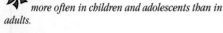 **AGE AWARE** *Diabetic ketoacidosis occurs more often in children and adolescents than in adults.*

Complications
- Cardiac arrhythmia
- Cerebral edema
- Hypoglycemia
- Myocardial infarction
- Pulmonary edema

Assessment

History
- Fatigue
- Increased thirst
- Increased urination
- Nausea
- Possible history of diabetes mellitus
- Vomiting

Physical assessment
- Acetone breath
- Evidence of acidosis
  - Abdominal pain
  - Altered level of consciousness
  - Shallow rapid breathing (Kussmaul's respirations)
- Evidence of dehydration

Test results
Laboratory
- Glucose and ketones in urine
- Blood glucose level higher than 250 mg/dl
- Ketones in serum
- Metabolic acidosis
- Increased serum potassium level
- Decreased serum sodium, chloride, and phosphorus levels
- Increased white blood cell count (even without infection)

Diagnostic procedures
- Electrocardiography may show T-wave changes that reflect disturbed potassium levels.

Nursing diagnoses
- Deficient fluid volume
- Deficient knowledge (diabetes mellitus and diabetic ketoacidosis)
- Imbalanced nutrition: less than body requirements
- Impaired gas exchange
- Ineffective coping
- Ineffective tissue perfusion: renal, cardiovascular, peripheral

Key outcomes
The patient will:
- have adequate respirations and ventilation
- be hemodynamically stable
- remain free from infection
- avoid complications
- verbalize understanding of the disorder and treatment
- demonstrate adaptive coping behaviors.

Interventions

General
- Serial laboratory tests and arterial blood gas (ABG) analyses
- Adequate oxygenation
- I.V. fluids

Nursing
- Give prescribed drugs.
- Give oxygen as ordered.
- Evaluate respiratory and neurologic status continuously.

○ Provide emotional support.
○ Encourage compliance with treatment program.

Drug therapy

○ Antibiotics (if infection present)
○ Correction of electrolyte imbalances
○ Insulin
○ Sodium bicarbonate

Monitoring

○ ABG analysis
○ Cardiac rhythm
○ Intake and output
○ Laboratory test results
○ Neurologic status
○ Respiratory status
○ Serial blood glucose levels
○ Vital signs

Patient teaching

Be sure to cover:
○ the disorder, diagnosis, and treatment
○ prescribed drugs, dosages, and possible adverse effects
○ signs of hyperglycemia and hypoglycemia and effective immediate treatment
○ when to contact a doctor or seek medical attention
○ how to test blood glucose levels at home.

Discharge planning

○ Refer the patient to a diabetic teaching class for more information.
○ Refer the patient to the Juvenile Diabetes Research Foundation, the American Association of Diabetes Educators, and the American Diabetes Association to obtain additional information.

Disseminated intravascular coagulation

Overview

Description

○ Syndrome of activated coagulation characterized by bleeding or thrombosis
○ Complicates diseases and conditions that accelerate clotting
  – occlusion of small blood vessels
  – organ necrosis
  – depletion of circulating clotting factors and platelets
  – activation of the fibrinolytic system
○ Also known as DIC, consumption coagulopathy, and defibrination syndrome

Pathophysiology

○ Typical accelerated clotting results in generalized activation of prothrombin and a consequent excess of thrombin.
○ Excess thrombin converts fibrinogen to fibrin, producing fibrin clots in the microcirculation.
○ This process consumes exorbitant amounts of coagulation factors (especially platelets, factor V, prothrombin, fibrinogen, and factor VIII), causing thrombocytopenia, deficiencies in factors V and VIII, hypoprothrombinemia, and hypofibrinogenemia.
○ Circulating thrombin activates the fibrinolytic system, which lyses fibrin clots into fibrinogen degradation products (FDPs).
○ The hemorrhage that occurs may result largely from the anticoagulant activity of FDPs and depletion of plasma coagulation factors.

Causes

○ Disorders that produce necrosis, such as extensive burns and trauma
○ Infection, sepsis
○ Neoplastic disease
○ Obstetric complications
○ Other disorders, such as acute respiratory distress syndrome, cardiac arrest, cardiopulmonary bypass, diabetic ketoacidosis, drug reactions, heatstroke, incompatible blood transfusion, pulmonary embolism, sickle cell anemia, and shock

Prevalence

○ Depends on the cause

Assessment

History

○ Abnormal bleeding (possibly at all body orifices) without a history of a serious hemorrhagic disorder
○ Possible bleeding from surgical or invasive procedure sites, such as incisions or venipuncture sites
○ Possible gastrointestinal (GI) bleeding, hematuria
○ Possible nausea and vomiting; severe muscle, back, and abdominal pain; chest pain; hemoptysis; epistaxis; seizures; and oliguria
○ Possible presence of a disorder that causes DIC
○ Possible signs of bleeding into the skin, such as cutaneous oozing, petechiae, ecchymoses, or hematomas

Physical assessment

○ Acrocyanosis
○ Dyspnea, tachypnea
○ Mental status changes, including confusion
○ Petechiae

Test results

Laboratory

○ Decreased serum platelet count (less than 150,000/mm^3)
○ Decreased serum fibrinogen level (less than 170 mg/dl)
○ Prolonged prothrombin time (more than 19 seconds)
○ Prolonged activated partial thromboplastin time (more than 40 seconds)
○ Increased FDPs (commonly greater than 45 mcg/ml, or positive at less than 1:100 dilution)
○ Positive D-dimer test (specific fibrinogen test for DIC) at less than 1:8 dilution
○ Prolonged thrombin time
○ Decreased levels of blood clotting factors V and VIII
○ Decreased hemoglobin levels (less than 10 g/dl)
○ Increased levels of blood urea nitrogen (greater than 25 mg/dl) and serum creatinine (greater than 1.3 mg/dl)

Nursing diagnoses

○ Acute pain
○ Anxiety
○ Fatigue
○ Fear
○ Impaired gas exchange
○ Ineffective tissue perfusion: GI, cerebral, renal
○ Risk for deficient fluid volume

Key outcomes

The patient will:
○ maintain balanced intake and output
○ maintain adequate ventilation

○ express feelings of increased comfort and decreased pain
○ have laboratory values return to normal
○ use available support systems to assist in coping with fears.

Interventions

General
○ Treatment for underlying condition
○ Possibly supportive care alone if the patient isn't actively bleeding
○ Activity, as tolerated

Nursing

▼ *ALERT Focus on early recognition of signs of abnormal bleeding, prompt treatment of the underlying disorders, and prevention of further bleeding.*

○ Provide emotional support.
○ Provide adequate rest periods.
○ Give prescribed drugs, including analgesics.
○ Reposition the patient every 2 hours, and provide meticulous skin care.
○ Give prescribed oxygen therapy.

▼ *ALERT To prevent clots from dislodging and causing fresh bleeding, don't vigorously rub the affected areas when bathing.*

○ Protect the patient from injury.
○ If bleeding occurs, use pressure and topical hemostatic agents to control bleeding.
○ Limit venipunctures whenever possible.
○ Watch for transfusion reactions and signs of fluid overload.
○ Measure the amount of blood lost, weigh dressings and linen, and record drainage.
○ Weigh the patient daily, particularly if there is renal involvement.

Drug therapy
In active bleeding
○ Antithrombin III and gabexate
○ Blood, fresh frozen plasma, platelets, or packed red blood cells
○ Cryoprecipitate
○ Fluid replacement

Monitoring
○ Intake and output, especially when giving blood products
○ Results of serial blood studies
○ Signs of shock
○ Vital signs

Patient teaching

Be sure to cover (for the patient and his family):
○ an explanation of the disorder
○ evidence of the problem, diagnostic procedures needed, and treatment that the patient is to receive.

Discharge planning

○ Refer the patient for follow-up care with a hematologist if appropriate.

Electric shock

Overview

Description

- Electric current passing through body
- Physical damage varies
  - Intensity of current
  - Resistance of tissues it passes through
  - Type of current
  - Frequency and duration of current flow
- Classified as lightning, low-voltage (less than 600 volts [V]), and high-voltage (more than 600 V)

Pathophysiology

- Electrical energy alters the resting potential of cell membranes, causing depolarization in muscles and nerves.
- Electric shock alters normal electrical activity of the heart and brain.
- High-frequency current generates more heat in tissues than a low-frequency current, resulting in burns and local tissue coagulation and necrosis.
- Electric shock causes muscle tetany, tissue destruction, and coagulative necrosis.

Causes

- Accidental contact with an exposed part of an electrical appliance or wiring
- Lightning
- Flash of electric arcs from high-voltage power lines or machines

Prevalence

- Causes more than 500 deaths annually
- More common in men ages 20 to 40

Complications

- Cardiac dysfunction
- Death
- Electrolyte abnormalities
- Neurologic dysfunction
- Peripheral nerve injuries
- Psychiatric dysfunction
- Renal failure
- Sepsis
- Thrombi
- Vascular disruption

Assessment

History

- Exposure to electricity or lightning
- Loss of consciousness
- Muscle pain
- Fatigue
- Headache
- Nervous irritability

Physical assessment

- Apnea
- Burns
- Cold skin
- Cyanosis
- Determined by voltage exposure
- Entrance and exit injuries
- Local tissue coagulation
- Markedly decreased blood pressure
- Numbness or tingling or sensorimotor deficits
- Unconsciousness

Test results

Laboratory

- Laboratory test results to evaluate internal damage and guide treatment:
  - Arterial blood gas analysis to determine respiratory status
  - Urine analysis and urine myoglobin tests to evaluate tissue damage
  - Complete blood count
  - Electrolyte status to show imbalances
  - Blood urea nitrogen and creatinine levels to show kidney damage

Imaging

- Chest X-rays, if chest injury or shortness of breath occurred, reveal internal damage.

Diagnostic procedures

- Electrocardiography (ECG) reveals arrhythmias, allows evaluation of internal damage, and guides treatment.

Nursing diagnoses

- Acute pain
- Anxiety
- Decreased cardiac output
- Impaired skin integrity
- Ineffective breathing pattern
- Ineffective tissue perfusion: cardiopulmonary
- Risk for imbalanced fluid volume
- Risk for post-trauma syndrome

Key outcomes

The patient will:
- maintain stable cardiac rhythm
- maintain cardiac output
- regain skin integrity
- have wounds and incisions that appear clean, pink, and free from purulent drainage
- maintain adequate fluid volume.

Interventions

General

○ Activity based on outcome of interventions
○ Cardiopulmonary resuscitation if needed
○ Emergency stabilizing measures
○ No dietary restrictions if swallowing ability intact
○ Separation of victim from source of electrical current
○ Stabilization of cervical spine
○ Treatment of acid-base imbalance
○ Vigorous fluid replacement

Nursing

○ Turn off the electricity to separate the victim from the source of current.
○ Provide emergency treatment.
○ Give rapid I.V. fluid infusion.
○ Obtain a 12-lead ECG.
○ Give prescribed drugs.

Drug therapy

○ Osmotic diuretic
○ Tetanus prophylaxis

Monitoring

○ Cardiac rhythm (continuously)
○ Intake and output (hourly)
○ Neurologic status
○ Peripheral neurovascular status
○ Sensorimotor deficits

Patient teaching

Be sure to cover:
○ information about the injury, diagnosis, and treatment
○ how to avoid electrical hazards at home and at work
○ electrical safety for children.

Discharge planning

○ Refer the patient to rehabilitation and specialist care in keeping with his injury and recovery.

Emphysema

Overview

Description

○ Chronic lung disease characterized by exertional dyspnea and permanent enlargement of air spaces distal to the terminal bronchioles
○ One of several diseases usually labeled collectively as chronic obstructive pulmonary disease or chronic obstructive lung disease

Pathophysiology

○ Recurrent inflammation caused by the release of proteolytic enzymes from lung cells causes abnormal, permanent enlargement of the air spaces distal to the terminal bronchioles.
○ This enlargement leads to the destruction of alveolar walls, which results in a breakdown of elasticity. (See *What happens in emphysema.*)

Causes

○ Cigarette smoking
○ Genetic deficiency of alpha$_1$-antitrypsin

Prevalence

○ Most common cause of death from respiratory disease in the United States
○ More common in men than women
○ About 2 million Americans affected
○ 1 in 3,000 neonates affected

Complications

○ Cor pulmonale
○ Peptic ulcer disease
○ Pneumomediastinum
○ Recurrent respiratory tract infections
○ Respiratory failure
○ Spontaneous pneumothorax

Assessment

History

○ Anorexia and weight loss
○ Chronic cough
○ Malaise
○ Shortness of breath
○ Smoking

Physical assessment

○ Barrel chest
○ Clubbed fingers and toes
○ Crackles
○ Cyanosis
○ Decreased breath sounds
○ Decreased chest expansion
○ Decreased tactile fremitus
○ Distant heart sounds
○ Hyperresonance
○ Inspiratory wheeze
○ Prolonged expiratory phase with grunting respirations
○ Pursed-lip breathing
○ Tachypnea
○ Use of accessory muscles

Test results

Laboratory
○ Decreased partial pressure of oxygen on arterial blood gas analysis
○ Normal partial pressure of carbon dioxide until late in the disease
○ Increased hemoglobin level late in the disease
Imaging
○ Chest X-rays may show several changes:
  – Flattened diaphragm
  – Reduced vascular markings at the lung periphery
  – Overaeration of the lungs
  – Vertical heart
  – Enlarged anteroposterior chest diameter
  – Large retrosternal air space.
Diagnostic procedures
○ Pulmonary function tests show typical changes:
  – Increased residual volume and total lung capacity
  – Reduced diffusing capacity
  – Increased inspiratory flow.
○ Electrocardiography may show changes:
  – Tall, symmetrical P waves in leads II, III, and aVF
  – Vertical QRS axis
  – Signs of right ventricular hypertrophy late in the disease.

Nursing diagnoses

○ Activity intolerance
○ Anxiety
○ Deficient knowledge (emphysema)
○ Fatigue
○ Impaired gas exchange
○ Ineffective airway clearance
○ Ineffective breathing pattern

Key outcomes

The patient will:
○ maintain a patent airway and adequate ventilation
○ use energy conservation techniques
○ express understanding of the illness
○ demonstrate effective coping strategies.

Interventions

General

○ Activity, as tolerated
○ Adequate hydration
○ Chest physiotherapy

- ○ Chest tube insertion for pneumothorax
- ○ High-protein, high-calorie diet
- ○ Possible transtracheal catheterization and home oxygen therapy

Nursing

- ○ Give prescribed drugs.
- ○ Provide supportive care.
- ○ Help the patient adjust to lifestyle changes caused by a chronic illness.
- ○ Encourage the patient to express fears and concerns.
- ○ Perform chest physiotherapy.
- ○ Provide a high-calorie, protein-rich diet.
- ○ Give small, frequent meals.
- ○ Encourage daily activity and diversional activities.
- ○ Provide frequent rest periods.

Drug therapy

- ○ Antibiotics
- ○ Anticholinergics
- ○ Bronchodilators
- ○ Corticosteroids
- ○ Mucolytics
- ○ Oxygen

Monitoring

- ○ Activity tolerance
- ○ Complications
- ○ Daily weight
- ○ Intake and output
- ○ Respiratory status
- ○ Vital signs

Patient teaching

Be sure to cover:
- ○ the disorder, diagnosis, and treatment
- ○ prescribed drugs, dosages, and possible adverse reactions
- ○ when to contact a doctor
- ○ the need to avoid smoking and areas where smoking is permitted
- ○ the need to avoid crowds and people with infections
- ○ home oxygen therapy, if indicated
- ○ transtracheal catheter care, if needed
- ○ coughing and deep-breathing exercises
- ○ proper use of handheld inhalers
- ○ high-calorie, protein-rich diet
- ○ adequate oral fluid intake
- ○ avoidance of respiratory irritants
- ○ signs and symptoms of pneumothorax.

> ▲ **ALERT** *Urge the patient to notify a doctor if he experiences a sudden onset of worsening dyspnea or sharp pleuritic chest pain worsened by chest movement, breathing, or coughing.*

What happens in emphysema

In a patient with emphysema, recurrent pulmonary inflammation damages and eventually destroys the alveolar walls, creating large air spaces and a reduced surface area for gas exchange. Damage to the alveoli leaves them unable to recoil normally after expanding, which traps air in the lungs. The patient must exhale forcefully to remove air from the lungs, which compresses the airways and may cause them to collapse.

Associated pulmonary capillary destruction usually allows a patient with severe emphysema to match ventilation to perfusion and thus avoid cyanosis.

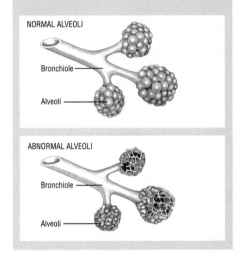

NORMAL ALVEOLI

Bronchiole

Alveoli

ABNORMAL ALVEOLI

Bronchiole

Alveoli

Discharge planning

- ○ Refer the patient to a smoking-cessation program if indicated.
- ○ Refer the patient for influenza and pneumococcal pneumonia immunizations as needed.
- ○ Refer the family of patients with familial emphysema for alpha$_1$-antitrypsin deficiency screening.

Esophageal cancer

Overview

Description
- Malignant esophageal tumor
  - Squamous cell carcinoma
  - Adenocarcinoma
- Usually fungating and infiltrating
- Commonly metastasizes to liver and lungs
- Nearly always fatal
- 5-year survival in fewer than 5% of cases
- Death common within 6 months of diagnosis

Pathophysiology
- Most esophageal cancers are poorly differentiated squamous cell carcinomas, with 50% occurring in the lower portion of the esophagus, 40% in the middle portion, and 10% in the upper or cervical esophagus.
- Adenocarcinomas are less common and are contained to the lower third of the esophagus.
- The tumor partially constricts the lumen of the esophagus.
- Regional metastasis occurs early by way of submucosal lymphatics, often fatally invading adjacent vital intrathoracic organs.
- If the patient survives primary extension, the liver and lungs are the usual sites of distant metastases; unusual metastasis sites include the bone, kidneys, and adrenal glands.

Risk factors
- Chronic irritation from heavy smoking
- Excessive use of alcohol
- Nutritional deficiency, as in untreated sprue and Plummer-Vinson syndrome
- Previous head and neck tumors
- Stasis-induced inflammation, as in achalasia or stricture

Causes
- Unknown

Prevalence
- Most common in men older than age 60
- Occurs worldwide, but most common in Japan, Russia, China, the Middle East, and the Transkei region of South Africa

Complications
- Direct invasion of adjoining structures
- Inability to control secretions
- Loss of lower esophageal sphincter control (may result in aspiration pneumonia)
- Obstruction of the esophagus

Assessment

History
- Anorexia, vomiting, and regurgitation of food
- Dysphagia of varying degrees depending on the extent of disease
- Feeling of fullness, pressure, indigestion, or substernal burning
- Hoarseness
- Pain on swallowing or pain that radiates to the back
- Weight loss

Physical assessment
- Cachexia and dehydration
- Chronic cough (possibly from aspiration)

Test results
Imaging
- X-rays of the esophagus, with barium swallow and motility studies, are used to delineate structural and filling defects and detect reduced peristalsis.
- Computed tomography scan may help diagnose and monitor esophageal lesions.
- Magnetic resonance imaging permits evaluation of esophagus and adjacent structures.

Diagnostic procedures
- Esophagoscopy, punch and brush biopsies, and exfoliative cytologic tests confirm esophageal tumors.
- Bronchoscopy (usually performed after an esophagoscopy) may reveal tumor growth in the tracheobronchial tree.
- Endoscopic ultrasonography of the esophagus combines endoscopy and ultrasound technology to measure the depth of penetration of the tumor.

Nursing diagnoses
- Acute pain
- Anxiety
- Fatigue
- Fear
- Deficient fluid volume
- Imbalanced nutrition: less than body requirements
- Impaired swallowing
- Risk for aspiration

Key outcomes
The patient will:
- maintain weight
- keep fluid volume in the normal range
- avoid aspiration
- express feelings of increased comfort and decreased pain.

Interventions

General

○ Surgery and other treatments to relieve disease effects
○ Palliative therapy to keep esophagus open
  – Dilation of the esophagus
  – Laser therapy
  – Radiation therapy
  – Installation of prosthetic tubes (such as Celestin's tube)
○ Liquid to soft diet, as tolerated
○ High-calorie supplements
○ Radical surgery to excise tumor and resect esophagus or stomach and esophagus
○ Gastrostomy or jejunostomy
○ Endoscopic laser treatment and bipolar electrocoagulation

Nursing

○ Provide support and encourage verbalization.
○ Position the patient properly to prevent aspiration.
○ Provide tube feedings, as ordered.
○ Give prescribed drugs.

Drug therapy

○ Chemotherapy and radiation therapy
○ Analgesics

Monitoring

○ Electrolyte levels
○ Hydration and nutritional status
○ Intake and output
○ Pain control
○ Postoperative complications
○ Swallowing ability
○ Vital signs

Patient teaching

Be sure to cover:
○ the disease process, treatment, and postoperative course
○ dietary needs
○ the need to rest between activities.

Discharge planning

○ Arrange for home care follow-up after discharge.
○ Refer the patient to the American Cancer Society.

Fanconi's syndrome

Overview

Description
○ Hereditary renal disorder producing malfunctions of the proximal tubules
○ Leads to electrolyte losses and, eventually, retarded growth and development, rickets, and osteomalacia
○ In children, onset usually during the first 6 months
○ May be secondary to another illness: acquired Fanconi's syndrome
○ Also known as de Toni-Fanconi syndrome

Pathophysiology
○ Characteristic changes occur in the proximal renal tubules, including shortening of the connection to the glomeruli by an abnormally narrow segment called a swan's neck.
○ Changes result from the atrophy of epithelial cells and loss of proximal tubular mass volume.
○ Changes in proximal renal tubules decrease tubular resorption of glucose, phosphate, amino acid, bicarbonate, potassium, and, occasionally, water.

Causes
○ Congenital
○ Idiopathic
Acquired Fanconi's syndrome
○ Certain drugs
○ Cystinosis
○ Dysproteinemias
○ Exposure to a toxic substance (heavy metal poisoning)
○ Galactosemia
○ Kidney transplant
○ Lowe's disease
○ Wilson's disease

 AGE AWARE Cystinosis is the most common cause of Fanconi's syndrome in children.

Prevalence
○ Most prevalent in children
○ Affects both sexes equally

Complications
○ Aminoaciduria
○ Bicarbonate wasting
○ End-stage renal disease
○ Glycosuria
○ Hyperkalemia
○ Hypernatremia
○ Phosphaturia
○ Retarded growth and development
○ Rickets
○ Uricosuria

Assessment

History

AGE AWARE An infant with Fanconi's syndrome appears normal at birth, although birth weight may be low.

Infants (at about age 6 months)
○ Anorexia
○ Constipation
○ Failure to thrive
○ Slow linear growth
○ Vomiting
○ Weakness
Adults
○ Osteomalacia
○ Weakness

Physical assessment
Infants
○ Cystine crystals in corneas and conjunctiva
○ Peripheral retinal pigment degeneration
○ Signs of dehydration
○ Yellow skin
Adults
○ Muscle weakness and paralysis
○ Signs of hypokalemia, hypophosphatemia, and glucosuria
○ Signs of metabolic acidosis

Test results
Laboratory
○ Excessive amounts of glucose, phosphate, amino acids, bicarbonate, and potassium in 24-hour urine specimen
○ Increased serum phosphate and androgen levels
○ Increased alkaline phosphatase level (with rickets)
○ Hyperchloremia
○ Hypokalemia

Nursing diagnoses

○ Activity intolerance
○ Anticipatory grieving
○ Impaired urinary elimination
○ Risk for deficient fluid volume
○ Risk for injury

Key outcomes
The patient will:
○ remain free from injury
○ maintain adequate fluid volume
○ keep electrolyte levels within normal limits
○ use positive coping mechanisms and available support systems
○ maintain or achieve optimal activity level.

Interventions

General

- Dialysis
- Symptomatic treatment to replace the patient's specific deficiencies
- With acquired Fanconi's syndrome, treatment of the underlying cause

Nursing

- Give prescribed electrolytes, mineral replacements, and drugs.
- Provide a nutritious diet.
- Maintain fluid therapy, as ordered.
- Provide adequate rest periods.
- Provide emotional support.

Drug therapy

- Cysteamine (for cystinosis)
- Dietary supplements
- D-penicillamine (for Wilson's disease)
- Electrolyte replacement

Monitoring

- Intake and output
- Laboratory test results
- Renal function
- Vital signs

Patient teaching

Be sure to cover:
- the disorder, diagnosis, and treatment plan
- dietary changes
- need to comply with treatment
- possible need for dialysis.

Discharge planning

- Refer patient and family for appropriate counseling.

Gastric cancer

Overview

Description

- Cancer of the gastrointestinal (GI) tract
- Classified according to gross appearance
  - Diffuse
  - Polypoid
  - Ulcerating
  - Ulcerating and infiltrating
- 5-year survival rate about 15%
- Prognosis based on stage of disease at time of diagnosis

Pathophysiology

- The most commonly affected areas of the stomach are the pylorus and antrum.
- Other affected areas in order of descending frequency are:
  - lesser curvature of the stomach
  - cardia
  - body of the stomach
  - greater curvature of the stomach.
- Cancer metastasizes rapidly to regional lymph nodes, omentum, liver, and lungs.

Risk factors

- Excessive alcohol consumption
- Family history of gastric cancer
- Gastritis with gastric atrophy
- Smoked foods, pickled vegetables, and salted fish and meat in the diet
- Smoking
- Type A blood (10% increased risk)

Causes

- Unknown

Prevalence

- Common worldwide in all races
- More common in men older than age 40
- Mortality high in Japan, Iceland, Chile, and Austria
- Occurrence decreased 50% over the past 25 years
- Death rate one-third the death rate of 30 years ago

Complications

- GI obstruction
- Iron-deficiency anemia
- Malnutrition
- Metastasis

Assessment

History

- Back, epigastric, or retrosternal pain not relieved by over-the-counter analgesics
- Vague feeling of fullness, heaviness, and moderate abdominal distention after meals
- Weight loss, nausea, vomiting
- Weakness and fatigue
- Dysphagia

Physical assessment

- Abdominal distention
- Palpable lymph nodes, especially supraclavicular and axillary nodes
- Palpable mass
- Other assessment findings corresponding to extent of disease and location of metastasis

Test results

Laboratory
- Iron-deficiency anemia
- Possible elevated liver function studies with metastasis to liver
- Possible elevated carcinoembryonic antigen radioimmunoassay

Imaging
- Barium X-rays of the GI tract with fluoroscopy show changes that suggest gastric cancer, including a tumor or filling defect in the outline of the stomach, loss of flexibility and distensibility, and abnormal gastric mucosa with or without ulceration.

Diagnostic procedures
- Gastroscopy with fiber-optic endoscopy helps rule out other diffuse gastric mucosal abnormalities by allowing direct visualization.
- Gastroscopic biopsy permits evaluation of gastric mucosal lesions.
- Gastric acid stimulation test discloses whether the stomach secretes acid properly.

Nursing diagnoses

- Acute pain
- Anxiety
- Fatigue
- Fear
- Imbalanced nutrition: less than body requirements
- Impaired oral mucous membrane
- Impaired swallowing
- Risk for deficient fluid volume
- Risk for infection

Key outcomes

The patient will:
- lose no more weight
- express feelings of increased energy
- report feeling less tension and pain
- avoid aspiration
- maintain fluid balance.

Interventions

General

○ Excision of lesion with appropriate margins (in more than one-third of patients)
○ Gastroduodenostomy
○ Gastrojejunostomy
○ Partial gastric resection
○ Total gastrectomy (including omentum and spleen if metastasis has occurred)
○ Radiation therapy with chemotherapy (not before surgery because it may damage viscera and impede healing)
○ Diet based on the patient's condition
○ Parenteral feeding if patient can't consume adequate calories

Nursing

○ Provide a high-protein, high-calorie diet with dietary supplements.
○ Give prescribed drugs.
○ Provide parenteral nutrition as appropriate.
○ After surgery, provide supportive care.

Drug therapy

○ Antiemetics
○ Chemotherapy
○ Opioid analgesics
○ Sedatives and tranquilizers

Monitoring

○ Effects of prescribed drugs
○ Hydration and nutritional status
○ Nasogastric tube function and drainage
○ Pain control
○ Postoperative complications
○ Vital signs
○ Wound site

Patient teaching

Be sure to cover (with the patient or his family):
○ the disorder, diagnosis, and treatment
○ prescribed drugs, dosages, and possible adverse effects
○ the diet plan
○ effective pulmonary toilet
○ the need to avoid crowds and people with infections
○ relaxation techniques.

Discharge planning

○ Direct the patient and his family to support services.
○ Refer the patient for home services if needed.
○ Refer the patient for physical or occupational therapy if needed.

Gastritis

Overview

Description
○ Inflammation of the gastric mucosa
○ May be acute or chronic
○ Most common stomach disorder (acute form)

Pathophysiology
Acute gastritis
○ The protective mucosal layer is altered.
○ Acid secretion produces mucosal reddening, edema, and superficial surface erosion.
Chronic gastritis
○ The gastric mucosa undergoes progressive thinning and degeneration.

Risk factors
○ Age older than 60 years
○ Exposure to toxic substances
○ Hemodynamic disorder

Causes
Acute gastritis
○ Complication of acute illness
○ Drugs
  – Antimetabolites
  – Aspirin and other nonsteroidal anti-inflammatory agents (in large doses)
  – Caffeine
  – Corticosteroids
  – Cytotoxic drugs
  – Indomethacin
  – Phenylbutazone
○ Endotoxins released from infecting bacteria, such as staphylococci, *Escherichia coli,* and salmonella
○ Ingested poisons
  – Ammonia
  – Carbon tetrachloride
  – Corrosive substances
  – Dichloro-diphenyl-trichloroethane (commonly known as DDT)
  – Mercury
○ Long-term ingestion of irritating foods and alcohol
Chronic gastritis
○ Diabetes mellitus
○ *Helicobacter pylori* infection (common cause of nonerosive gastritis)
○ Pernicious anemia
○ Recurring exposure to irritating substances, such as drugs, alcohol, cigarette smoke, and environmental agents
○ Renal disease

Prevalence
○ Occurs equally in men and women
○ May occur at any age
○ Increased presence of *H. pylori* in people older than age 60
○ 8 of 1,000 people affected by acute gastritis
○ 2 of 10,000 people affected by chronic gastritis

Complications
○ Gastric cancer
○ Hemorrhage
○ Obstruction
○ Perforation
○ Peritonitis

Assessment

History
○ Anorexia
○ Coffee-ground emesis or melena with GI bleeding
○ Cramping
○ Epigastric discomfort
○ Indigestion
○ Nausea, hematemesis, and vomiting
○ Presence of one or more causative factors
○ Rapid onset of symptoms (acute gastritis)

Physical assessment
○ Abdominal distention, tenderness, and guarding
○ Grimacing
○ Hypotension
○ Normoactive to hyperactive bowel sounds
○ Pallor
○ Possible normal appearance
○ Restlessness
○ Tachycardia

Test results
Laboratory
○ Occult blood in vomitus, stool, or both if the patient has gastric bleeding
○ Decreased hemoglobin level and hematocrit
Diagnostic procedures
○ Urea breath test shows the presence of *H. pylori.*
○ Upper-GI endoscopy reveals gastritis when performed within 24 hours of bleeding.
○ Biopsy reveals inflammatory process.

Nursing diagnoses

○ Acute pain
○ Deficient knowledge (gastritis)
○ Imbalanced nutrition: less than body requirements
○ Ineffective coping
○ Risk for deficient fluid volume

Key outcomes
The patient will:
○ express feelings of increased comfort
○ maintain weight
○ express concerns about current condition

○ maintain adequate fluid balance
○ verbalize understanding of the disorder and treatment regimen.

Interventions

General

○ Elimination of cause
○ For massive bleeding, blood transfusion, iced saline lavage, angiography with vasopressin
○ Nothing by mouth if bleeding occurs
○ Elimination of irritating foods
○ Activity, as tolerated (encourage mobilization)
○ If conservative treatment fails, vagotomy, pyloroplasty, or partial or total gastrectomy (rarely)

Nursing

○ Provide physical and emotional support.
○ Give prescribed drugs and I.V. fluids.
○ Assist the patient with diet modification.
○ If surgery is needed, prepare the patient beforehand and provide appropriate postoperative care.
○ Consult a dietitian as needed.

Drug therapy

○ Antacids
○ Histamine (H_2) blockers
○ Proton pump inhibitors
○ Prostaglandins
○ Vitamin B_{12}
○ Triple therapy—two antibiotics and bismuth subsalicylate
○ Dual therapy—antibiotic and proton pump inhibitor

Monitoring

○ Electrolyte and hemoglobin levels
○ Fluid intake and output
○ Pain control
○ Response to drug therapy
○ Returning symptoms as food is reintroduced
○ Vital signs

Patient teaching

Be sure to cover:
○ the disorder, diagnosis, and treatment
○ lifestyle and diet modifications
○ preoperative teaching if surgery is needed
○ stress-reduction techniques
○ drugs, dosages, and possible adverse effects.

Discharge planning

○ Refer the patient to a smoking-cessation program if indicated.

Gastroenteritis

Overview

Description

- Self-limiting inflammation of the stomach and small intestine
- Also known as intestinal flu, traveler's diarrhea, viral enteritis, and food poisoning (See *Preventing traveler's diarrhea.*)

Pathophysiology

- The bowel reacts to the various causes of gastroenteritis with increased luminal fluid that can't be absorbed.
- This results in severe diarrhea with abdominal pain, vomiting, and depletion of intracellular fluid.
- Dehydration and electrolyte loss develop.

Causes

- Amoebae, especially *Entamoeba histolytica*
- Bacteria, such as *Staphylococcus aureus, Salmonella, Shigella, Clostridium botulinum, Clostridium perfringens,* and *Escherichia coli*
- Drug reactions from antibiotics
- Enzyme deficiencies
- Food allergens
- Ingestion of toxins, such as poisonous plants and toadstools
- Parasites, such as *Ascaris, Enterobius,* and *Trichinella spiralis*
- Viruses, such as adenoviruses, echoviruses, and coxsackieviruses

Prevalence

- Occurs at any age
- Major cause of illness and death in developing nations
- Ranks second to common cold as cause of lost work time in the United States
- Fifth most common cause of death among young children
- May be life-threatening in elderly and debilitated patients

Complications

- Electrolyte imbalance
- Severe dehydration

Assessment

History

- Abdominal pain and discomfort
- Acute onset of diarrhea
- Exposure to contaminated food
- Malaise and fatigue
- Nausea, vomiting
- Recent travel

Physical assessment

- Decreased blood pressure
- Hyperactive bowel sounds
- Poor skin turgor (with dehydration)
- Slight abdominal distention

Test results

Laboratory
- Causative bacteria revealed by Gram's stain, stool culture (by direct rectal swab), or blood culture

Nursing diagnoses

- Acute pain
- Diarrhea
- Imbalanced nutrition: less than body requirements
- Risk for deficient fluid volume

Key outcomes

The patient will:
- maintain weight without further loss
- express feelings of increased comfort
- maintain adequate fluid volume
- maintain normal vital signs.

Preventing traveler's diarrhea

If your patient travels, especially to developing nations, discuss precautions he can take to reduce his risk of traveler's diarrhea. Explain that this condition is caused by ingestion of bacteria-contaminated food or water in areas of inadequate sanitation. Organisms attach to the lining of the small intestine, where they release a toxin that causes cramps and diarrhea. To minimize this risk, advise taking the following steps.

- Drink water only if it's chlorinated or bottled. Chlorination protects water from bacterial contaminants such as *Escherichia coli.* Brush your teeth with chlorinated water as well.
- Don't drink out of glasses that may have been washed in contaminated water.
- Don't use ice cubes that may have been made from contaminated water.
- Drink only beverages made with boiled water, such as coffee and tea, or those in bottles or cans.
- Sanitize impure water by adding 2% tincture of iodine (5 drops/L of clear water; 10 drops/L of cloudy water) or by adding liquid laundry bleach (about 2 drops/L of clear water; 4 drops/L of cloudy water)
- Don't eat uncooked vegetables, unpeeled fresh fruits, salads, unpasteurized milk, and other dairy products.
- Don't eat foods offered by street vendors.
- If traveler's diarrhea occurs despite precautions, try relieving the symptoms by taking loperamide (Imodium), bismuth subsalicylate (Pepto Bismol), or diphenoxylate with atropine (Lomotil).

Interventions

General

○ Activity, as tolerated (encourage mobilization)
○ Avoidance of milk products
○ Electrolyte solutions
○ Initially, clear liquids as tolerated
○ Rehydration
○ Supportive treatment for nausea, vomiting, and diarrhea

Nursing

○ Allow uninterrupted rest periods.
○ Replace lost fluids and electrolytes through diet or I.V. fluids.
○ Give prescribed drugs.

Drug therapy

○ Antidiarrheal therapy
○ Antiemetics
○ Antibiotics
○ I.V. fluids

Monitoring

○ Electrolytes
○ Intake and output
○ Signs of dehydration
○ Vital signs

Patient teaching

Be sure to cover:
○ the disorder, diagnosis, and treatment
○ diet modifications
○ prescribed drugs, dosages, and possible adverse effects
○ preventive measures
○ how to perform warm sitz baths three times daily to relieve anal irritation.

Discharge planning

○ Refer the patient for dietary follow-up as needed.

Goodpasture's syndrome

Overview

Description
○ Pulmonary-renal syndrome characterized by hemoptysis and rapidly progressive glomerulonephritis

Pathophysiology
○ Abnormal production and deposition of antibodies against glomerular basement membrane (GBM) and alveolar basement membrane activate the complement and inflammatory responses.
○ Glomerular and alveolar tissue damage result.

Causes
○ Unknown
○ May be related to exposure to hydrocarbons or type II hypersensitivity reaction
○ Possible genetic predisposition

Prevalence
○ Occurs at any age
○ Most common in men between ages 20 and 30

Complications
○ Pulmonary edema and hemorrhage
○ Renal failure

Assessment

History
○ Possible complaint of malaise, fatigue, and pallor
○ Possible pulmonary bleeding for months or years before developing overt hemorrhage and signs of renal disease

Physical assessment
○ Decreased urine output
○ Dyspnea, tachypnea, orthopnea
○ Hematuria
○ Hemoptysis, ranging from a cough with blood-tinged sputum to frank pulmonary hemorrhage
○ Pulmonary crackles and rhonchi
○ Restlessness

Test results
Laboratory
○ Circulating serum anti-GBM antibodies, which distinguish Goodpasture's syndrome from other pulmonary-renal syndromes, such as Wegener's granulomatosis, polyarteritis, and systemic lupus erythematosus
○ Increased serum creatinine and blood urea nitrogen (BUN) levels (typically two to three times normal)
○ Possible red blood cells and cellular casts in urine, which typify glomerular inflammation
○ Possible proteinuria and granular casts in urine
Imaging
○ Chest X-rays reveal pulmonary infiltrates in a diffuse, nodular pattern.
Diagnostic procedures
○ Immunofluorescence of the alveolar basement membrane shows linear deposition of immunoglobulins as well as C3 and fibrinogen.
○ Immunofluorescence of the GBM shows linear deposition of immunoglobulins.
○ Lung biopsy shows interstitial and intra-alveolar hemorrhage with hemosiderin-laden macrophages.
○ Renal biopsy usually shows focal necrotic lesions and cellular crescents.

Nursing diagnoses

○ Activity intolerance
○ Anxiety
○ Excess fluid volume
○ Fatigue
○ Impaired gas exchange
○ Impaired oral mucous membrane
○ Impaired urinary elimination
○ Ineffective airway clearance
○ Ineffective breathing pattern
○ Risk for injury

Key outcomes
The patient will:
○ maintain a patent airway and adequate ventilation
○ maintain adequate fluid balance
○ express feelings of increased energy
○ maintain intact mucous membranes
○ avoid complications
○ use available support systems.

Interventions

General
○ Activity, as tolerated
○ Dialysis
○ Low-protein, low-sodium diet
○ Kidney transplantation
○ Plasmapheresis

Nursing
○ Elevate the head of the bed, and give humidified oxygen, as ordered.
○ Encourage the patient to conserve energy.
○ Assist with range-of-motion exercises.
○ Assist with activities of daily living, and provide frequent rest periods.
○ Transfuse blood and give corticosteroids, as ordered. Watch closely for adverse reactions.

Drug therapy
○ High-dose I.V. corticosteroids

Monitoring
○ Arterial blood gas levels
○ Creatinine clearance, BUN, and serum creatinine
  levels
○ Daily weight
○ Hematocrit and coagulation studies
○ Intake and output
○ Respiratory status
○ Vital signs

Patient teaching

Be sure to cover:
○ the disorder, diagnosis, and treatment
○ the importance of conserving energy
○ the possible need for fluid restriction
○ prescribed drugs, dosages, and possible adverse effects
○ how to deep-breathe and cough
○ how to recognize respiratory and genitourinary
  bleeding and the need to report them to the doctor
  at once.

Discharge planning

○ If the patient needs dialysis or kidney transplantation, refer him to a renal support group.
○ Encourage regular follow-up care.

Gout

Overview

Description

○ Inflammatory arthritis caused by uric acid and crystal deposits
○ Red, swollen, acutely painful joints
○ Mostly affects feet, great toe, ankle, and midfoot

Primary gout
○ Patient symptom-free for years between attacks
○ Sudden first acute attack that peaks quickly
○ Delayed attacks with olecranon bursitis

Chronic polyarticular gout
○ Final, unremitting stage of the disease marked by persistent painful polyarthritis

Pathophysiology

○ Uric acid crystallizes in blood or body fluids, and the precipitate accumulates in connective tissue, creating tophi.
○ Crystals trigger an immune response.
○ Neutrophils secrete lysosomes for phagocytosis.
○ Lysosomes damage tissue and worsen the immune response.

Causes

○ Decreased renal excretion of uric acid
○ Exact cause unknown
○ Genetic defect in purine metabolism (hyperuricemia)

Recognizing gouty tophi

In advanced gout, urate crystal deposits develop into hard, irregular, yellow-white nodules called tophi. These bumps commonly protrude from the great toe and ear.

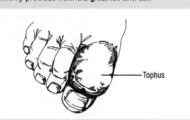

Tophus

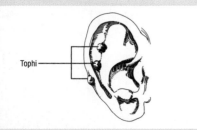

Tophi

○ Secondary gout that develops with other diseases
  – Diabetes mellitus
  – Hypertension
  – Leukemia
  – Myeloma
  – Obesity
  – Polycythemia
  – Renal disease
  – Sickle cell anemia
○ Secondary gout that follows treatment with drugs
  – Hydrochlorothiazide
  – Pyrazinamide

Prevalence

○ Primary gout typically in men older than age 30 and postmenopausal women who take diuretics

Complications

○ Atherosclerotic disease
○ Cardiovascular lesions
○ Cerebrovascular accident
○ Coronary thrombosis
○ Hypertension
○ Infection when tophi rupture
○ Renal calculi

Assessment

History

○ Sedentary lifestyle
○ Hypertension
○ Renal calculi
○ Waking during the night with pain in great toe
○ Initial moderate pain that grows intense
○ Chills, mild fever

Physical assessment

○ Swollen, dusky red or purple joint
○ Limited movement of joint
○ Tophi, especially in the outer ears, hands, and feet (See *Recognizing gouty tophi.*)
○ Skin over tophi that may ulcerate and release chalky white exudate or pus
○ Secondary joint degeneration
○ Erosions, deformity, and disability
○ Warmth over joint
○ Extreme tenderness
○ Fever
○ Hypertension

Test results

Laboratory
○ Increased serum uric acid levels during an attack
○ Increased white blood cell count during acute attack
○ Increased urine uric acid level in 20% of patients

Imaging
○ X-ray of articular cartilage and subchondral bone shows evidence of chronic gout.

Diagnostic procedures
○ Needle aspiration of synovial fluid shows needlelike intracellular crystals.

Nursing diagnoses

○ Acute pain
○ Anxiety
○ Deficient knowledge: gout
○ Impaired physical mobility
○ Risk for imbalanced fluid volume
○ Risk for injury

Key outcomes
The patient will:
○ express feelings of increased comfort and decreased pain
○ maintain joint mobility and range of motion
○ perform activities of daily living within the confines of the disease
○ express knowledge of the condition and treatment
○ maintain adequate fluid volume.

Interventions

General
Initial interventions
○ Termination of acute attack
○ Bed rest in acute attack
○ Immobilization of joint
○ Local application of cold
○ Protection of inflamed, painful joints
Ongoing interventions
○ Avoidance of alcohol
○ Prevention of recurrent gout
○ Prevention of renal calculi
○ Sparing consumption of purine-rich foods (such as anchovies, liver, and sardines)
○ Treatment for hyperuricemia
○ Weight loss program, if indicated

Nursing
○ Institute bed rest.
○ Use a bed cradle, if appropriate.
○ Apply cold packs to affected areas.
○ Give analgesics as needed.
○ Give anti-inflammatories and other drugs as prescribed.
○ Identify techniques and activities that promote rest and relaxation.
○ Allow adequate time for self-care.
○ Provide a purine-poor diet.

Drug therapy
○ Allopurinol
○ Analgesics
○ Colchicine
○ Nonsteroidal anti-inflammatory drugs
○ Probenecid or sulfinpyrazone

Monitoring
○ For 24 to 96 hours after surgery, development of acute gout attacks
○ Intake and output
○ Serum uric acid levels

Patient teaching

Be sure to cover:
○ the disorder, diagnosis, and treatment
○ the need to drink plenty of fluids (up to 2 L daily)
○ relaxation techniques
○ prescribed drugs, dosages, and possible adverse effects
○ compliance with prescribed drug regimen
○ dietary adjustments
○ the need to control hypertension.

Discharge planning

○ Refer the patient to a weight-reduction program if appropriate.

Graft rejection syndrome

Overview

Description
○ Rejection of a donated organ when the host's immune responses are directed against the graft
○ Three subtypes based on time of onset and mechanisms involved:
  – Hyperacute rejection
  – Acute rejection
  – Chronic rejection

Pathophysiology
○ Hyperacute rejection occurs minutes to hours after graft transplantation.
○ Circulating host antibodies recognize and bind to graft antigens.
○ Binding of these antibodies starts the complement cascade, recruitment of neutrophils, platelet activation, damage to graft endothelial cells, and stimulation of coagulation reactions.
○ Acute rejection may occur hours, days, or even weeks after transplantation.
○ Alloantigen-reactive T cells from the host infiltrate the graft and are activated by contact with foreign, graft-related proteins on antigen-presenting cells.
○ These T cells may damage graft tissue.
○ In chronic rejection, blood vessel lumens become occluded through progressive thickening of the intimal layers of medium and large arterial walls.
○ Large amounts of intimal matrix are produced, leading to increasingly occlusive vessel wall thickening.
○ A slowly progressing reduction in blood flow results in regional tissue ischemia, cell death, and tissue fibrosis.

Causes
○ Immune system response to a graft

Prevalence
○ *Hyperacute rejection:* rare; affects less than 1% of transplant recipients
○ *Acute rejection:* occurs in 50% of transplant patients; loss of graft in 10%
○ *Chronic rejection:* occurs in 50% of transplant patients within 10 years after transplantation

Complications
○ Rapid thrombosis
○ Loss of graft function

Assessment

History
○ Signs and symptoms that vary markedly with type of rejection, underlying illnesses, and type of organ transplanted

Physical assessment
○ *Kidney transplant:* oliguria and increasing serum creatinine and blood urea nitrogen levels
○ *Liver transplant:* increased transaminase levels, decreased albumin levels, and hypocoagulability
○ *Heart transplant:* hypotension, heart failure, and edema

Test results
Laboratory
○ *Hyperacute rejection:* large numbers of polymorphonuclear leukocytes in the graft blood vessels, widespread microthrombi, platelet accumulation, and interstitial hemorrhage, with little or no interstitial inflammation
Diagnostic procedures
○ Biopsy of the transplanted tissue confirms rejection.

Nursing diagnoses

○ Activity intolerance
○ Disturbed body image
○ Fatigue
○ Imbalanced nutrition: less than body requirements
○ Impaired urinary elimination
○ Ineffective coping
○ Interrupted family processes
○ Risk for deficient fluid volume
○ Risk for infection

Key outcomes
The patient will:
○ experience no fever, chills, or other evidence of illness
○ use support systems to assist with coping
○ express his feelings about the condition
○ comply with the treatment regimen
○ maintain fluid volume balance.

Interventions

General
○ Activity, as tolerated
○ Close monitoring of function of grafted organ
○ Diet restrictions based on organ system affected
○ Surveillance, with preventive measures against opportunistic infections

Nursing

○ Give prescribed antibiotics for infection.
○ Give prescribed antirejection therapies.
○ Give prescribed immunosuppressants.

Drug therapy

○ Antibiotics
○ Antirejection therapies
○ Immunosuppressants

Monitoring

○ Function of the transplanted organ
○ Signs and symptoms of infection
○ Signs and symptoms of rejection
○ Vital signs

Patient teaching

Be sure to cover:
○ the disorder, diagnosis, and treatment
○ prescribed drugs, dosages, and possible adverse effects
○ how to recognize organ dysfunction
○ the need to immediately report fever, chills, and other symptoms of infection
○ the need for lifelong compliance with the drug regimen.

Discharge planning

○ Refer the patient and his family to social support, including psychological support services, as indicated.

Guillain-Barré syndrome

Overview

Description
- A form of polyneuritis
- Acute, rapidly progressive, and potentially fatal
- Three phases
  - *Acute:* beginning from first symptom, ending in 1 to 3 weeks
  - *Plateau:* lasting several days to 2 weeks
  - *Recovery:* coincides with remyelination and axonal process regrowth and typically lasts 4 months to 3 years, although recovery may never be complete

Pathophysiology
- Peripheral nerves undergo segmented demyelination, preventing normal transmission of electrical impulses.
- Sensorimotor nerve roots are affected; autonomic nerve transmission also may be affected. (See *Understanding sensorimotor nerve degeneration.*)

Risk factors
- Hodgkin's or some other malignant disease
- Lupus erythematosus
- Rabies or swine influenza vaccination
- Surgery
- Viral illness

Causes
- Unknown

Understanding sensorimotor nerve degeneration

Guillain-Barré syndrome attacks the peripheral nerves, disrupting the transmission of messages to the brain. Here's what goes wrong:
- The myelin sheath degenerates for unknown reasons. This sheath covers the nerve axons and conducts electrical impulses along the nerve pathways.
- With degeneration come inflammation, swelling, and patchy demyelination.
- As this disorder destroys myelin, the nodes of Ranvier (at the junctures of the myelin sheaths) widen. This delays and impairs impulse transmission along the dorsal and ventral nerve roots.
- The dorsal nerve roots are responsible for sensory function, so the patient may experience tingling, numbness, or other sensations when the nerve root is impaired.
- The ventral nerve roots are responsible for motor function, so the patient may experience varying amounts of weakness, immobility, and paralysis when the nerve root is impaired.

Prevalence
- Occurs equally in both sexes
- Occurs between ages 30 and 50

Complications
- Aspiration
- Contractures
- Life-threatening respiratory and cardiac compromise
- Muscle wasting
- Pressure ulcers
- Respiratory tract infections
- Thrombophlebitis

Assessment

History
- Minor febrile illness 1 to 4 weeks before current symptoms
- Paresthesia in the legs
- Progression of symptoms to arms, trunk and, finally, face
- Stiffness and pain in the calves

Physical assessment
- Difficulty talking, chewing, and swallowing
- Diminished or absent deep tendon reflexes
- Loss of position sense
- Muscle weakness (the major neurologic sign)
- Paralysis of ocular, facial, and oropharyngeal muscles
- Sensory loss, usually in the legs (spreads to arms)

Test results
Laboratory
- Normal white blood cell count and increased protein level in cerebrospinal fluid
- Increased cerebrospinal fluid pressure in severe disease

Diagnostic procedures
- Electromyography may show repeated firing of the same motor unit instead of widespread sectional stimulation.
- Nerve conduction studies show marked slowing of nerve conduction velocities.

Nursing diagnoses

- Anxiety
- Fear
- Imbalanced nutrition: less than body requirements
- Impaired gas exchange
- Impaired physical mobility
- Impaired urinary elimination
- Impaired verbal communication
- Ineffective breathing pattern
- Ineffective coping
- Risk for imbalanced fluid volume

Key outcomes

The patient will:
○ maintain a patent airway and adequate ventilation
○ develop alternate means of communication
○ maintain required caloric intake daily
○ maintain joint mobility and range of motion
○ develop and use effective coping mechanisms
○ use available support systems
○ maintain adequate fluid volume.

Interventions

General

○ Adequate caloric intake
○ Emotional support
○ Exercise program to prevent contractures
○ Fluid volume replacement
○ Maintenance of skin integrity
○ Plasmapheresis
○ Possible endotracheal intubation or tracheotomy
○ Possible gastrostomy or jejunotomy feeding tube insertion
○ Possible tracheostomy
○ Possible tube feedings with endotracheal intubation
○ Supportive measures

Nursing

○ Establish a means of communication before the patient needs intubation, if possible.
○ Turn and reposition the patient.
○ Encourage coughing and deep breathing.
○ Provide meticulous skin care.
○ Perform passive range-of-motion exercises.
○ In case of facial paralysis, provide eye and mouth care.
○ Provide emotional support.
○ Give prescribed drugs.

Drug therapy

○ I.V. beta blockers
○ I.V. immune globulin
○ Parasympatholytics

Monitoring

○ Arterial blood gas measurements
○ Level of consciousness
○ Pulse oximetry
○ Respiratory status
○ Response to drug therapy
○ Signs of thrombophlebitis
○ Signs of urine retention
○ Skin integrity
○ Vital signs

Patient teaching

Be sure to cover:
○ the disorder, diagnosis, and treatment

○ effective means of communication
○ the appropriate home care plan
○ prescribed drugs, dosages, and possible adverse effects.

Discharge planning

○ Refer the patient to physical rehabilitation as needed.
○ Refer the patient to occupational and speech rehabilitation resources as indicated.
○ Refer the patient to the Guillain-Barré Syndrome Foundation.

Heart failure

Overview

Description
- Fluid buildup in the heart because the myocardium can't provide sufficient cardiac output
- Usually occurs in a damaged left ventricle
- May occur mainly in right ventricle
- May be secondary to left-sided heart failure

Pathophysiology
Left-sided heart failure
- The pumping ability of the left ventricle fails and cardiac output falls.
- Blood backs up into the left atrium and lungs, causing pulmonary congestion.

Right-sided heart failure
- Ineffective contraction of the right ventricle leads to blood backing up into the right atrium and peripheral circulation.
- Peripheral edema results, along with engorgement of the kidneys and other organs.

Causes
- Anemia
- Arrhythmias
- Atherosclerosis with myocardial infarction
- Constrictive pericarditis
- Emotional stress
- Hypertension
- Increased salt or water intake
- Infection
- Mitral or aortic insufficiency
- Mitral stenosis secondary to rheumatic heart disease, constrictive pericarditis, or atrial fibrillation
- Myocarditis
- Pregnancy
- Pulmonary embolism
- Thyrotoxicosis
- Ventricular and atrial septal defects

Prevalence
- Affects 1% of people older than age 50
- Affects 10% of people older than age 80

Complications
- Myocardial infarction
- Pulmonary edema
- Organ failure, especially the brain and kidneys

Assessment

History
- A disorder or condition that can cause heart failure
- Anorexia
- Dyspnea or paroxysmal nocturnal dyspnea
- Fatigue
- Insomnia
- Nausea
- Peripheral edema
- Sense of abdominal fullness (particularly in right-sided heart failure)
- Substance abuse (alcohol, drugs, tobacco)
- Weakness

Physical assessment
- Ascites
- Cool, clammy, pale skin
- Cough that produces pink, frothy sputum
- Cyanosis of the lips and nail beds
- Decreased pulse oximetry
- Decreased pulse pressure
- Decreased urinary output
- Diaphoresis
- Hepatomegaly and, possibly, splenomegaly
- Jugular vein distention
- Moist, bibasilar crackles, rhonchi, and expiratory wheezing
- Peripheral edema
- Pulsus alternans
- S_3 and S_4 heart sounds
- Tachycardia

Test results
Laboratory
- Elevated B-type natriuretic peptide immunoassay

Imaging
- Chest X-rays show increased pulmonary vascular markings, interstitial edema, or pleural effusion and cardiomegaly.

Diagnostic procedures
- Electrocardiography reflects heart strain, enlargement or ischemia. It also may reveal atrial enlargement, tachycardia, extrasystole, or atrial fibrillation.
- Pulmonary artery pressure monitoring typically shows elevated pulmonary artery and pulmonary artery wedge pressures, left ventricular end-diastolic pressure in left-sided heart failure, and elevated right atrial or central venous pressure in right-sided heart failure.

Nursing diagnoses
- Activity intolerance
- Decreased cardiac output
- Excess fluid volume
- Fatigue
- Imbalanced nutrition: less than body requirements
- Ineffective gas exchange
- Ineffective tissue perfusion: cardiopulmonary

Key outcomes
The patient will:
- maintain hemodynamic stability
- maintain adequate cardiac output

- carry out activities of daily living without excess fatigue or decreased energy
- maintain adequate ventilation
- maintain adequate fluid balance.

Interventions

General

- Activity, as tolerated
- Antiembolism stockings
- Calorie restriction, if indicated
- Elevation of legs
- Fluid restriction
- Heart transplantation
- Low-fat diet, if indicated
- Sodium-restricted diet
- Stent placement
- Surgical replacement (valvular dysfunction with recurrent acute heart failure)
- Ventricular assist device
- Walking program

Nursing

- Place the patient in Fowler's position, and give supplemental oxygen.
- Provide continuous cardiac monitoring during acute and advanced stages.
- Assist the patient with range-of-motion exercises.
- Apply antiembolism stockings. Check for calf pain and tenderness.

Drug therapy

- Anticoagulants
- Angiotensin-converting enzyme inhibitors
- Angiotensin receptor blockers
- Beta blockers
- Cardiac glycosides
- Diuretics
- Inotropic drugs
- Oxygen
- Potassium supplements
- Vasodilators

Monitoring

- Blood urea nitrogen and serum creatinine, potassium, sodium, chloride, and magnesium levels
- Cardiac rhythm
- Daily weight for peripheral edema and other signs and symptoms of fluid overload
- Intake and output
- Mental status
- Peripheral edema
- Response to treatment
- Vital signs

 ALERT Auscultate for abnormal heart and breath sounds, and report changes immediately.

Patient teaching

Be sure to cover:
- the disorder, diagnosis, and treatment
- signs and symptoms of worsening heart failure
- when to contact a doctor
- prescribed drugs, dosages, potential adverse effects, and monitoring needs
- the need to avoid high-sodium foods
- the need to avoid fatigue
- instructions about fluid restrictions
- the need to weigh himself every morning, at the same time, before eating, and after urinating; keeping a record of his weight, and reporting a weight gain of 3 to 5 lb (1.5 to 2.5 kg) in 1 week
- the importance of smoking cessation, if appropriate
- weight reduction, as needed
- the importance of follow-up care.

Discharge planning

- Encourage follow-up care.
- Refer the patient to a smoking-cessation program, if appropriate.

Heat syndrome

Overview

Description
○ Heat exhaustion—acute heat injury with hyperthermia caused by dehydration
○ Heatstroke—extreme hyperthermia with thermoregulatory failure

Pathophysiology
○ Normally, temperature is regulated by evaporation (30% of body's heat loss) or vasodilation.
○ When heat is generated or gained by the body faster than it can dissipate, the thermoregulatory mechanism is stressed and eventually fails.
○ Hyperthermia accelerates.
○ Cerebral edema and cerebrovascular congestion occurs.
○ Cerebral perfusion pressure increases and cerebral perfusion decreases.
○ Tissue damage occurs when temperature exceeds 107.6° F (42° C), resulting in tissue necrosis, organ dysfunction, and failure.

Risk factors
○ Age
○ Alcohol use
○ Obesity
○ Poor physical condition
○ Salt and water depletion
○ Socioeconomic status

Causes
○ Behavior
○ Dehydration
○ Drugs, such as phenothiazines, anticholinergics, and amphetamines
○ Endocrine disorders
○ Excessive clothing
○ Excessive physical activity
○ Heart disease
○ Hot environment without ventilation
○ Illness
○ Inadequate fluid intake
○ Infection (fever)
○ Lack of acclimatization
○ Neurologic disorder
○ Sudden discontinuation of Parkinson's disease medications

Prevalence
○ Affects men and women equally
○ More common among elderly patients and neonates during excessively hot summer days

Complications
○ Cardiac arrhythmias
○ Cardiogenic shock
○ Disseminated intravascular coagulation
○ Hepatic failure
○ Hypovolemic shock
○ Renal failure

Assessment

History
Heat exhaustion
○ Fatigue
○ Headache
○ Muscle cramps
○ Nausea and vomiting
○ Prolonged activity in a very warm or hot environment
○ Thirst
○ Weakness

Heatstroke
○ Same signs as heat exhaustion
○ Blurred vision
○ Confusion
○ Decreased muscle coordination
○ Exposure to high temperatures and humidity without air circulation
○ Hallucinations
○ Syncope

Physical assessment
Heat exhaustion
○ Cool, moist skin
○ Decreased blood pressure
○ Hyperventilation
○ Impaired judgment
○ Irritability
○ Pale skin
○ Rectal temperature over 100° F (37.8° C)
○ Syncope
○ Thready, rapid pulse

Heatstroke
○ Altered mental status
○ Anhydrosis (late sign)
○ Cheyne-Stokes respirations
○ Decreased blood pressure in later stages
○ Gray, dry, hot skin in later stages
○ Hyperpnea
○ Rectal temperature of at least 104° F (40° C)
○ Red, diaphoretic, hot skin in early stages
○ Signs of central nervous system dysfunction
○ Slightly elevated blood pressure in early stages
○ Tachycardia

Test results
Laboratory
○ Elevated serum electrolyte levels
○ Possible hyponatremia and hypokalemia
○ Possible respiratory alkalosis on arterial blood gas measurements
○ Leukocytosis

- Thrombocytopenia
- Increased bleeding and clotting times
- Possible concentrated urine
- Possible proteinuria with tubular casts and myoglobinuria
- Possible increased blood urea nitrogen level
- Possible decreased serum calcium level
- Possible decreased serum phosphorus level

Nursing diagnoses

- Decreased cardiac output
- Deficient fluid volume
- Deficient knowledge (heat syndrome)
- Hyperthermia
- Impaired gas exchange

Key outcomes
The patient will:
- maintain adequate ventilation
- maintain a normal body temperature
- prevent recurrent episodes of hyperthermia
- express understanding of the need to maintain adequate fluid intake.

Interventions

General
Heat exhaustion
- Cool environment
- Oral or I.V. fluid administration

Heatstroke
- Avoidance of caffeine and alcohol
- Evaporation, hypothermia blankets, and ice packs to the groin, axillae, and neck
- Increased hydration; cool liquids only
- Lowering body temperature as rapidly as possible
- Rest periods, as needed
- Supportive respiratory and cardiovascular measures

Nursing
- Perform rapid cooling procedures.
- Provide supportive measures.
- Provide adequate fluid intake.
- Give prescribed drugs.

Monitoring
- Cardiac rhythm
- Complications
- Intake and output
- Level of consciousness
- Myoglobin test results
- Pulse oximetry readings
- Vital signs

Patient teaching

Be sure to cover:
- the disorder, diagnosis, and treatment
- how to avoid reexposure to high temperatures
- the need to maintain adequate fluid intake
- the need to wear loose clothing
- limiting activity in hot weather.

Discharge planning

- Refer the patient to social services, if appropriate.

Hemolytic uremic syndrome

Overview

Description

○ Syndrome characterized by acute renal failure, hemolytic anemia, fever and thrombocytopenia
○ Usually affects children

Pathophysiology

○ A toxin produced by *Escherichia coli, Shigella dysenteriae,* or a virus (such as varicella) causes endothelial damage.
○ Microvascular lesions develop with microthrombi.
○ Arterioles and capillaries in the renal microvasculature become occluded.
○ Thrombocytopenia and microangiopathic hemolytic anemia develop.

Risk factors

○ Eating rare hamburger
○ Visiting a petting zoo
○ Visiting someone with diarrhea

Causes

○ Prodromal infectious disease
○ Upper respiratory infection

Prevalence

 AGE AWARE Hemolytic uremic syndrome usually affects children 6 months to 4 years of age.

○ In adults, usually women who take oral contraceptives, recently gave birth, or have obstetric complications
○ More common among patients who have received chemotherapy with 5-fluorouracil

Complications

○ Acute renal failure
○ Cerebrovascular accident
○ Disseminated intravascular coagulation
○ Chronic renal failure
○ Hypertension
○ Neurologic deficits

Assessment

History

○ Acute diarrhea a few weeks before the onset of symptoms
○ Bloody stool
○ Decreased urine output
○ Fatigue

Physical assessment

Early symptoms

○ Bloody stool
○ Diarrhea
○ Fever
○ Irritability
○ Lethargy
○ Vomiting
○ Weakness

Later symptoms

○ Anuria
○ Bruising
○ Decreased consciousness
○ Jaundice
○ Low urine output
○ Pallor
○ Petechiae
○ Seizures (rare)

Test results

Laboratory

○ Schistocytes and giant platelets in peripheral smear
○ Increased lactate dehydrogenase level
○ Increased indirect bilirubin level
○ Increased blood urea nitrogen level
○ Increased creatinine level
○ Red blood cells in urine
○ Proteinuria
○ Disseminated intravascular coagulation panel within normal range
○ Increased reticulocyte count

Nursing diagnoses

○ Acute pain
○ Impaired urinary elimination
○ Risk for imbalanced fluid volume

Key outcomes

The patient will:
○ maintain hemodynamic stability
○ maintain balanced electrolytes and fluid status
○ express understanding of disorder and treatment.

Interventions

General

○ Dialysis
○ Initially, fluid replacement
○ Plasmapheresis
○ Supportive care

Nursing

○ Give fluids as prescribed.
○ Give prescribed drugs.
○ Provide emotional support.
○ Antibiotics may be avoided.

Drug therapy
○ Antihypertensives

Monitoring
○ Intake and output
○ Laboratory test results
○ Renal status
○ Vital signs

Patient teaching

Be sure to cover:
○ the disorder, diagnosis, and treatment
○ the need to refrain from eating rare beef
○ the need to wash hands thoroughly.

Discharge planning

○ Encourage follow-up care with a nephrologist and hematologist.

Hepatorenal syndrome

Overview

Description

- Renal failure in patients with chronic liver disease
- Liver disease progressed to portal hypertension and ascites
- Two types
  - *Type 1:* rapid and progressive renal impairment caused by spontaneous bacterial peritonitis
  - *Type 2:* moderate and stable reduction in the glomerular filtration rate

Pathophysiology

- Advanced liver disease causes vasoconstriction in the renal circulation and intense systemic arteriolar vasodilatation.
- This results in reduced systemic vascular resistance and arterial hypotension.
- Renal perfusion is affected.
- Renal failure eventually occurs.

Causes

- Chronic liver disease with marked sodium and water retention

Prevalence

- Affects both sexes equally
- Ages 40 to 80 in most adults with chronic liver failure

Complications

- Death

Assessment

History

- Chronic liver disease
- Decreased urine output
- Fatigue
- Malaise

Physical assessment

- Clubbing
- Decreased urine output
- Evidence of chronic advanced liver disease
  - Asterixis
  - Scleral icterus
  - Muscle wasting
  - Spider nevi
  - Ascites
  - Peripheral edema

Test results

Laboratory

- Increased serum creatinine level
- Creatinine clearance less than 40 ml/minute in 24-hour urine test
- Proteinuria
- Low urine sodium level
- Bacteria in ascites fluid

Nursing diagnoses

- Anticipatory grieving
- Anxiety
- Deficient knowledge (hepatorenal syndrome)
- Impaired urinary elimination
- Ineffective coping
- Risk for imbalanced fluid volume

Key outcomes

The patient will:
- maintain adequate fluid balance
- express understanding of the disease process and treatment
- use positive coping mechanisms
- use available support systems
- express desires for end-of-life care.

Interventions

General

- Liver transplant
- Low-sodium diet
- Peritoneovenous shunting (type 2)
- Supportive care
- Surgical shunts

Nursing

- Give drugs and fluids as prescribed.
- Provide supportive care.
- Provide emotional support.
- Encourage a low-sodium diet.

Drug therapy

- Antibiotics
- Antioxidants
- Plasma expanders
- Vasoconstrictors
- Vasodilators
- Vasopressin analogues

Monitoring

- Intake and output
- Laboratory test results
- Renal status
- Vital signs

Patient teaching

Be sure to cover:
○ the disorder, diagnosis, and treatment
○ low-sodium diet
○ liver transplantation
○ end-of-life issues.

Discharge planning

○ Refer the patient to social services for appropriate counseling.

Hydronephrosis

Overview

Description

- Abnormal dilation of the renal pelvis and calyces of one or both kidneys
- Caused by obstruction of urine flow in the genitourinary tract
- May be acute or chronic

Pathophysiology

- With obstruction in the urethra or bladder, hydronephrosis is usually bilateral.
- With obstruction in a ureter, hydronephrosis is usually unilateral.
- Obstruction distal to the bladder causes the bladder to dilate, acting as a buffer zone, delaying hydronephrosis.
- Total obstruction of urine flow with dilation of the collecting system ultimately causes complete cortical atrophy, and glomerular filtration ceases.

Causes

- Benign prostatic hyperplasia (BPH)
- Bladder, ureteral, or pelvic tumors
- Blood clots
- Congenital abnormalities
- Gram-negative infection
- Neurogenic bladder
- Renal calculi
- Strictures or stenosis of the ureter or bladder outlet
- Tuberculosis
- Ureterocele
- Urethral strictures

Prevalence

- About 1 in 100 people affected by unilateral hydronephrosis
- About 1 in 200 people affected by bilateral hydronephrosis

Complications

- Infection
- Obstructive nephropathy
- Paralytic ileus
- Pyelonephritis
- Renal calculi
- Renal failure
- Renovascular hypertension
- Sepsis

Assessment

History

- Abdominal fullness
- Alternating oliguria and polyuria, anuria
- Change in voiding pattern
- Dribbling
- Dysuria
- Hematuria
- No symptoms or only mild pain and slightly decreased urine flow
- Pain on urination
- Possibly no initial symptoms, but eventual renal dysfunction as pressure increases behind the obstruction
- Pyuria
- Severe, colicky, renal pain or dull flank pain that radiates to the groin
- Nausea
- Urinary hesitancy
- Varies with cause of obstruction
- Vomiting

Physical assessment

- Costovertebral angle tenderness
- Distended bladder
- Hematuria
- Leg edema
- Palpable kidney
- Pyuria
- Urinary tract infection

Test results

Laboratory
- Abnormal results on renal function study
- Inability to concentrate urine
- Decreased glomerular filtration rate
- Pyuria if infection is present
- Leukocytosis, indicating infection

Imaging
- Radionuclide scan may show the site of obstruction.
- Computed tomography may indicate the cause.

Diagnostic procedures
- Excretory urography, retrograde pyelography, and renal ultrasonography confirm diagnosis.
- I.V. urogram may show site of obstruction.
- On a nephrogram, the apearance of contrast material may be delayed.

Nursing diagnoses

- Acute pain
- Anxiety
- Deficient fluid volume
- Imbalanced nutrition: less than body requirements
- Impaired urinary elimination
- Risk for infection

Key outcomes

The patient will:
- avoid or minimize complications
- maintain fluid balance
- report increased comfort

- maintain hemodynamic stability
- demonstrate skill in managing urinary elimination.

Interventions

General

- Dilatation for urethral stricture
- For inoperable obstructions, decompression and drainage of the kidney using a nephrostomy tube placed temporarily or permanently in the renal pelvis
- If renal function affected, low-protein, low-sodium, and low-potassium diet
- Placement of percutaneous nephrostomy tube
- Prostatectomy for BPH
- Urinary catheterization

Nursing

- Give prescribed drugs.
- Give prescribed I.V. fluids.
- Allow the patient to express his fears and anxieties.

Drug therapy

- Analgesics
- Antibiotic therapy
- Oral alkalinization therapy (for uric acid calculi)
- Corticosteroid therapy (for retroperitoneal fibrosis)

Monitoring

- Fluid and electrolyte status
- Intake and output
- Nephrostomy tube function and drainage, if appropriate
- Renal function studies
- Vital signs
- Wound site (postoperatively)

Patient teaching

Be sure to cover:
- the disorder, diagnosis, and treatment
- the procedure and postoperative care, if surgery is scheduled
- nephrostomy tube care, if appropriate
- prescribed drugs, dosages, and possible adverse effects
- diet changes
- how to recognize and when to report hydronephrosis symptoms.

Discharge planning

- Follow-up imaging studies may be required to evaluate the patient's recovery.
- Follow-up laboratory studies may be needed to assess renal function.

Hyperaldosteronism

Overview

Description
- Hypersecretion of the mineralocorticoid aldosterone by the adrenal cortex
- Excessive reabsorption of sodium and water
- Excessive renal excretion of potassium
- May be primary (uncommon) or secondary

Pathophysiology
Primary hyperaldosteronism (Conn's syndrome)
- Chronic excessive secretion of aldosterone is independent of the renin-angiotensin system and suppresses plasma renin activity.
- This aldosterone excess enhances sodium and water reabsorption and potassium loss by the kidneys, which leads to mild hypernatremia and, simultaneously, hypokalemia and increased extracellular fluid volume.
- Expansion of intravascular fluid volume results in volume-dependent hypertension and increased cardiac output.

▼ *ALERT Excessive consumption of English black licorice or licorice-like substances can produce a syndrome similar to primary hyperaldosteronism because of the mineralocorticoid action of glycyrrhizic acid.*

Secondary hyperaldosteronism
- An extra-adrenal abnormality stimulates the adrenal gland to increase aldosterone production.

Causes
- Bartter's syndrome
- Benign aldosterone-producing adrenal adenoma (in 70% of patients)
- Bilateral adrenocortical hyperplasia (in children) or carcinoma (rarely)
- Conditions that produce a sodium deficit (Wilms' tumor)
- Conditions that reduce renal blood flow and extracellular fluid volume (renal artery stenosis)
- Heart failure
- Hepatic cirrhosis with ascites
- Nephrotic syndrome

Prevalence
- Most common between ages 30 and 50
- Three times more common in women than in men

Complications
- Left ventricular hypertrophy, heart failure, death
- Metabolic alkalosis, nephropathy, azotemia
- Neuromuscular irritability, tetany, paresthesia
- Seizures

Assessment

History
- Fatigue
- Headaches
- Nocturnal polyuria
- Polydipsia
- Vision disturbances

Physical assessment
- High blood pressure
- Intermittent flaccid paralysis
- Muscle weakness
- Paresthesia

Test results
Laboratory
- Persistently low serum potassium levels
- Low plasma renin level that fails to increase appropriately during volume depletion (upright posture, sodium depletion) and a high plasma aldosterone level during volume expansion by salt loading (confirmation of primary hyperaldosteronism in a hypertensive patient without edema)
- Increased serum bicarbonate level
- Markedly increased urine aldosterone level
- Increased plasma aldosterone level
- Increased plasma renin level (secondary)
- Suppression test to differentiate between primary and secondary hyperaldosteronism
Imaging
- Chest X-rays show left ventricular hypertrophy from chronic hypertension.
Diagnostic procedures
- Electrocardiography shows signs of hypokalemia (ST-segment depression and U waves).
- Adrenal angiography or computed tomography scan localize tumor.

Nursing diagnoses
- Acute pain
- Decreased cardiac output
- Deficient knowledge (hyperaldosteronism)
- Impaired urinary elimination
- Ineffective coping
- Ineffective tissue perfusion: renal

Key outcomes
The patient will:
- maintain hemodynamic stability
- express feelings of increased comfort
- maintain adequate fluid balance
- express understanding of the condition and treatment.

Interventions

General

○ Treatment of underlying cause (secondary)
○ Low-sodium, high-potassium diet
○ Unilateral adrenalectomy (primary)

Nursing

○ Watch for signs of tetany (muscle twitching, Chvostek's sign, Trousseau's sign).
○ Give potassium replacement, and keep I.V. calcium gluconate available.
○ After adrenalectomy, watch for weakness, hyponatremia, rising serum potassium levels, and signs of adrenal hypofunction, especially hypotension.

Drug therapy

○ Potassium-sparing diuretics (primary)

Monitoring

○ Cardiac arrhythmias
○ Intake and output
○ Serum electrolyte levels
○ Vital signs
○ Weight

Patient teaching

Be sure to cover:
○ adverse effects of spironolactone, including hyperkalemia, impotence, and gynecomastia, if needed
○ the importance of wearing medical identification jewelry while taking steroid hormone replacement therapy.

Discharge planning

○ Refer the patient to an endocrinologist as needed.

Hypercalcemia

Overview

Description
○ Excessive serum calcium level

Pathophysiology
○ Together with phosphorus, calcium is responsible for the formation and structure of bones and teeth.
○ Calcium helps maintain cell structure and function.
○ It plays a role in cell membrane permeability and impulse transmission.
○ It affects the contraction of cardiac muscle, smooth muscle, and skeletal muscle.
○ It participates in the blood-clotting process.

Causes
○ Certain cancers
○ Certain drugs (See *Drugs that cause hypercalcemia.*)
○ Hyperparathyroidism
○ Hypervitaminosis D
○ Multiple fractures
○ Prolonged immobilization

Prevalence
○ Considerably more common in women than in men
○ No gender predominance when related to cancer
○ Increases with age

Complications
○ Cardiac arrest
○ Coma
○ Renal calculi

Assessment

History
○ Anorexia
○ Constipation
○ Lethargy
○ Nausea, vomiting
○ Polyuria
○ Underlying cause
○ Weakness

Drugs that cause hypercalcemia

These drugs can cause or contribute to hypercalcemia:
● antacids that contain calcium
● calcium preparations (oral or I.V.)
● lithium
● thiazide diuretics
● vitamin A
● vitamin D.

Physical assessment
○ Confusion
○ Decreased muscle tone (See *Effects of hypercalcemia.*)
○ Hyporeflexia
○ Muscle weakness

Test results
Laboratory
○ Serum calcium levels greater than 10.5 mg/dl
○ Ionized calcium levels less than 5.3 mg/dl
Imaging
○ Electrocardiogram shows a shortened QT interval and ventricular arrhythmias.

Nursing diagnoses

○ Decreased cardiac output
○ Deficient knowledge (hypercalcemia)
○ Impaired gas exchange
○ Ineffective tissue perfusion: cardiopulmonary

Key outcomes
The patient will:
○ maintain stable vital signs
○ maintain adequate cardiac output
○ express an understanding of the disorder and treatment regimen.

Interventions

General
○ Activity, as tolerated
○ Treatment of the underlying cause

Nursing
○ Provide safety measures.
○ Institute seizure precautions, if appropriate.
○ Give prescribed I.V. solutions.
○ Watch for evidence of heart failure.

Drug therapy
○ Loop diuretics
○ Normal saline solution

Monitoring
○ Calcium levels
○ Cardiac rhythm
○ Seizures

Patient teaching

Be sure to cover:
○ the need to avoid over-the-counter drugs that are high in calcium
○ the need to increase fluid intake
○ the need to follow a low-calcium diet.

Effects of hypercalcemia

Body system	Effects
Cardiovascular	• Cardiac arrest • Hypertension • Signs of heart block
Gastrointestinal	• Anorexia • Constipation • Dehydration • Nausea and vomiting • Polydipsia
Musculoskeletal	• Bone pain • Muscle flaccidity • Pathologic fractures • Weakness
Neurologic	• Confusion • Depression or apathy • Drowsiness • Headaches • Irritability • Lethargy
Other	• Eventual azotemia • Flank pain • Renal polyuria

Discharge planning

○ Refer the patient to a dietitian and social services, if indicated.

Hyperchloremia

Overview

Description
○ Excessive serum levels of the chloride anion
○ Usually accompanied by sodium and water retention

Pathophysiology
○ Chloride accounts for two-thirds of all serum anions.
○ Chloride is secreted by the stomach mucosa as hydrochloric acid; it provides an acid medium that aids digestion and activates enzymes.
○ Chloride helps to maintain acid-base and body water balances, influences the osmolality or tonicity of extracellular fluid, plays a role in the exchange of oxygen and carbon dioxide in red blood cells, and helps activate salivary amylase (which, in turn, activates digestion).
○ An inverse relationship exists between chloride and bicarbonate. (See *Anion gap and metabolic acidosis.*)

Risk factors
○ Therapy with drugs known to increase the chloride level

Causes
○ Certain drugs (See *Drugs that cause hyperchloremia.*)

Anion gap and metabolic acidosis

The anion gap is the difference between measurements of cations and anions. Because concentrations of positive and negative electrolytes balance in the body, you might think the difference should be zero. However, because not all electrolytes are routinely measured, there's an anion gap. Plus, the patient may have small amounts of anions — such as lactate, phosphates, sulfates, and proteins — in his blood. Usually, the anion gap is considered normal if it's 8 to 16 mEq/L if potassium is included in the calculation (8 to 12 mEq/L if it isn't).

The anion gap can be used to help identify metabolic acidosis. That's because, as acids accumulate in the bloodstream, bicarbonate levels decline to regulate blood pH. When bicarbonate levels decline, the anion gap increases. That's why metabolic acidosis usually is reflected in an increased anion gap. Metabolic alkalosis usually is reflected in a decreased anion gap.

Hyperchloremia relates to the anion gap because chloride and bicarbonate have an inverse relationship. As chloride levels rise, bicarbonate levels decline. If a patient with metabolic acidosis has a normal anion gap, the acidosis probably results from a loss of bicarbonate ions by the kidneys or the gastrointestinal tract. Or the acidosis could result from an accumulation of chloride ions as acidifying salts. In these cases, chloride ion levels rise, causing hyperchloremia — with a normal anion gap.

○ Hypernatremia
○ Hyperparathyroidism
○ Loss of pancreatic secretion
○ Metabolic acidosis
○ Prolonged diarrhea
○ Renal tubular acidosis

Complications
○ Coma

Assessment

History
○ Altered level of consciousness

Physical assessment
○ Agitation
○ Dyspnea
○ Hypertension
○ Pitting edema
○ Rapid deep breathing (Kussmaul's respirations)
○ Tachypnea
○ Weakness

Test results
Laboratory
○ Serum chloride level above 108 mEq/L
○ With metabolic acidosis, serum pH below 7.35, serum carbon dioxide level below 22 mEq/L, and normal anion gap
○ Serum sodium level above 145 mEq/L

Nursing diagnoses

○ Anxiety
○ Deficient fluid volume
○ Deficient knowledge (hyperchloremia)
○ Ineffective breathing pattern
○ Ineffective tissue perfusion: cardiopulmonary

Key outcomes
The patient will:
○ maintain adequate cardiac output
○ maintain stable vital signs
○ maintain adequate fluid volume
○ avoid complications.

Interventions

General
○ Activity, as tolerated
○ Restoration of fluid, electrolyte, and acid-base balance
○ Restricted sodium and chloride intake
○ Treatment of underlying cause

Drugs that cause hyperchloremia

These drugs can cause or contribute to hyperchloremia:
- acetazolamide
- ammonium chloride
- phenylbutazone
- salicylates (overdose)
- sodium polystyrene sulfonate (Kayexalate)
- triamterene.

Nursing
○ Provide a safe environment.
○ Give prescribed I.V. fluids.
○ Evaluate muscle strength.
○ Adjust activity level.
○ Reorient a confused patient when needed.

Drug therapy
○ Diuretics
○ Lactated Ringer's solution
○ Sodium bicarbonate I.V.

Monitoring
○ Arterial blood gas levels
○ Cardiac rhythm
○ Intake and output
○ Neurologic status
○ Respiratory status
○ Serum electrolyte levels
○ Signs of metabolic alkalosis

Patient teaching

Be sure to cover:
○ the disorder, diagnosis, and treatment
○ dietary or fluid restrictions, as indicated
○ prescribed drugs, dosages, and possible adverse effects.

Discharge planning

○ Refer the patient to a nutritionist for diet restrictions as appropriate.

Hyperkalemia

Overview

Description
○ Excessive serum levels of the potassium anion
○ Commonly induced by other treatments

Pathophysiology
○ Potassium facilitates contraction of skeletal and smooth muscles, including myocardial contraction.
○ Potassium figures prominently in nerve impulse conduction, acid-base balance, enzyme action, and cell membrane function.
○ Slight changes in serum levels can produce profound clinical consequences.
○ Potassium imbalance can lead to muscle weakness and flaccid paralysis because of an ionic imbalance in neuromuscular tissue excitability.

Causes
○ Adrenal gland insufficiency
○ Burns
○ Certain drugs (See *Drugs that cause hyperkalemia.*)
○ Crush injuries
○ Decreased urinary excretion of potassium
○ Dehydration
○ Diabetic acidosis
○ Increased potassium intake
○ Large quantities of transfused blood
○ Renal dysfunction or failure
○ Severe infection
○ Use of potassium-sparing diuretics, such as triamterene, by patients with renal disease

Prevalence
○ Affects males and females equally
○ Diagnosed in up to 8% of hospitalized patients in the United States

Complications
○ Cardiac arrest
○ Cardiac arrhythmia
○ Metabolic acidosis

Drugs that cause hyperkalemia

These drugs may increase potassium levels:
● angiotensin-converting enzyme inhibitors
● antibiotics
● beta blockers
● chemotherapeutic drugs
● nonsteroidal anti-inflammatory drugs
● potassium (in excessive amounts)
● spironolactone.

Assessment

History
○ Abdominal cramps
○ Diarrhea
○ Irritability
○ Muscle weakness
○ Nausea
○ Paresthesia

Physical assessment
○ Hypotension
○ Irregular heart rate
○ Possible cardiac arrhythmia (See *Effects of hyperkalemia.*)

Test results
Laboratory
○ Serum potassium levels greater than 5 mEq/L
○ Decreased arterial pH
Imaging
○ Electrocardiogram shows a tall, tented T wave.

Nursing diagnoses
○ Decreased cardiac output
○ Deficient knowledge (hyperkalemia)

Effects of hyperkalemia

Type of dysfunction	Effects
Acid-base balance	● Metabolic acidosis
Cardiovascular	● Cardiac arrest (with levels > 7.0 mEq/L) ● Electrocardiogram changes (tented and elevated T waves, widened QRS complex, prolonged PR interval, flattened or absent P waves, depressed ST segment) ● Tachycardia and later bradycardia
Gastrointestinal	● Abdominal cramps ● Diarrhea ● Nausea
Genitourinary	● Anuria ● Oliguria
Musculoskeletal	● Flaccid paralysis ● Muscle weakness
Neurologic	● Flaccid paralysis ● Hyperreflexia progressing to weakness ● Numbness ● Tingling

Avoiding false results

When your patient gets a laboratory test result indicating a high potassium level, and the result doesn't make sense, make sure it's a true result. If the sample was drawn using poor technique, the results may be falsely high. Some of the causes of falsely high potassium levels are:

- drawing the sample above the site of an I.V. infusion that contains potassium
- using a recently exercised arm or leg for the venipuncture site
- causing hemolysis (cell damage) as the specimen is obtained.

○ Diarrhea
○ Fluid volume deficit

Key outcomes

The patient will:
○ maintain hemodynamic stability
○ maintain a normal potassium level
○ understand potential adverse effects of prescribed drugs.

Interventions

General

○ Activity, as tolerated
○ Hemodialysis or peritoneal dialysis
○ Treatment of the underlying cause

Nursing

○ Check the serum sample. (See *Avoiding false results.*)
○ Give prescribed drugs.
○ Insert an indwelling urinary catheter.
○ Implement safety measures.
○ Be alert for signs of hypokalemia after treatment.

Drug therapy

○ Insulin and 10% to 50% glucose I.V.
○ Rapid infusion of 10% calcium gluconate (decreases myocardial irritability)
○ Sodium polystyrene sulfonate with 70% sorbitol

Monitoring

○ Cardiac rhythm
○ Intake and output
○ Serum potassium levels

Patient teaching

Be sure to cover:
○ prescribed drugs and potential adverse effects
○ the need to monitor intake and output
○ preventing future episodes of hyperkalemia
○ the need for a potassium-restricted diet.

Discharge planning

○ Refer the patient to a nutritionist for a low-potassium diet as appropriate.

Hypermagnesemia

Overview

Description

○ Excessive serum levels of the magnesium cation

Pathophysiology

○ Magnesium enhances neuromuscular integration and stimulates parathyroid hormone secretion, thus regulating intracellular fluid calcium levels.
○ Magnesium may also regulate skeletal muscles through its influence on calcium utilization by depressing acetylcholine release at synaptic junctions.
○ Magnesium activates many enzymes needed for carbohydrate and protein metabolism, aids in cell metabolism and the transport of sodium and potassium across cell membranes, and influences sodium, potassium, calcium, and protein levels.
○ About one-third of magnesium consumed is absorbed through the small intestine and eventually is excreted in the urine; the remaining unabsorbed magnesium is excreted in stool.

Risk factors

○ Advanced age
○ Pregnancy
○ Neonates whose mothers received magnesium sulfate during labor
○ Receiving magnesium sulfate to control seizures

Causes

○ Addison's disease
○ Adrenocortical insufficiency
○ Chronic renal insufficiency
○ Overcorrection of hypomagnesemia
○ Overuse of magnesium-containing antacids
○ Severe dehydration (resulting oliguria can cause magnesium retention)
○ Untreated diabetic ketoacidosis
○ Use of magnesium-containing laxatives (magnesium sulfate, Milk of Magnesia, and magnesium citrate solutions), especially with renal insufficiency (See *Drugs and supplements that cause hypermagnesemia.*)

Drugs and supplements that cause hypermagnesemia

Monitor your patient's magnesium level closely if he's receiving:
● an antacid (Di-Gel, Gaviscon, Maalox)
● a laxative (Milk of Magnesia, Haley's M-O, magnesium citrate)
● a magnesium supplement (magnesium oxide, magnesium sulfate).

Prevalence

○ Rarely occurs in the United States

Complications

○ Cardiac arrest
○ Cardiac arrhythmia
○ Respiratory depression

Assessment

History

○ Confusion
○ Drowsiness
○ Nausea
○ Vomiting

Physical assessment

○ Flushed appearance
○ Hyporeflexia (See *Effects of hypermagnesemia* and *Testing the patellar reflex.*)
○ Hypotension
○ Muscle weakness
○ Weak pulse

Test results

Laboratory
○ Serum magnesium levels greater than 2.5 mEq/L
Diagnostic procedures
○ Electrocardiogram (ECG) shows prolonged PR interval, widened QRS complex, and tall T waves.

Nursing diagnoses

○ Anxiety
○ Deficient knowledge (hypermagnesemia)
○ Impaired gas exchange
○ Ineffective tissue perfusion: renal
○ Risk for deficient fluid volume

Effects of hypermagnesemia

Body system	Effects
Cardiovascular	● Bradycardia ● Cardiac arrest ● Heart block ● Hypotension ● Weak pulse
Neurologic	● Confusion ● Diminished sensorium ● Drowsiness ● Flushing ● Lethargy
Neuromuscular	● Diminished reflexes ● Flaccid paralysis ● Muscle weakness ● Respiratory muscle paralysis that may cause respiratory compromise

---

Testing the patellar reflex

One way to gauge your patient's magnesium status is to test his patellar reflex, one of the deep tendon reflexes affected by magnesium level. To test the reflex, strike the patellar tendon just below the patella with the patient sitting or lying in a supine position, as shown. Look for leg extension or contraction of the quadriceps muscle in the front of the thigh.

If the patellar reflex is absent, notify the doctor immediately. This finding may mean your patient's magnesium level is 7 mEq/L or higher.

Sitting
Test the reflex with the patient sitting on the side of the bed, legs dangling freely, as shown here.

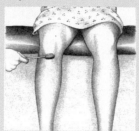

Supine position
Test the reflex after flexing the patient's knee at a 45-degree angle with nondominant hand behind it for support.

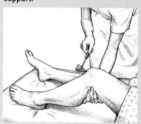

Key outcomes

The patient will:
- maintain hemodynamic stability
- attain and maintain a normal magnesium level
- understand the causes of high magnesium levels
- have a normal ECG
- maintain fluid volume balance.

Interventions

General
- Identification and correction of the underlying cause
- Increased fluid intake
- Peritoneal dialysis or hemodialysis

Nursing
- Provide sufficient fluids for adequate hydration and maintenance of renal function.
- Give prescribed drugs.
- Report abnormal serum electrolyte levels immediately.
- Watch patients receiving both a cardiac glycoside and calcium gluconate because calcium excess enhances the cardiac glycoside.

Drug therapy
- Calcium gluconate (10%)
- Loop diuretics, such as furosemide, with impaired renal function

Monitoring
- Cardiac rhythm
- Electrolyte levels
- Intake and output
- Level of consciousness
- Magnesium levels
- Neuromuscular system
- Respiratory status
- Vital signs

Patient teaching

Be sure to cover:
- the need not to abuse laxatives and antacids containing magnesium, particularly by the elderly or patients with compromised renal function
- hydration requirements
- prescribed drugs.

Discharge planning

None.

Hypernatremia

Overview

Description
○ Excessive serum levels of the sodium cation relative to body water

Pathophysiology
○ Sodium is the major cation (90%) in extracellular fluid; potassium, the major cation in intracellular fluid.
○ During repolarization, the sodium-potassium pump continually shifts sodium into the cells and potassium out of the cells; during depolarization, it does the reverse.
○ Sodium cation functions include maintaining tonicity and concentration of extracellular fluid, acid-base balance (reabsorption of sodium ion and excretion of hydrogen ion), nerve conduction and neuromuscular function, glandular secretion, and water balance.
○ Increased sodium causes high serum osmolality (increased solute concentrations in the body), which stimulates the hypothalamus to create the sensation of thirst.

Risk factors
○ Inability to drink voluntarily

Causes
○ Antidiuretic hormone deficiency (diabetes insipidus)
○ Certain drugs (See *Drugs that cause hypernatremia.*)
○ Decreased water intake
○ Excess adrenocortical hormones, as in Cushing's syndrome
○ Excessive I.V. administration of sodium solutions
○ Salt intoxication (less common), which may be produced by excessive consumption of table salt

Prevalence
○ Occurs in about 1% of hospitalized patients
○ Usually occurs in elderly patients
○ Affects males and females equally

Drugs that cause hypernatremia

Ask your patient if he has received or is taking any of these drugs, all of which can elevate his sodium level:
● anatacids with sodium bicarbonate
● antibiotics, such as ticarcillin disodium–clavulanate potassium (Timentin)
● I.V. sodium chloride preparations
● salt tablets
● sodium bicarbonate injections (such as those given during cardiac arrest)
● sodium polystyrene sulfonate (Kayexalate).

Complications
○ Coma
○ Permanent neurologic damage
○ Seizures

Assessment

History
○ Disorientation
○ Fatigue
○ Lethargy
○ Restlessness, agitation
○ Weakness

Physical assessment
○ Dry, swollen tongue
○ Flushed skin
○ Hypertension, dyspnea (with hypervolemia)
○ Low-grade fever
○ Orthostatic hypotension and oliguria (with hypovolemia) (See *Effects of hypernatremia.*)
○ Sticky mucous membranes
○ Twitching

Test results
Laboratory
○ Serum sodium level greater than 145 mEq/L
○ Urine sodium level less than 40 mEq/24 hours, with high serum osmolality

Nursing diagnoses

○ Deficient knowledge (hypernatremia)
○ Disturbed thought processes
○ Ineffective tissue perfusion: cardiopulmonary
○ Risk for deficient fluid volume
○ Risk for injury

Key outcomes
The patient will:
○ maintain adequate fluid volume
○ maintain a normal sodium level
○ maintain stable vital signs
○ remain alert and oriented to the environment.

Interventions

General
○ Activity, as tolerated
○ Administration of salt-free solutions (such as dextrose in water) followed by infusion of half-normal saline solution to prevent hyponatremia
○ Discontinuation of drugs that promote sodium retention
○ Sodium-restricted diet
○ Treatment of underlying cause

Effects of hypernatremia

Body system	Effects
Cardiovascular	• Excessive weight gain • Hypertension • Pitting edema • Tachycardia
Gastrointestinal	• Dry, sticky membranes • Flushed skin
Genitourinary	• Intense thirst • Rough, dry tongue
Musculoskeletal	• Oliguria
Neurologic	• Agitation • Fever • Restlessness • Seizures
Respiratory	• Death (from dramatic rise in osmotic pressure) • Dyspnea • Respiratory arrest

Nursing

○ Obtain a drug history to check for drugs that promote sodium retention.
○ Assist with oral hygiene.
○ Watch for signs of cerebral edema during fluid replacement therapy.

Drug therapy

○ Diuretics
○ Vasopressin if the patient has diabetes insipidus.

Monitoring

○ Intake and output
○ Neurologic status
○ Serum sodium levels

Patient teaching

Be sure to cover:
○ the disorder and treatment
○ the importance of sodium restriction
○ low-sodium diet
○ prescribed drugs, dosages, and possible adverse effects
○ signs and symptoms of hypernatremia
○ the need to avoid over-the-counter drugs that contain sodium.

Discharge planning

○ Refer the patient to a nutritionist or dietitian for diet restrictions as appropriate.

Hyperosmolar hyperglycemic nonketotic syndrome

Overview

Description
○ Metabolic condition characterized by hyperglycemia and hyperosmolarity without ketoacidosis
○ Occurs in adult-onset diabetes mellitus

Pathophysiology
○ Fluid intake decreases in a diabetic patient, usually because of a secondary illness.
○ Hyperglycemia and hyperosmolarity lead to osmotic diuresis and intracellular dehydration.
○ Ketoacidosis doesn't occur, for unknown reasons.

Causes
○ Certain drugs (such as diuretics and beta blockers)
○ Illness in a person with diabetes mellitus
○ Noncompliance with diabetic drug therapy
○ Stress

Prevalence
○ Occurs slightly more in women than men
○ Mean age of occurrence is the early 40s

Complications
○ Coma

Assessment

History
○ Diabetes mellitus
○ Drowsiness
○ Secondary illness, acute or chronic
○ Seizures
○ Sensory deficits
○ Visual changes

Physical assessment
○ Hypotension
○ Signs of dehydration
○ Signs of infection (See *Comparing hyperosmolar hyperglycemic nonketotic syndrome and diabetic ketoacidosis.*)
○ Tachycardia

Test results
Laboratory
○ Increased serum glucose level
○ Abnormal sodium level
○ Elevated blood urea nitrogen and creatinine levels
○ Increased serum osmolarity
○ Negative ketone test
○ pH usually above 7.25
○ Increased urine specific gravity
○ Glycosuria
○ Possible evidence of urinary tract infection

Nursing diagnoses
○ Deficient fluid volume
○ Deficient knowledge (hyperosmolar hyperglycemic nonketotic syndrome)
○ Disturbed thought processes
○ Ineffective coping
○ Risk for injury

Key outcomes
The patient will:
○ maintain adequate fluid volume
○ express understanding of disorder
○ remain safe from injury
○ remain alert and oriented
○ use positive coping mechanisms and available support systems.

Interventions

General
○ Airway maintenance
○ I.V. fluids
○ Supportive care
○ Treatment for concurrent illness

Nursing
○ Give drugs and I.V. fluids as ordered.
○ Provide emotional support.

Drug therapy
○ Antibiotics (if infection present)
○ Insulin

Monitoring
○ Blood glucose levels
○ Intake and output
○ Hydration status
○ Neurological status
○ Vital signs

Patient teaching

Be sure to cover:
○ the disorder, diagnosis, and treatment
○ the need to follow the appropriate diabetic diet
○ when to notify the doctor
○ prescribed drugs, and possible adverse effects.

Comparing hyperosmolar hyperglycemic nonketotic syndrome and diabetic ketoacidosis

Hyperosmolar hyperglycemic nonketotic syndrome (HHNS) and diabetic ketoacidosis (DKA), both acute complications of diabetes, share some similarities, but they're two distinct conditions. Use this flowchart to help determine which condition your patient is experiencing.

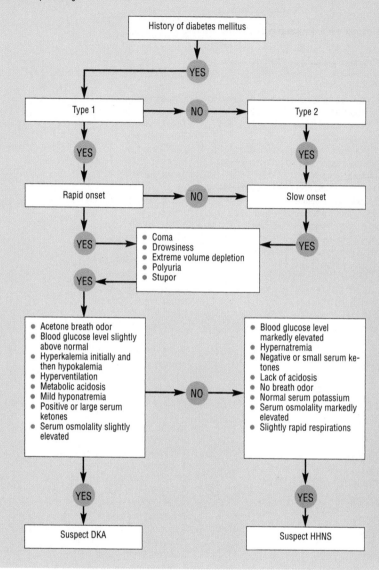

Discharge planning

○ Refer the patient for diabetic teaching if needed.

Hyperparathyroidism

Overview

Description
- Increased secretion of parathyroid hormone (PTH)
- Classified as either primary or secondary

Pathophysiology
- *Primary:* One or more of the parathyroid glands enlarges, increasing PTH secretion and elevating serum calcium levels; or an adenoma secretes PTH, unresponsive to negative feedback of serum calcium.
- *Secondary:* Excessive compensatory production of PTH stems from a hypocalcemia-producing abnormality outside the parathyroid gland that isn't responsive to PTH, such as decreased intestinal absorption of calcium or vitamin D.
- Increased PTH levels act directly on bone and renal tubules, increasing extracellular calcium levels.
- Renal excretion and uptake into the soft tissues or skeleton can't compensate for increased calcium.

Causes
- Adenoma
- Certain drugs, such as phenytoin
- Chronic renal failure
- Decreased intestinal absorption of vitamin D or calcium
- Dietary vitamin D or calcium deficiency
- Genetic disorders
- Idiopathic
- Laxative use
- Multiple endocrine neoplasia
- Osteomalacia

Prevalence
- More common in women than men
- More common in postmenopausal women
- Onset usually between ages 35 and 65

Complications
- Cardiac arrhythmias
- Cholelithiasis
- Depression
- Heart failure
- Muscle atrophy
- Osteoporosis
- Peptic ulcers
- Renal calculi and colic
- Renal insufficiency and failure
- Subchondral fractures
- Traumatic synovitis
- Vascular damage

Assessment

History
- Abdominal pain
- Anemia
- Anorexia, nausea, and vomiting
- Cataracts
- Chronic lower back pain
- Constant, severe epigastric pain that radiates to the back
- Constipation
- Depression
- Easy fracturing
- Hematuria
- Lethargy
- Muscle weakness, particularly in the legs
- Osteoporosis
- Overt psychosis
- Personality disturbances
- Polydipsia
- Polyuria
- Recurring nephrolithiasis

Physical assessment
- Muscle weakness and atrophy
- Psychomotor disturbances
- Stupor, possibly coma
- Skin necrosis
- Subcutaneous calcification

Test results
Primary disease
- Increased alkaline phosphatase level
- Increased osteocalcin level
- Increased tartrate-resistant acid phosphatase level
- Increased serum PTH level
- Increased serum calcium level
- Decreased serum phosphorus level
- Increased urine and serum calcium level
- Increased serum chloride level
- Possible increased creatinine level
- Possible increased basal acid secretion
- Possible increased serum amylase level

Secondary disease
- Normal or slightly decreased serum calcium level
- Variable serum phosphorus level
- Increased serum PTH level
- Changes on imaging tests
  - X-rays show diffuse bone demineralization, bone cysts, outer cortical bone absorption, and subperiosteal erosion of the phalanges and distal clavicles in primary disease.
  - X-ray spectrophotometry shows increased bone turnover in primary disease.
  - Esophagography, thyroid scan, parathyroid thermography, ultrasonography, thyroid angiography, computed tomography scan, and magnetic resonance imaging may show the location of parathyroid lesions.

Nursing diagnoses

○ Activity intolerance
○ Decreased cardiac output
○ Disturbed body image
○ Disturbed thought processes
○ Excess fluid volume
○ Fear
○ Imbalanced nutrition: less than body requirements

Key outcomes

The patient will:
○ maintain current weight
○ express feelings of increased comfort
○ maintain adequate cardiac output
○ maintain balanced fluid volume status
○ perform activities of daily living without excessive fatigue
○ express positive feelings about self.

Interventions

General

○ Activity, as tolerated
○ Increased oral fluid intake
○ In renal failure, dialysis
○ In primary disease, treatment to decrease calcium levels
○ In primary disease, removal of adenoma or all but half of one gland
○ In secondary disease, treatment to correct underlying cause of parathyroid hypertrophy

Nursing

○ Obtain baseline serum potassium, calcium, phosphate, and magnesium levels before treatment.
○ Provide at least 3 L of fluid daily.
○ Institute safety precautions.
○ Schedule frequent rest periods.
○ Provide comfort measures.
○ Give prescribed drugs.
○ Help the patient turn and reposition every 2 hours.
○ Support affected limbs with pillows.
○ Offer emotional support.
○ Help the patient develop effective coping strategies.
After parathyroidectomy
○ Keep a tracheotomy tray and endotracheal tube setup at the bedside.
○ Maintain seizure precautions.
○ Place the patient in semi-Fowler's position.
○ Support the patient's head and neck with sandbags.
○ Have the patient ambulate as soon as possible.

▶ **ALERT** *Listen for complaints of tingling in the hands and around the mouth. If these symptoms don't subside quickly, they may be prodromal*

signs of tetany, so keep I.V. calcium gluconate or calcium chloride available for emergency use.

Drug therapy

Primary disease
○ Bisphosphonates
○ Calcitonin
○ Oral sodium or potassium phosphate
○ Plicamycin if primary disease is metastatic
Secondary disease
○ Aluminum hydroxide
○ Glucocorticoids
○ Vitamin D therapy
After surgery
○ I.V. magnesium and phosphate
○ Sodium phosphate
○ Supplemental calcium
○ Vitamin D or calcitriol

Monitoring

○ Cardiovascular status
○ Intake and output
○ Respiratory status
○ Serum calcium levels
○ Vital signs
After parathyroidectomy
○ Chvostek's sign
○ Complications
○ Increased neuromuscular irritability
○ Neck edema
○ Trousseau's sign

Patient teaching

Be sure to cover:
○ the disorder, diagnosis, and treatment
○ prescribed drugs, dosages, and possible adverse effects
○ when to notify a doctor
○ the signs and symptoms of tetany, respiratory distress, and renal dysfunction
○ the need for periodic blood tests
○ avoidance of calcium-containing antacids and thiazide diuretics
○ the need for medical identification.

Discharge planning

○ Refer the patient to an endocrinologist, as appropriate.

Hyperphosphatemia

Overview

Description
- Excessive serum phosphate levels
- Reflects the kidney's inability to excrete excess phosphorus

Pathophysiology
- Phosphorus exists mainly in inorganic combination with calcium in teeth and bones.
- In extracellular fluid, phosphate ions support several metabolic functions: use of B vitamins, acid-base homeostasis, bone formation, nerve and muscle activity, cell division, transmission of hereditary traits, and metabolism of carbohydrates, proteins, and fats.
- Renal tubular reabsorption of phosphate is inversely regulated by calcium levels — an increase in phosphorus causes a decrease in calcium. An imbalance causes hypophosphatemia or hyperphosphatemia.

Risk factors
- Chemotherapy
- Heatstroke
- Infection
- Muscle necrosis
- Trauma

Causes
- Acid-base imbalance
- Certain drugs (See *Drugs and supplements that cause hyperphosphatemia.*)
- Hypervitaminosis D
- Hypocalcemia
- Hypoparathyroidism
- Overuse of laxatives with phosphates or phosphate enemas
- Renal failure

Prevalence
- Occurs most commonly in children, who tend to consume more phosphorus-rich foods and beverages than adults
- More common in children and adults with renal insufficiency

---

Drugs and supplements that cause hyperphosphatemia

These drugs may cause hyperphosphatemia:
- enemas, such as Fleet enemas
- laxatives that contain phosphorus or phosphate
- oral phosphorus supplements
- parenteral phosphorus supplements (sodium phosphate, potassium phosphate)
- vitamin D supplements.

Complications
- Acute hyopcalcemia
- Tetany
- Calcium-phosphate deposits in major organs, bones, joints, subcutaneous tissue, soft tissue, or eyes

Assessment

History
- Anorexia
- Decreased mental status
- Nausea and vomiting

Physical assessment
- Abdominal spasm
- Conjunctivitis
- Hyperreflexia
- Hypocalcemic electrocardiogram changes
- Muscle weakness and cramps
- Papular eruptions
- Paresthesia
- Presence of Chvostek's or Trousseau's sign
- Tetany
- Visual impairment

Test results
Laboratory
- Serum phosphorus level higher than 4.5 mg/dl
- Serum calcium level lower than 8.9 mg/dl
- Increased blood urea nitrogen level
- Increased creatinine level

Imaging
- X-ray studies may reveal skeletal changes caused by osteodystrophy in chronic hyperphosphatemia.

Diagnostic procedures
- Electrocardiography may show changes characteristic of hypercalcemia.

Nursing diagnoses

- Anxiety
- Deficient knowledge (hyperphosphatemia)
- Impaired gas exchange
- Risk for deficient fluid volume

Key outcomes
The patient will:
- maintain a patent airway
- maintain adequate vital signs
- have a normal phosphorus level
- express understanding of the condition and treatment
- maintain a low-phosphorus diet
- maintain fluid volume balance.

Foods high in phosphorus

These foods have a high phosphorus content:
- beans
- bran
- cheese
- chocolate
- dark-colored sodas
- ice cream
- lentils
- milk
- nuts
- peanut butter
- seeds
- yogurt.

Discharge planning

○ Refer the patient to a dietitian and social services, if indicated.

Interventions

General

○ Activity, as tolerated
○ Discontinuation of drugs linked to hyperphosphatemia
○ I.V. saline solution
○ Low-phosphorus diet
○ Peritoneal dialysis or hemodialysis (if severe)
○ Treatment of the underlying cause

Nursing

○ Provide safety measures.
○ Be alert for signs of hypocalcemia.
○ Give prescribed drugs.
○ Give antacids with meals to increase their effectiveness.
○ Prepare the patient for dialysis, if appropriate.
○ Assist with selecting a low-phosphorus diet.

Drug therapy

○ Aluminum
○ Calcium gel
○ Magnesium
○ Phosphate-binding antacids

Monitoring

○ Calcium and phosphorus levels
○ Intake and output
○ Renal studies
○ Vital signs

Patient teaching

Be sure to cover:
○ the disorder and treatment
○ prescribed drugs, dosages, and possible adverse effects
○ avoidance of products that contain phosphorus
○ avoidance of high-phosphorus foods. (See *Foods high in phosphorus.*)

Hypertension

Overview

Description

- Intermittent or sustained increase in systolic blood pressure, diastolic blood pressure, or both
- Usually begins as benign disease, slowly progressing to accelerated or malignant state
- Two major types
  - Essential hypertension, also called primary or idiopathic hypertension
  - Secondary hypertension, which results from renal disease or another identifiable cause
- Occurs in stages
  - *Prehypertension:* systolic blood pressure 120 to 139 mm Hg or diastolic blood pressure 80 to 89 mm Hg
  - *Stage 1:* systolic blood pressure 140 to 159 mm Hg or diastolic blood pressure 90 to 99 mm Hg
  - *Stage 2:* systolic blood pressure 160 mm Hg or higher or diastolic blood pressure 100 mm Hg or higher
- Malignant hypertension
  - A medical emergency
  - A severe, fulminant form of hypertension
  - Commonly arises from essential and secondary hypertension

Pathophysiology

- Several theories:
  - Changes in the arteriolar bed increase peripheral vascular resistance.
  - Abnormally increased tone in the sympathetic nervous system (originating in the vasomotor system centers) increases peripheral vascular resistance.
  - Renal or hormonal dysfunction causes increased blood volume.
  - An increase in arteriolar thickening (caused by genetic factors) increases peripheral vascular resistance.
  - Abnormal renin release causes formation of angiotensin II, which constricts arterioles and increases blood volume.

Risk factors

- Aging
- Excessive alcohol intake
- Family history
- High-sodium, high–saturated-fat diet
- Hormonal contraceptive use
- Obesity
- Sedentary lifestyle
- Smoking
- Stress

Causes

- Unknown

Prevalence

- Affects 15% to 20% of adults in the United States
- Essential hypertension: 90% to 95% of cases

Complications

- Blindness
- Cardiac disease
- Cerebrovascular accident
- Renal failure

Assessment

History

- Commonly no symptoms
- Discovered incidentally during evaluation for another disorder or during a routine blood pressure screening program
- Symptoms that reflect the effect of hypertension on the organ systems
- Awakening with a headache in the occipital region, which subsides spontaneously after a few hours
- Dizziness, fatigue, confusion
- Palpitations, chest pain, dyspnea
- Epistaxis
- Hematuria
- Blurred vision

Physical assessment

- Bounding pulse
- Bruits over the abdominal aorta and femoral arteries or the carotids
- Elevated blood pressure readings on at least two consecutive occasions after initial screenings
- Hemorrhages, exudates, and papilledema of the eye in late stages if hypertensive retinopathy present
- Peripheral edema (late stages)
- Pulsating abdominal mass, suggesting an abdominal aneurysm
- S_4 sound

Test results

Laboratory

- Protein, red blood cells, or white blood cells in urine, suggesting renal disease
- Glucose in urine, suggesting diabetes mellitus
- Serum potassium levels less than 3.5 mEq/L, possibly indicating adrenal dysfunction (primary hyperaldosteronism)

▼ **ALERT** *If the patient has serum potassium levels less than 3.5 mEq/L, monitor electrocardiogram tracings because these levels may potentiate cardiac arrhythmias.*

- Blood urea nitrogen levels normal or higher than 20 mg/dl, suggesting renal disease
- Serum creatinine levels normal or higher than 1.5 mg/dl, suggesting renal disease

Imaging
○ Excretory urography may reveal renal atrophy, indicating chronic renal disease; one kidney more than 5/8″ (1.6 cm) shorter than the other suggests unilateral renal disease.
○ Chest X-rays may show cardiomegaly.

Diagnostic procedures
○ Electrocardiography may show left ventricular hypertrophy or ischemia.
○ Renal arteriography may show renal artery stenosis.
○ An oral captopril challenge may be done to test for renovascular hypertension.
○ Ophthalmoscopy reveals arteriovenous nicking and, in hypertensive encephalopathy, edema.

Nursing diagnoses

○ Decreased cardiac output
○ Ineffective tissue perfusion: cardiopulmonary, peripheral, renal, cerebral, gastrointestinal
○ Noncompliance with medication regimen
○ Risk for activity intolerance

Key outcomes
The patient will:
○ maintain adequate cardiac output
○ maintain hemodynamic stability
○ develop no arrhythmias
○ express feelings of increased energy
○ comply with the therapy regimen.

Interventions

General
○ For a patient with secondary hypertension, correction of the underlying cause and control of hypertensive effects
○ Diet containing adequate calcium, magnesium, and potassium
○ Diet low in saturated fat and sodium
○ Lifestyle modification, such as weight control, limiting alcohol, regular exercise, and smoking cessation

Nursing
○ Give prescribed drugs.
○ Encourage dietary changes, as needed.
○ Help the patient identify risk factors and modify his lifestyle, as appropriate.

Drug therapy
○ Aldosterone antagonist
○ Alpha blockers
○ Angiotensin-converting enzyme inhibitors
○ Angiotensin II–receptor blockers
○ Beta blockers
○ Calcium channel blockers
○ Diuretics
○ Vasodilators

Monitoring
○ Adverse effects of antihypertensive drugs
○ Complications
○ Signs and symptoms of target end-organ damage
○ Response to treatment
○ Risk factor modification
○ Vital signs, especially blood pressure

Patient teaching

Be sure to cover:
○ the disorder, diagnosis, and treatment
○ how to use a self-monitoring blood pressure cuff and record the reading in a journal for review by a doctor
○ importance of compliance with antihypertensive therapy and establishing a daily routine for taking prescribed drugs
○ the need to report adverse drug effects
○ the need to avoid high-sodium antacids and over-the-counter cold and sinus medications containing vasoconstrictors
○ examining and modifying lifestyle, including diet
○ the need for a routine exercise program, particularly aerobic walking
○ dietary restrictions
○ the importance of follow-up care.

Discharge planning

○ Refer the patient to stress-reduction therapies, support groups, and smoking cessation programs as needed.
○ Refer the patient to a nutritionist, if indicated.

Hypocalcemia

Overview

Description
○ Calcium level below 8.9 mg/dl or ionized calcium level below 4.5 mg/dl

Pathophysiology
○ Together with phosphorous, calcium is responsible for the formation and structure of bones and teeth.
○ Calcium helps maintain cell structure and function.
○ It plays a role in cell membrane permeability and impulse transmission.
○ It affects the contraction of cardiac muscle, smooth muscle, and skeletal muscle.
○ It also participates in the blood-clotting process.

Causes
○ Hypomagnesemia
○ Hypoparathyroidism
○ Inadequate dietary intake of calcium and vitamin D
○ Malabsorption or loss of calcium from the gastrointestinal tract
○ Overcorrection of acidosis
○ Pancreatic insufficiency
○ Renal failure
○ Severe infections or burns
○ Drugs such as calcitonin and mithramycin that decrease calcium resorption from the bone

Prevalence
○ Occurs equally in males and females
○ Affects all ages

Complications
○ Cardiac arrhythmia
○ Laryngeal spasm
○ Respiratory arrest
○ Seizures

Assessment

History
○ Anxiety
○ Brittle nails, dry skin and hair
○ Diarrhea
○ Fractures
○ Irritability
○ Muscle cramps
○ Seizures
○ Underlying cause

Physical assessment
○ Carpopedal spasm
○ Confusion
○ Hypotension
○ Perioral paresthesia
○ Positive Chvostek's and Trousseau's signs (See *Checking for Trousseau's and Chvostek's signs.*)
○ Tetany
○ Twitching

Test results
Laboratory
○ Serum calcium levels less than 8.5 mg/dl
○ Ionized calcium levels less than 4.5 mg/dl
Diagnostic procedures
○ Depending on cause, electrocardiography may show arrhythmias.

Checking for Trousseau's and Chvostek's signs

Trousseau's and Chvostek's signs can aid in the diagnosis of tetany and hypocalcemia. Here's how to assess your patient for these important signs.

Trousseau's sign
To check for Trousseau's sign, apply a blood pressure cuff to the patient's upper arm and inflate it to 20 mm Hg above the patient's systolic pressure. Trousseau's sign may appear after 1 to 4 minutes. The patient will experience an adducted thumb, flexed wrist and metacarpophalangeal joints, and extended interphalangeal joints (with fingers together) — carpopedal spasm — indicating tetany, a major sign of hypocalcemia.

Chvostek's sign
You can induce Chvostek's sign by tapping the patient's facial nerve next to the ear. A brief contraction of the upper lip, nose, or side of the face indicates Chvostek's sign.

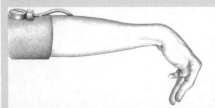

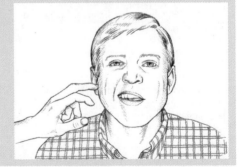

Nursing diagnoses

○ Acute confusion
○ Anxiety
○ Decreased cardiac output
○ Disturbed thought process
○ Risk for deficient fluid volume
○ Risk for falls

Key outcomes

The patient will:
○ maintain stable vital signs
○ maintain adequate cardiac output
○ express an understanding of the disorder and its treatment
○ maintain fluid volume balance.

Interventions

General

○ Treatment of the underlying cause
○ Diet high in calcium and vitamin D

AGE AWARE A breast-fed infant may have low calcium and vitamin D levels if his mother's intake is inadequate. Assess the mother for adequate intake and exposure to sunlight.

○ Activity, as tolerated

Nursing

○ Provide safety measures.
○ Institute seizure precautions, if appropriate.
○ Reorient the patient as needed.
○ Give prescribed calcium replacement.

ALERT Dilute I.V. calcium preparations in dextrose 5% in water because normal saline solution can increase renal calcium loss. Dilution in a bicarbonate solution will cause precipitation. Give calcium slowly because rapid delivery may cause syncope, hypotension, and arrhythmias.

○ Assess I.V. sites if giving calcium I.V. because infiltration causes necrosis and sloughing.
○ Assess the patient's ability to perform activities of daily living, and assist as needed.

Drug therapy

○ Calcium gluconate I.V.
○ Oral calcium and vitamin D supplements

Monitoring

○ Cardiac rhythm
○ Respiratory status
○ Seizures
○ Serum calcium levels

Patient teaching

Be sure to cover:
○ taking calcium supplements 1 to 1½ hours after meals
○ the need to follow a high-calcium diet
○ foods high in calcium
○ warning signs and symptoms and when to report them
○ the importance of exercise to prevent calcium loss from bones.

Discharge planning

○ Refer the patient to a nutritionist and social services, if indicated.

Hypochloremia

Overview

Description
○ Serum chloride levels below 98 mEq/L
○ Possible changes in levels of sodium, potassium, calcium, and other electrolytes
○ Possible metabolic alkalosis if bicarbonate levels rise to compensate for decreased chloride levels (See *How hypochloremia can lead to metabolic alkalosis.*)

Pathophysiology
○ Chloride accounts for two-thirds of all serum anions.
○ Chloride is secreted by the stomach's mucosa as hydrochloric acid; it provides an acid medium that aids digestion and activation of enzymes.
○ It helps maintain acid-base and body water balances, influences the osmolality or tonicity of extracellular fluid, plays a role in the exchange of oxygen and carbon dioxide in red blood cells, and helps activate salivary amylase (which, in turn, activates the digestive process).

Risk factors
○ Cystic fibrosis
○ Draining fistula
○ Heart failure
○ Ileostomy
○ Pyloric obstruction

Causes
○ Addison's disease
○ Administration of dextrose I.V. without electrolytes
○ Certain drugs
○ Loss of hydrochloric acid in gastric secretions from vomiting, gastric suctioning, or gastric surgery
○ Prolonged diarrhea or diaphoresis
○ Prolonged use of mercurial diuretics
○ Salt-restricted diets

✳ *AGE AWARE Chloride-deficient formula can be a cause of this disorder in infants.*
○ Untreated diabetic ketoacidosis

Prevalence
○ Depends on underlying cause

Complications
○ Coma
○ Respiratory arrest
○ Seizures

Assessment

History
○ Agitation
○ Irritability
○ Risk factors for low chloride levels

Physical assessment
○ Cardiac arrhythmias, tachycardia
○ Hyperactive deep tendon reflexes
○ Muscle cramps
○ Muscle weakness and twitching
○ Shallow, depressed breathing (with metabolic alkalosis)
○ Tetany

Test results
Laboratory
○ Serum chloride level less than 98 mEq/L
○ Serum sodium level below 135 mEq/L
○ pH above 7.45
○ Carbon dioxide level above 32 mEq/L

Nursing diagnoses

○ Decreased cardiac output
○ Impaired gas exchange
○ Ineffective breathing pattern

How hypochloremia can lead to metabolic alkalosis

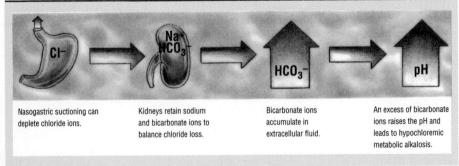

Nasogastric suctioning can deplete chloride ions.

Kidneys retain sodium and bicarbonate ions to balance chloride loss.

Bicarbonate ions accumulate in extracellular fluid.

An excess of bicarbonate ions raises the pH and leads to hypochloremic metabolic alkalosis.

- Risk for deficient fluid volume
- Risk for falls

Key outcomes

The patient will:
- maintain adequate cardiac output
- maintain adequate fluid volume
- maintain stable vital signs
- avoid complications.

Interventions

General

- Activity, as tolerated
- High-sodium diet
- Treatment of metabolic acidosis or electrolyte imbalances
- Treatment of underlying condition

Nursing

- Offer foods high in chloride.
- Ensure a safe environment.
- Give prescribed I.V. fluids, drugs, and supplements.

Drug therapy

- Ammonium chloride
- Normal saline solution I.V.
- Potassium chloride (for metabolic acidosis)

Monitoring

- Arterial blood gas levels
- Cardiac rhythm
- Level of consciousness
- Muscle strength and movement
- Respiratory status
- Serum electrolyte levels
- Signs of metabolic alkalosis
- Vital signs

Patient teaching

Be sure to cover:
- the disorder, diagnosis, and treatment
- signs and symptoms of electrolyte imbalance
- dietary supplements
- prescribed drugs.

Discharge planning

- Refer the patient to a physical therapist and nutritionist, as needed.

Hypokalemia

 ALERT *Before giving digoxin, check the patient's serum digoxin and potassium levels. Hypokalemia can potentiate digoxin toxicity.*

Overview

Description

○ Serum potassium level less than 3.5 mEq/L
○ Narrow normal range for serum potassium level: 3.5 to 5 mEq/L

 ALERT *A slight decrease in potassium levels can have profound clinical consequences.*

Pathophysiology

○ Potassium facilitates contraction of skeletal and smooth muscles, including myocardial muscle.
○ This anion figures prominently in nerve impulse conduction, acid-base balance, enzyme action, and cell membrane function.
○ Potassium imbalance can lead to muscle weakness and flaccid paralysis because of an ionic imbalance in neuromuscular tissue excitability.

Causes

○ Acid-base imbalances
○ Certain drugs
  – Corticosteroids
  – Potassium-wasting diuretics
  – Some sodium-containing antibiotics (such as carbenicillin)
○ Chronic renal disease and tubular potassium wasting
○ Cushing's syndrome
○ Excessive ingestion of licorice
○ Excessive gastrointestinal or urinary losses
  – Anorexia
  – Chronic laxative abuse
  – Dehydration
  – Diarrhea
  – Gastric suction
  – Vomiting
○ Hyperglycemia
○ Low-potassium diet
○ Primary hyperaldosteronism
○ Prolonged potassium-free I.V. therapy
○ Severe serum magnesium deficiency
○ Trauma, as from injury, burns, or surgery

Prevalence

○ Affects up to 20% of hospitalized patients (significant in about 4% to 5% of these patients)
○ Affects up to 14% of outpatients mildly
○ Affects about 80% of patients who receive diuretics
○ Males and females affected equally

Complications

○ Cardiac arrest
○ Cardiac arrhythmia
○ Digoxin toxicity
○ Rhabdomyolysis

Assessment

History

○ Abdominal cramps
○ Anorexia
○ Constipation
○ Muscle weakness
○ Nausea, vomiting
○ Paresthesia
○ Polyuria

Physical assessment

○ Decreased bowel sounds
○ Hyporeflexia
○ Orthostatic hypotension
○ Weak, irregular pulse

Test results

Laboratory

○ Serum potassium levels less than 3.5 mEq/L
○ Increased pH and bicarbonate levels
○ Slightly increased serum glucose level

Diagnostic procedures

○ Characteristic electrocardiogram changes include a flattened T wave, depressed ST segment, and U wave.

Nursing diagnoses

○ Constipation
○ Decreased cardiac output
○ Nausea
○ Risk for activity intolerance
○ Risk for deficient fluid volume

Key outcomes

The patient will:
○ maintain hemodynamic stability
○ maintain a normal potassium level
○ understand potential adverse effects of medications
○ express understanding of high-potassium foods
○ maintain fluid volume balance.

Interventions

General

○ Activity, as tolerated
○ High-potassium diet
○ Treatment of the underlying cause

Nursing

○ Give prescribed drugs.
○ Implement safety measures.

Guidelines for I.V. potassium administration

Following are some guidelines for giving I.V. potassium and for monitoring patients receiving it. Remember that potassium only needs to be replaced I.V. if hypokalemia is severe or the patient can't take oral potassium supplements.

Administration

- When adding the potassium preparation to an I.V. solution, mix it well. Don't add it to a hanging container; the potassium will pool, and the patient will receive a highly concentrated bolus. Use premixed potassium when possible.
- To prevent or reduce toxic effects, I.V. infusion concentrations shouldn't exceed 40 to 60 mEq/L. Rates are usually 10 mEq/hour. More rapid infusions may be used in severe cases; they demand closer monitoring of the patient's cardiac status. The maximum adult dose typically shouldn't exceed 200 mEq/24 hours unless prescribed.
- Use an infusion device to control the flow rate.
- Never give potassium by I.V. push or bolus; doing so can cause cardiac arrhythmias and cardiac arrest.

Patient monitoring

- Monitor the patient's cardiac rhythm during rapid I.V. potassium delivery to prevent toxic effects from hyperkalemia. Report any irregularities immediately.
- Evaluate the results of treatment by checking serum potassium levels and assessing the patient for evidence of a toxic reaction, such as muscle weakness and paralysis.
- Watch the I.V. site for evidence of infiltration, phlebitis, or tissue necrosis.
- Monitor the patient's urine output, and notify the doctor if volume is inadequate. To avoid hyperkalemia, urine output should exceed 30 ml/hour.

○ Be alert for signs of hyperkalemia after treatment.
○ Give I.V. fluids.

Drug therapy

○ Potassium chloride (I.V. or P.O.)

ALERT I.V. potassium supplements must be diluted and given with caution to prevent serious complications, such as cardiac arrest. (See Guidelines for I.V. potassium administration.)

ALERT A patient taking a potassium-wasting diuretic may be switched to a potassium-sparing diuretic to prevent excessive urinary loss of potassium.

Monitoring

○ Cardiac rhythm
○ Intake and output
○ Respiratory status
○ Serum potassium levels
○ Vital signs

Patient teaching

Be sure to cover:
○ the disorder, diagnosis, and treatment
○ prescribed drugs, dosages, and possible adverse effects
○ monitoring of intake and output
○ prevention of future episodes of hypokalemia
○ need for and components of a high-potassium diet
○ warning signs and symptoms to report to the doctor.

Discharge planning

○ Refer the patient to a nutritionist, if needed.

Hypomagnesemia

Overview

Description
○ Serum magnesium levels less than 1.5 mEq/L

Pathophysiology
○ Magnesium enhances neuromuscular integration and stimulates parathyroid hormone secretion, thus regulating intracellular fluid calcium levels.
○ It also may regulate skeletal muscles through its influence on calcium use by depressing acetylcholine release at synaptic junctions.
○ Magnesium activates many enzymes for carbohydrate and protein metabolism, aids in cell metabolism and the transport of sodium and potassium across cell membranes, and influences sodium, potassium, calcium, and protein levels.
○ About one-third of magnesium taken into the body is absorbed through the small intestine and is eventually excreted in urine; the remaining unabsorbed magnesium is excreted in stool.

Causes
○ Administration of parenteral fluids without magnesium salts
○ Certain drugs
  – Aminoglucoside antibiotics
  – Amphotericin B
  – Cisplatin
  – Insulin
  – Laxatives
  – Loop or thiazide diuretics
  – Pentamidine isethionate
○ Chronic alcoholism
○ Chronic diarrhea
○ Diabetic acidosis
○ Excessive release of adrenocortical hormones
○ Hyperaldosteronism
○ Hypercalcemia
○ Hyperparathyroidism
○ Hypoparathyroidism
○ Malabsorption syndrome
○ Nasogastric suctioning
○ Postoperative complications after bowel resection
○ Prolonged diuretic therapy
○ Severe dehydration
○ Starvation or malnutrition

Prevalence
○ Occurs in 10% to 20% of hospitalized patients
○ Occurs in 50% to 60% of patients in the intensive care unit
○ Occurs in 25% of outpatients with diabetes
○ Occurs in 30% to 80% of alcoholics
○ Affects males and females equally

Complications
○ Cardiac arrest
○ Cardiac arrhythmia
○ Laryngeal stridor
○ Respiratory depression
○ Seizures

Assessment

History
○ Altered level of consciousness
○ Anorexia
○ Drowsiness
○ Dysphagia
○ Leg and foot cramps
○ Nausea
○ Vomiting

Physical assessment
○ Cardiac arrhythmia
○ Chvostek's and Trousseau's signs
○ Hyperactive deep tendon reflexes
○ Hypertension
○ Muscle weakness, tremors, twitching
○ Tachycardia

Test results
Laboratory
○ Serum magnesium levels less than 1.5 mEq/L
○ Other electrolyte abnormalities, such as decreased potassium or calcium levels
Diagnostic procedures
○ Electrocardiography shows abnormalities, such as a prolonged QT interval and atrioventricular block.

Nursing diagnoses

○ Acute confusion
○ Imbalanced nutrition: less than body requirements
○ Impaired swallowing
○ Risk for activity intolerance
○ Risk for fluid volume deficit

Key outcomes
The patient will:
○ maintain hemodynamic stability
○ maintain a normal magnesium level
○ understand the causes of high magnesium levels
○ swallow effectively
○ maintain adequate nutritional intake
○ maintain fluid volume balance.

Interventions

General

○ Activity, as tolerated
○ Dietary replacement of magnesium
○ Treatment of the underlying cause

Nursing

○ Institute seizure precautions.
○ Give prescribed drugs.
○ Report abnormal serum electrolyte levels right away.

▼ **ALERT** *A low magnesium level may increase the body's retention of a cardiac glycoside. Be alert for signs of digoxin toxicity if your patient takes digoxin.*

○ Ensure patient safety.
○ Reorient the patient as needed.
○ Keep emergency equipment nearby for airway protection.

Drug therapy

○ Magnesium oxide
○ Magnesium sulfate (I.M. or I.V.)

▼ **ALERT** *Infuse magnesium sulfate I.V. at no more than 150 mg/minute. Infusing it too rapidly can lead to cardiac arrest.*

Monitoring

○ Aspiration risk
○ Cardiac rhythm
○ Deep tendon reflexes (See *Grading deep tendon reflexes.*)
○ Electrolyte levels
○ Intake and output
○ Level of consciousness
○ Magnesium levels
○ Respiratory status
○ Vital signs

Patient teaching

Be sure to cover:
○ the disorder, diagnosis, and treatment
○ prescribed drugs
○ the need to avoid drugs that deplete magnesium, such as diuretics and laxatives
○ the need to adhere to a high-magnesium diet
○ food high in magnesium
○ danger signs and when to report them.

Grading deep tendon reflexes

If you think your patient has hypomagnesemia, you'll want to test his deep tendon reflexes (DTRs) to determine whether his neuromuscular system is irritable — a clue that his magnesium level is too low. When grading your patient's DTRs, use the following scale:

0	Absent
+	Present but diminished
++	Normal
+++	Increased but not necessarily abnormal
++++	Hyperactive, clonic

To record the patient's reflex activity, draw a stick figure and mark the strength of the response at the proper locations. This figure shows normal DTR activity.

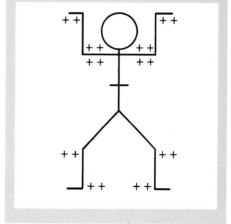

Discharge planning

○ Refer the patient to Alcoholics Anonymous if appropriate.
○ Refer the patient to a nutritionist and for a swallowing evaluation and exercises, if needed.

Hyponatremia

Overview

Description
○ Serum sodium level less than 135 mEq/L

Pathophysiology
○ Sodium is the major cation (90%) in extracellular fluid.
○ During repolarization, the sodium-potassium pump continually shifts sodium into the cells and potassium out of the cells; during depolarization, it does the reverse.
○ Sodium cations have many functions, including maintaining:
   – the tonicity and concentration of extracellular fluid
   – acid-base balance (reabsorption of sodium ions and excretion of hydrogen ions)
   – nerve conduction
   – neuromuscular function
   – glandular secretion
   – water balance.

Causes
○ Adrenal gland insufficiency (Addison's disease) or hypoaldosteronism
○ Burns
○ Certain drugs
   – Chlorpropamide
   – Clofibrate
○ Cirrhosis of the liver with ascites
○ Diarrhea
○ Excessive sweating
○ Excessive water intake
○ Fever
○ Infusion of I.V. dextrose in water without other solutes
○ Low-sodium diet, usually with one of the other causes
○ Malnutrition or starvation
○ Suctioning
○ Surgery, including wound drainage
○ Syndrome of inappropriate antidiuretic hormone (SIADH) from various causes
   – Brain tumor
   – Cerebrovascular accident
   – Pulmonary disease
   – Neoplasm with ectopic antidiuretic hormone production
○ Tap water enemas
○ Traumatic injury
○ Use of potent diuretics
○ Vomiting

Prevalence
○ Occurs in about 1% of hospitalized patients
○ More common in the very young and very old
○ Affects males and females equally

Complications
○ Coma
○ Permanent neurological damage
○ Respiratory difficulty
○ Seizures

Assessment

History
○ Abdominal cramps
○ Altered level of consciousness
○ Headache
○ Muscle weakness and twitching
○ Nausea

Physical assessment
○ Dry mucous membranes
○ Orthostatic hypotension
○ Poor skin turgor
○ Rales or crackles
○ Rapid, bounding pulse

Test results
Laboratory
○ Serum sodium level lower than 135 mEq/L
○ Urine specific gravity less than 1.010
○ Serum osmolality less than 280 mOsm/kg (dilute blood)
○ In SIADH: increased urine specific gravity and elevated urine sodium level (0.20 mEq/L)

Nursing diagnoses

○ Acute confusion
○ Decreased cardiac output
○ Impaired oral mucous membrane
○ Ineffective breathing pattern
○ Nausea
○ Risk for injury

Key outcomes
The patient will:
○ maintain adequate fluid volume
○ maintain a normal sodium level
○ maintain stable vital signs
○ remain alert and oriented to the environment.

Interventions

General
○ Activity, as tolerated
○ High-sodium diet
○ Restricted fluid intake
○ Treatment of the underlying cause

Nursing

- ○ Restrict fluid intake.
- ○ Give prescribed I.V. fluids.
- ○ Provide a safe environment.
- ○ Institute seizure precautions, if needed.

Drug therapy

- ○ Demeclocycline or lithium
- ○ Hypertonic (3% or 5%) saline solutions (with serum sodium levels below 110 mEq/L)
- ○ Normal saline solution
- ○ Oral sodium supplements

▼ **ALERT** *Monitor the patient carefully while giving hypertonic saline solutions. They can cause water to shift out of cells, which may lead to intravascular volume overload and serious brain damage.*

Monitoring

- ○ Daily weights
- ○ Intake and output
- ○ Neurological status
- ○ Serum sodium levels
- ○ Urine specific gravity
- ○ Vital signs

Patient teaching

Be sure to cover:
- ○ the disorder, diagnosis, and treatment
- ○ drug therapy, dosages, and possible adverse effects
- ○ dietary changes and fluid restrictions
- ○ monitoring daily weight
- ○ signs and symptoms to report to the doctor.

Discharge planning

- ○ Refer the patient to a nutritionist, if needed.

Hypoparathyroidism

Overview

Description

- Deficiency of parathyroid hormone (PTH) secretion by the parathyroid glands or decreased action of PTH in the periphery
- Neuromuscular symptoms ranging from paresthesia to tetany (because parathyroid glands mainly regulate calcium balance)
- May be acute or chronic
- Classified as idiopathic, acquired, or reversible

Pathophysiology

- PTH normally maintains serum calcium levels by increasing bone resorption and by stimulating renal conversion of vitamin D to its active form, which enhances gastrointestinal absorption of calcium and bone resorption.
- PTH also maintains the inverse relationship between serum calcium and phosphate levels by inhibiting phosphate reabsorption in the renal tubules and enhancing calcium reabsorption.
- Abnormal PTH production in hypoparathyroidism disrupts this delicate balance.

Causes

Idiopathic
- Autoimmune genetic disorder
- Congenital absence or malformation of the parathyroid glands

Acquired
- Accidental removal of or injury to one or more parathyroid glands during surgery
- Amyloidosis
- Hemochromatosis
- Ischemia or infarction of the parathyroid glands during surgery
- Neoplasms
- Sarcoidosis
- Traumatic injury to one or more parathyroid glands
- Tuberculosis

Acquired, reversible
- Hypomagnesemia-induced impairment of hormone secretion
- Suppression of normal gland function by hypercalcemia
- Delayed maturation of parathyroid function
- Abnormalities of the calcium-sensor receptor

Prevalence

- Idiopathic and reversible forms most common in children
- Acquired form most common in older patients who have undergone thyroid surgery

Complications

- Bone deformities

 AGE AWARE *Hypoparathyroidism that develops during childhood results in malformed teeth.*

- Cataracts
- Death
- Heart failure
- Increased intracranial pressure
- Irreversible calcification of basal ganglia
- Laryngospasm, respiratory stridor, anoxia
- Seizures
- Tetany
- Vocal cord paralysis

Assessment

History

- Alcoholism
- Constipation or diarrhea
- Difficulty walking and a tendency to fall
- Dysphagia
- Fatigue
- Feeling of throat constriction
- Malabsorption disorders
- Muscle tension and spasms
- Nausea, vomiting, abdominal pain
- Neck surgery or irradiation
- Personality changes
- Tingling in the fingertips, around the mouth, and, occasionally, in the feet

Physical assessment

- Brittle nails
- Coarse hair, alopecia
- Dry skin
- Increased deep tendon reflexes
- Irregular, slow or rapid pulse
- Loss of eyelashes and fingernails
- Positive Chvostek's and Trousseau's signs
- Stained, cracked, and decayed teeth
- Tetany
- Transverse and longitudinal ridges in the fingernails

Test results

Laboratory
- Decreased radioimmunoassay for PTH
- Decreased serum and urine calcium levels
- Increased serum phosphate levels
- Decreased urine creatinine levels

Imaging
- Computed tomography scan may show frontal lobe and basal ganglia calcifications.
- X-rays may show increased bone density and bone malformation.

Diagnostic procedures
- Electrocardiography shows a prolonged QT and ST interval.

Nursing diagnoses

- Decreased cardiac output
- Ineffective breathing pattern
- Risk for imbalanced fluid volume
- Risk for impaired skin integrity
- Risk for injury

Key outcomes

The patient will:
- maintain normal cardiac output
- maintain stable vital signs
- maintain adequate ventilation
- maintain intact skin integrity
- verbalize an understanding of the disorder and treatment regimen
- maintain adequate fluid volume.

Interventions

General

- Activity, as tolerated
- High-calcium, low-phosphorus diet
- Restoration of calcium and related mineral balance
- Supportive care for an acute, life-threatening attack or hypoparathyroid tetany

▼ **ALERT** *If a patient with acute, life-threatening tetany is awake and alert, help raise his serum calcium level by having him breathe into a paper bag and inhale his own carbon dioxide.*

- Surgery to treat an underlying cause such as a tumor

Nursing

- Give prescribed drugs.
- Maintain patent I.V. line.
- Keep emergency equipment readily available.
- Maintain seizure precautions.
- Provide meticulous skin care.
- Institute safety precautions.
- Keep a tracheostomy tray and endotracheal tube by the bedside.
- Encourage the patient to express his feelings.
- Offer emotional support.
- Help the patient develop effective coping strategies.

Drug therapy

- Anticonvulsants
- Calcitriol
- Calcium supplementation

▼ **ALERT** *Acute, life-threatening tetany requires I.V. administration of 10% calcium gluconate, 10% calcium glucepate, or 10% calcium chloride to raise serum calcium levels.*

- Sedatives
- Vitamin D

Monitoring

- Chvostek's sign
- Electrocardiogram for QT interval changes and arrhythmias
- Intake and output
- Serum calcium, phosphorus, and, if appropriate, digoxin levels

▼ **ALERT** *Closely monitor a patient receiving digoxin and calcium because calcium potentiates the effect of digoxin. Stay alert for signs of digoxin toxicity.*

- Signs and symptoms of decreased cardiac output
- Trousseau's sign
- Vital signs

Patient teaching

Be sure to cover:
- the disorder, diagnosis, and treatment
- prescribed drugs, dosages, and possible adverse effects
- when to consult a doctor
- follow-up care
- complications
- follow-up monitoring of serum calcium level.

Discharge planning

- Refer the patient to a mental health professional for additional counseling, if needed.

Hypophosphatemia

Overview

Description

- Serum phosphate levels less than 1.7 mEq/L or 2.5 mg/dl

Pathophysiology

- Phosphorus exists mainly in inorganic combination with calcium in teeth and bones.
- In extracellular fluid, phosphate ions support several metabolic functions, including these:
  - utilization of B vitamins
  - acid-base homeostasis
  - bone formation
  - nerve and muscle activity
  - cell division
  - transmission of hereditary traits
  - metabolism of carbohydrates, proteins, and fats.
- Renal tubular reabsorption of phosphate is inversely regulated by calcium levels—an increase in phosphorus causes a decrease in calcium. An imbalance causes hypophosphatemia or hyperphosphatemia.

Causes

- Chronic diarrhea
- Diabetic acidosis
- Hyperparathyroidism and resulting hypercalcemia
- Hypomagnesemia
- Inadequate dietary intake
- Intestinal malabsorption
- Long-term use of antacids containing aluminum hydroxide
- Malnutrition from a prolonged catabolic state or chronic alcoholism
- Renal tubular defects
- Tissue damage in which phosphorus is released by injured cells
- Use of parenteral nutrition solution with inadequate phosphate content
- Vitamin D deficiency

AGE AWARE *Elderly patients have an increased risk of altered electrolyte levels for two main reasons. First, they have a decreased ratio of lean body mass to total body mass, which places them at risk for water deficit. Second, their thirst response is decreased and renal function is decreased, which makes maintaining electrolyte balance more difficult.*

Prevalence

- Varies according to the underlying cause

Complications

- Arrhythmias
- Coma
- Heart failure
- Rhabdomyolysis
- Seizures
- Shock

Assessment

History

- Anorexia
- Chest pain
- Fractures
- Memory loss
- Muscle and bone pain

Physical assessment

- Bruising and bleeding
- Confusion
- Muscle weakness
- Paresthesia
- Peripheral hypoxia
- Tremor and weakness in speaking voice
- Tremors

Test results

Laboratory

- Serum phosphorus levels less than 1.7 mEq/L or 2.5 mg/dl
- Urine phosphorus levels above 1.3 g/24 hours

Nursing diagnoses

- Acute pain
- Impaired memory
- Impaired nutrition: less than body requirements
- Ineffective breathing pattern
- Risk for deficient fluid volume
- Risk for injury

Key outcomes

The patient will:

- maintain a patent airway
- maintain adequate vital signs
- maintain a normal phosphorus level
- maintain fluid volume balance.

Interventions

General

- Activity, as tolerated
- High-phosphorus diet
- Stopping drugs that may cause hypophosphatemia
- Treatment of the underlying cause

Nursing

- Provide safety measures.
- Give prescribed phosphorus replacement.
- Assist with ambulation and activities of daily living.

Drug therapy

○ Phosphate salt tablets or capsules
○ Potassium or sodium phosphate I.V.

Monitoring

○ Calcium level
○ Intake and output
○ Neurological status
○ Phosphorus level
○ Respiratory status

Patient teaching

Be sure to cover:
○ proper administration of phosphorus supplements
○ the need to follow a high-phosphorus diet
○ sources of phosphorus.

Discharge planning

○ Refer the patient to a nutritionist and social services, if indicated.

Kidney cancer

Overview

Description
- Proliferation of cancer cells in the kidney
- 85%: origination in kidneys
- 15%: metastasis from a primary site
- Also called nephrocarcinoma, renal carcinoma, hypernephroma, and Grawitz's tumor

Pathophysiology
- Most kidney tumors share certain characteristics, including these:
  - large size
  - firm texture
  - nodular
  - encapsulated
  - unilateral
  - solitary.
- Kidney cancer may affect either kidney; occasionally, tumors are bilateral or multifocal.
- Renal cancers arise from the tubular epithelium.
- Tumor margins are usually clearly defined.
- Tumors can include areas of ischemia, necrosis, and focal hemorrhage.
- Tumor cells may be well differentiated to anaplastic.
- Kidney cancer can be separated histologically into several types, including these:
  - clear cell type
  - granular cell type
  - spindle cell type.
- Prognosis depends more on the cancer's stage than on its type.
- Typically, patients with the clear cell type have a better prognosis than patients with the other types.
- The overall prognosis has improved considerably in recent years, with a 5-year survival rate of about 50%.

Risk factors
- Heavy cigarette smoking
- Regular hemodialysis treatments

Causes
- Unknown

Prevalence
- Accounts for about 2% of all adult cancers
- Twice as common in men as in women
- Usually occurs in older adults

✳ *AGE AWARE Kidney cancer is most common in people between ages 50 and 60. Renal pelvic tumors and Wilms' tumor are most common in children.*

Complications
- Hemorrhage
- Metastasis

Assessment

History
- Hematuria
- Dull, aching flank pain
- Nausea and vomiting (advanced disease)

Physical assessment
- Edema in the legs (advanced disease)
- Fever
- Hypertension
- Palpable, smooth, firm, nontender abdominal mass
- Urine retention

Test results
Laboratory
- Increased alkaline phosphatase, bilirubin, and transaminase levels
- Prolonged prothrombin time
- Possible hypercalcemia from ectopic parathyroid hormone production by the tumor

Imaging
- Renal ultrasonography and computed tomography scans can be used to verify renal cancer.
- Excretory urography, nephrotomography, and kidney-ureter-bladder radiography are used to aid diagnosis and help in staging.

Nursing diagnoses
- Chronic pain
- Effective therapeutic regimen management
- Excess fluid volume
- Impaired gas exchange

Key outcomes
The patient will:
- maintain fluid balance
- report increased comfort
- communicate understanding of medical regimen, prescribed drugs, diet, and activity restrictions
- maintain ventilation
- use support services.

Interventions

General
- Low-protein diet
- Radiation (because of radiation resistance, only when cancer has spread into perinephric region or lymph nodes or when primary tumor or metastatic sites can't be completely excised)

○ Radical nephrectomy, with or without regional lymph node dissection (the only chance of cure)

Nursing

○ Give prescribed drugs.
○ Encourage verbalization.
○ Provide support.
○ Prepare patient for diagnostic tests.
○ Provide comfort measures.

Drug therapy

○ Analgesics
○ Biotherapy
  – Lymphokine-activated killer cells
  – Recombinant interleukin-2
○ Chemotherapy (erratically effective)
○ Interferon

Monitoring

○ Adverse drug effects
○ Complete blood count; serum chemistry results
○ Daily weights
○ Intake and output
○ Pain control
○ Wound site

Patient teaching

Be sure to cover:
○ the disorder, diagnosis, and treatment
○ prescribed drugs, dosages, and possible adverse effects
○ need for a healthy, well-balanced diet and regular exercise
○ importance of checking with the doctor before taking vitamins or other dietary supplements
○ importance of follow-up care
○ importance of monitoring weight.

Discharge planning

○ Refer the patient to support services.
○ Refer the patient to a weight-reduction program, if needed.
○ Refer the patient to a smoking-cessation program, if needed.

Legionnaires' disease

Overview

Description
- Acute bronchopneumonia caused by the gram-negative bacillus *Legionella pneumophila*
- Varies from mild illness with or without pneumonitis to serious multilobed pneumonia fatal in up to 15% of affected patients
- May occur in epidemic outbreaks (usually in late summer and early fall) or just a few cases

Pathophysiology
- *Legionella* bacteria enter the lungs after aspiration or inhalation.
- Although alveolar macrophages phagocytize the bacteria, they aren't killed, and they proliferate inside the macrophages.
- The macrophages rupture, releasing the *Legionella* bacteria, and the cycle starts again.
- Lesions develop a nodular appearance, and alveoli become filled with fibrin, neutrophils, and alveolar macrophages.

Risk factors
- Alcoholism
- Chronic underlying disease
- Immunosuppression
- Old age
- Smoking

Causes
- *L. pneumophila,* an aerobic, gram-negative bacillus that's most likely transmitted through air
- Water distribution systems (such as whirlpool spas and decorative fountains) that serve as a primary reservoir for the organism

Prevalence
- More likely to affect men than women

Complications
- Arrhythmias
- Heart failure
- Pneumonia
- Renal failure
- Respiratory failure
- Shock (usually fatal)

Assessment

History
- Presence at a suspected source of infection
- Prodromal symptoms
  – Anorexia

- Diarrhea
- Headache
- Malaise
- Myalgia

Physical assessment
- Altered level of consciousness (LOC)
- Bradycardia (about half of patients)
- Dullness over areas of secretions, consolidation, or pleural effusions
- Fine crackles that develop into coarse crackles as the disease progresses
- Grayish or rust-colored nonpurulent, occasionally blood-streaked, sputum
- Rapidly rising fever with chills
- Tachypnea

Test results
Laboratory
- Numerous neutrophils but no organism under Gram's staining
- Isolation of the organism from respiratory secretions
- *L. pneumophila* detected in direct immunofluorescence and indirect fluorescent serum antibody tests
- Leukocytosis
- Increased erythrocyte sedimentation rate
- Decreased partial pressure of arterial oxygen
- Initially decreased partial pressure of arterial carbon dioxide
- Hyponatremia (serum sodium level less than 131 mg/L)

Imaging
- Chest X-rays typically show patchy, localized infiltration, which progresses to multilobed consolidation (usually involving the lower lobes) and pleural effusion.
- In fulminant disease, chest X-rays reveal opacification of the entire lung.

Diagnostic procedures
- Bronchial washing or thoracentesis may be used to obtain specimens to isolate the organism, the only definitive diagnostic evidence.

Nursing diagnoses

- Acute pain
- Diarrhea
- Excess fluid volume
- Imbalanced nutrition: less than body requirements
- Impaired gas exchange
- Ineffective airway clearance

Key outcomes
The patient will:
- cough effectively
- expectorate sputum effectively
- express feelings of increased comfort in maintaining air exchange

- ○ regain and maintain normal fluid and electrolyte balance
- ○ have normal breath sounds.

Interventions

General
- ○ Fluid replacement
- ○ Oxygen administration

Nursing
- ○ Give tepid sponge baths or use hypothermia blankets to lower fever.
- ○ Provide frequent mouth care.
- ○ If needed, apply cream to irritated nostrils.
- ○ Replace fluids and electrolytes, as needed.
- ○ Institute seizure precautions.
- ○ Give prescribed drugs.
- ○ Encourage coughing and deep breathing.
- ○ Maintain infection control precautions.

Drug therapy
- ○ Antibiotics (when diagnosis is suspected but not necessarily confirmed)
- ○ Antipyretics
- ○ Diuretics
- ○ Pressor drugs

Monitoring
- ○ Arterial blood gases
- ○ LOC
- ○ Respiratory status
- ○ Vital signs

Patient teaching

Be sure to cover:
- ○ the disorder, diagnosis, and treatment
- ○ prevention of infection
- ○ the importance of disinfecting the water supply
- ○ the purpose of postural drainage
- ○ how to perform coughing and deep-breathing exercises
- ○ proper hand-washing and disposal of soiled tissues to prevent disease transmission.

Discharge planning

- ○ Refer the patient to a pulmonologist, chest physiotherapist, or both, if needed.

Liver failure

Overview

Description

- Severe deterioration in liver function that leads to end-stage dysfunction (See *Understanding liver functions.*)
- Two conditions occurring in liver failure:
  - Hepatic encephalopathy
  - Hepatorenal syndrome

Pathophysiology

- A large portion of the liver must be damaged before liver failure occurs.
- Once damaged, the liver fails to meet the demands placed on it and fails to function.
- Liver failure may develop rapidly over days or weeks (acute liver failure) or gradually over months or years (chronic liver failure).

Hepatic encephalopathy

- The liver can no longer detoxify the blood.
- Liver dysfunction and collateral vessels that shunt blood around the liver to the systemic circulation permit toxins absorbed from the gastrointestinal tract to circulate freely to the brain.
- Short-chain fatty acids, serotonin, tryptophan, and false neurotransmitters may also accumulate in the blood.

Hepatorenal syndrome

- Renal failure accompanies liver disease; the kidneys appear to be normal but abruptly cease functioning.
- Blood volume expands, hydrogen ions accumulate, and electrolyte disturbances occur.
- The cause may be an accumulation of vasoactive substances that cause inappropriate constriction of renal arterioles, leading to decreased glomerular filtration and oliguria.
- Vasoconstriction also may be a compensatory response to portal hypertension and the pooling of blood in the splenic circulation.

Causes

- Biliary atresia
- Cirrhosis
- Hepatitis (viral and nonviral)
- Liver cancer
- Liver damage from toxins (alcohol or such drugs as acetaminophen)
- Metabolic liver disease

Prevalence

- Fatal to more than 60,000 Americans each year

 AGE AWARE *Patients younger than age 10 and older than age 40 fare poorly.*

Complications

- Coma
- Death
- Hemorrhage

Assessment

History

- Abdominal swelling and edema
- Anorexia
- Clay-colored stools
- Fatigue
- Existing disease or condition
- Exposure to hepatitis
- Nausea
- Pruritus
- Tendency to bruise or bleed easily

Physical assessment

- Ammonia-scented breath
- Ascites
- Asterixis
- Hematemesis or rectal bleeding
- Hepatomegaly
- Icteric sclera
- Jaundice
- Mental status changes from encephalopathy
- Oliguria and dark brown urine
- Tremors
- Weakness

Test results

Laboratory

- Increased serum liver enzymes, bilirubin levels, ammonia level, and lactic acid level
- Decreased serum albumin, total protein, globulin, sodium, and glucose levels
- Prolonged prothrombin time
- Confirmed hepatitis in hepatitis serology studies

Imaging

- Abdominal ultrasound shows hepatic blood flow and ascites.
- Computed tomography scan gives a detailed view of the liver and the presence of tumors and damaged hepatic tissue.

Diagnostic procedures

- A liver biopsy confirms the diagnosis and determines the underlying disease process.
- Endoscopy reveals esophageal varices (large, torturous veins).
- Paracentesis confirms the presence of ascites.
- Swan-Ganz catheter readings indicate portal hypertension.

Nursing diagnoses

- Acute confusion
- Anticipatory grieving

- Death anxiety
- Excess fluid volume
- Fatigue
- Impaired gas exchange
- Nausea
- Risk for infection
- Risk for injury

Key outcomes

The patient will:
- show no signs and symptoms of bleeding
- remain alert and oriented
- maintain normal fluid volume and electrolyte balance
- maintain adequate ventilation
- maintain a patent airway.

Interventions

General

- Administration of packed red blood cells to combat blood loss or fresh frozen plasma or platelets to help prevent bleeding
- Balloon tamponade to control bleeding varices
- Fluid restriction
- Low-protein, low-sodium, high-calorie diet
- Mechanical ventilation
- Paracentesis
- Plasmapheresis
- Shunt placement between the portal vein and another systemic vein to control pulmonary hypertension
- Liver transplantation, which is the only cure

Nursing

- Give all prescribed drugs.
- Provide a safe environment.
- Maintain bleeding precautions.
- Observe universal precautions.
- Provide emotional support for the patient and family.
- Reorient the patient as needed.
- Elevate the legs to prevent edema.
- Encourage activity as tolerated.

Drug therapy

- Albumin I.V.
- Antibiotics
- Antipruritics
- Antivirals
- Dextrose 50%, if hypoglycemia occurs
- Diuretics
- Lactulose by mouth or rectum
- Vasoconstrictor drugs
- Vitamin K

Monitoring

- Blood tests to check liver enzymes, clotting times, blood sugar levels, ammonia levels, and renal function
- Daily weight

Understanding liver functions

To understand how liver disease affects the body, you need to understand its main functions. The liver:
- detoxifies poisonous chemicals (including alcohol) and drugs (prescribed and over-the-counter as well as illegal substances)
- makes bile to help digest food
- stores energy by stockpiling carbohydrates, glucose, and fat until needed
- stores iron reserves as well as vitamins and minerals
- manufactures new proteins
- produces plasma proteins needed for blood coagulation, including prothrombin and fibrinogen
- serves as a site for hematopoiesis during fetal development.

- Intake and output
- Neurologic status
- Respiratory status
- Signs and symptoms of bleeding
- Vital signs

Patient teaching

Be sure to cover:
- the diagnosis, prognosis, and treatment
- infection control precautions
- diet and fluid restrictions
- importance of checking weight daily
- signs and symptoms of ascites
- signs and symptoms of bleeding, and when to contact a doctor
- signs and symptoms of encephalopathy, and when to contact a doctor
- the importance of taking all prescribed drugs.

ALERT *Explain to the patient that he must notify a doctor immediately if he thinks he has ascites. Ascites fluid can lead to spontaneous bacterial peritonitis.*

ALERT *Lactulose promotes excretion of the byproducts of protein breakdown (ammonia) through bowel movements. Instruct the patient not to stop lactulose if he develops diarrhea. Explain that this is the desired effect and that he should contact a doctor before making any changes in the drug regimen.*

Discharge planning

- Refer the patient to Alcoholics Anonymous or a drug rehabilitation program as needed.
- Refer the patient to a nutritionist, if needed.
- Refer the patient and family to pastoral care and social services if the prognosis is poor.

Lung cancer

Overview

Description

○ Malignant tumors arising from the respiratory epithelium
○ Most common types:
  – Epidermoid (squamous cell)
  – Adenocarcinoma
  – Small-cell (oat cell)
  – Large-cell (anaplastic)
○ Most common site: wall or epithelium of bronchial tree
○ Poor prognosis for most patients
○ Depends on extent of cancer when diagnosed and cells' growth rate

Pathophysiology

○ Lung cancer causes bronchial epithelial changes progressing from squamous cell alteration or metaplasia to carcinoma in situ.
○ Tumors originating in the bronchi are thought to produce more mucus.
○ Partial or complete airway obstruction occurs with tumor growth, resulting in lobar collapse distal to the tumor.
○ Early metastasis occurs to other thoracic structures, such as hilar lymph nodes or the mediastinum.
○ Distant metastasis occurs to the brain, liver, bone, and adrenal glands.

Risk factors

○ Exposure to carcinogenic and industrial air pollutants
  – Arsenic
  – Asbestos
  – Chromium
  – Coal dust
  – Iron oxides
  – Nickel
  – Radioactive dust
  – Uranium
○ Genetic predisposition
○ Smoking

Causes

○ Exact cause unknown

Prevalence

○ Family susceptibility
○ 5-year survival rate after diagnosis: about 14%

✺ *AGE AWARE Lung cancer is the most common cause of cancer death for men and women ages 50 to 75.*

Complications

○ Anorexia and weight loss, sometimes leading to cachexia, digital clubbing, and hypertrophic osteoarthropathy
○ Esophageal compression with dysphagia
○ Hypoxemia
○ Lymphatic obstruction with pleural effusion
○ Neoplastic and paraneoplastic syndromes, including Pancoast's syndrome and syndrome of inappropriate secretion of antidiuretic hormone
○ Phrenic nerve paralysis with hemidiaphragm elevation and dyspnea
○ Spinal cord compression
○ Spread of primary tumor to intrathoracic structures
○ Sympathetic nerve paralysis with Horner's syndrome
○ Tracheal obstruction

Assessment

History

○ Possibly no symptoms

Epidermoid and small-cell tumors
○ Chest pain
○ Dyspnea
○ Hemoptysis
○ Hoarseness
○ Smoker's cough
○ Wheezing

Adenocarcinoma and large-cell tumors
○ Anorexia
○ Fever
○ Shoulder pain
○ Weakness
○ Weight loss

Physical assessment

○ Decreased breath sounds
○ Dilated chest and abdominal veins (superior vena cava syndrome)
○ Dyspnea on exertion
○ Edema of the face, neck, and upper torso
○ Enlarged lymph nodes
○ Enlarged liver
○ Finger clubbing
○ Pleural friction rub
○ Weight loss
○ Wheezing

Test results

Laboratory
○ Evidence of pulmonary malignancy in cytologic sputum analysis
○ Abnormal liver function test results, especially with metastasis

Imaging
○ Chest X-rays show advanced lesions and can show a lesion up to 2 years before signs and symptoms appear; findings may indicate tumor size and location.

- Contrast studies of the bronchial tree (chest tomography, bronchography) show size and location as well as spread of lesion.
- Bone scan is used to detect metastasis.
- Computed tomography (CT) of the chest is used to detect malignant pleural effusion.
- CT of the brain is used to detect metastasis.
- Positron emission tomography aids in the diagnosis of primary and metastatic sites.
- Gallium scans of the liver and spleen help to detect metastasis.

Diagnostic procedures
- Bronchoscopy identifies the tumor site.
- Bronchial washings provide material for cytologic and histologic study.
- Needle biopsy of the lungs (relies on biplanar fluoroscopic visual control to locate peripheral tumors before withdrawing a tissue specimen for analysis) allows firm diagnosis in 80% of patients.
- Tissue biopsy of metastatic sites (including supraclavicular and mediastinal nodes and pleura) is used to stage the disease and establishes prognosis and treatment.
- Thoracentesis allows chemical and cytologic examination of pleural fluid.
- Exploratory thoracotomy is performed to obtain biopsy.

Nursing diagnoses

- Acute pain
- Anticipatory grieving
- Death anxiety
- Imbalanced nutrition: less than body requirements
- Ineffective airway clearance
- Ineffective breathing pattern
- Risk for deficient fluid volume

Key outcomes
The patient will:
- maintain normal fluid volume
- maintain adequate ventilation
- maintain a patent airway
- express feelings of increased comfort and decreased pain.

Interventions

General
- Activity, as tolerated according to breathing capacity
- Laser therapy (experimental)
- Palliative (most treatments)
- Preoperative and postoperative radiation therapy
- Surgery
  - Partial removal of lung (wedge resection, segmental resection, lobectomy, radical lobectomy)
  - Total removal of lung (pneumonectomy, radical pneumonectomy)

- Various combinations of surgery, radiation therapy, and chemotherapy to improve prognosis and possibly prolong survival
- Well-balanced diet

Nursing
- Provide supportive care.
- Encourage verbalization.
- Give prescribed drugs.

Drug therapy
- Antidiarrheals and antiemetics, as needed, with chemotherapy and radiation
- Chemotherapy drug combinations
- Immunotherapy (investigational)

Monitoring
- Chest tube function and drainage
- Hydration and nutrition
- Oxygenation
- Pain control
- Postoperative complications
- Sputum production
- Vital signs
- Wound site

Patient teaching

Be sure to cover:
- postoperative procedures and equipment
- chest physiotherapy
- exercises to prevent shoulder stiffness
- prescribed drugs, dosages, administration, and possible adverse effects
- risk factors for recurrent cancer.

Discharge planning

- Refer smokers to local branches of the American Cancer Society or Smokenders.
- Provide information about group therapy, individual counseling, and hypnosis.
- Refer the patient to available resources and support services.

Medullary sponge kidney

Overview

Description
- A congenital defect of the kidney
- May affect a single pyramid in one kidney or all pyramids in both kidneys
- Leads to cystic dilation of the collecting tubules
- A benign condition

Pathophysiology
- The collecting ducts of the renal pyramids dilate.
- Cavities, clefts, and cysts form in the medulla.
- Urinary stasis occurs, which may lead to renal calculi or kidney infection.
- The kidneys are usually somewhat enlarged but may be of normal size; they appear spongy.

Causes
- Congenital abnormality
- Possibly transmitted as an autosomal dominant trait

Prevalence
- Occurs in 1 in every 5,000 to 20,000 persons

 AGE AWARE Medullary sponge kidney occurs mainly in men ages 40 to 70.

Complications
- Formation of calcium oxylate stones
- Infection (especially lower urinary tract infections and pyelonephritis)

Assessment

History
- Burning on urination
- Frequency
- Pain
- Urgency

Physical assessment
- Fever
- Hematuria
- Possibly edema and rales in fluid overload

Test results
Laboratory
- Possible slight reduction in urine-concentrating ability
- Possible hypercalciuria

Imaging
- Excretory urography shows a characteristic flower-like appearance of the pyramidal cavities when they fill with contrast material and renal calculi.

Nursing diagnoses
- Acute pain
- Excess fluid volume
- Impaired urinary elimination
- Ineffective tissue perfusion: renal
- Risk for infection
- Risk for injury

Key outcomes
The patient will:
- maintain normal fluid volume
- maintain adequate intake and output
- remain free from infection
- report increased comfort
- avoid or minimize complications
- maintain hemodynamic stability
- identify risk factors that worsen ineffective tissue perfusion, and modify his lifestyle accordingly.

Interventions

General
- Increasing fluid intake
- Low-calcium diet
- Preventing and treating complications caused by calculi and infection

Nursing
- Give drugs as prescribed.
- Emphasize the need for fluids.
- Strain urine for calculi.
- Collect clean-catch urine specimen for culture.
- Check for allergy to excretory urography dye.

Drug therapy
- Analgesics if the patient has calculi
- Antibiotics if the patient has an infection
- Drugs to acidify urine

Monitoring
- Calculi from strained urine
- Daily weight
- Intake and output
- Urine culture results
- Vital signs including temperature
- White blood cell count

Patient teaching

Be sure to cover:
○ the disorder, diagnosis, and treatment
○ the importance of frequent bathing and proper toilet hygiene
○ the need to complete the prescribed course of antibiotics if an infection occurs
○ the importance of adequate fluid intake
○ preprocedural and postprocedural teaching for excretory urography
○ how to strain urine
○ sign and symptoms of infection
○ the importance of and components of a low-calcium diet.

Discharge planning

○ Refer the patient to a nutritionist, if needed.

Metabolic acidosis

Overview

Description
○ Blood pH below 7.35 and bicarbonate (HCO_3^-) level below 22 mEq/L

Pathophysiology
○ Hydrogen ions begin to accumulate in the body, and chemical buffers in the cells and extracellular fluid bind with them.
○ Excess hydrogen ions that the buffers can't bind with decrease the pH and stimulate chemoreceptors in the medulla to increase the respiratory rate.
○ The increased respiratory rate lowers the partial pressure of carbon dioxide ($Paco_2$), which allows more hydrogen ions to bind with bicarbonate ions (HCO_3^-).
○ Healthy kidneys try to compensate for the acidosis by secreting excess hydrogen ions into the renal tubules.
○ Each time a hydrogen ion is secreted into the renal tubules, a sodium ion and a bicarbonate ion are absorbed from the tubules and returned to the blood.
○ Excess hydrogen ions in the extracellular fluid diffuse into cells.
○ To maintain the balance of the charge across the membrane, the cells release potassium ions into the blood.
○ Excess hydrogen ions alter the normal balance of potassium, sodium, and calcium ions, leading to reduced excitability of nerve cells.

Causes
○ Decreased tissue oxygenation or perfusion
○ Excessive bicarbonate loss
 – Gastrointestinal loss: diarrhea, intestinal suction
 – Renal loss: renal failure, hyperaldosteronism
○ Excessive production of metabolic acids
 – Chronic alcoholism
 – Diabetic ketoacidosis
 – Lactic acidosis
 – Malnutrition
 – Starvation
○ Exogenous poisoning
○ Salicylate intoxication

Prevalence
○ Affects all age groups
○ Equally common in males and females

Complications
○ Shock
○ Death

Assessment

History
○ Diabetes mellitus type I
○ Ingestion of toxic substances
○ Kidney failure
○ Shock

Physical assessment
○ Confusion
○ Decreased deep tendon reflexes
○ Dull headache
○ Dyspnea
○ Hyperventilation
○ Hypotension
○ Kussmaul's respirations
○ Lethargy
○ Signs of hyperkalemia
 – Abdominal cramping
 – Diarrhea
 – Muscle weakness
 – Electrocardiogram changes
○ Warm, dry skin

Test results
Laboratory
○ pH below 7.35, $Paco_2$ less than 35 mm Hg, and HCO_3^- less than 22 mEq/L
○ Increased blood glucose and serum ketone levels in patients with diabetic ketoacidosis
○ Increased serum potassium levels
○ Increasing plasma lactate levels in patients with lactic acidosis
○ Increased anion gap
Diagnostic procedures
○ Electrocardiography shows tall P waves, prolonged PR intervals, and wide QRS complexes.

Nursing diagnoses

○ Acute confusion
○ Decreased cardiac output
○ Ineffective breathing pattern

Key outcomes
The patient will:
○ maintain a normal pH
○ maintain hemodynamic stability
○ maintain respiratory stability.

Interventions

General
○ Correction of acidosis
○ Mechanical ventilation
○ Dialysis in patients with renal failure

Nursing

○ Maintain the patient's safety.
○ Assist the patient with activities as needed.
○ Give prescribed drugs.
○ Prepare for mechanical ventilation or dialysis, as needed.
○ Insert an I.V. line, as ordered, and maintain patent I.V. access.
○ Position the patient to promote chest expansion and facilitate breathing.

Drug therapy

○ I.V. fluids to replace fluid loss
○ Rapid-acting insulin to reverse diabetic ketoacidosis in diabetic patients
○ Sodium bicarbonate I.V.

Monitoring

○ Arterial blood gas analysis
○ Cardiac status
○ Deep tendon reflexes and muscle strength
○ Intake and output
○ Level of consciousness
○ Respirations
○ Serum electrolytes
○ Vital signs

Patient teaching

Be sure to cover:
○ the disorder, diagnosis, and treatment
○ testing of blood glucose levels, if indicated
○ need for strict adherence to antidiabetic therapy, if appropriate
○ prescribed drugs
○ avoidance of ingestion of toxic substances
○ avoidance of alcohol
○ warning signs and symptoms and when to report them.

Discharge planning

○ Refer the patient to a nutritionist or social services, if needed.

Metabolic alkalosis

Overview

Description
○ Blood pH above 7.45 and a bicarbonate (HCO_3^-) level above 26 mEq/L.
○ HCO_3^- level as high as 50 mEq/L in acute metabolic alkalosis

Pathophysiology
○ Underlying mechanisms include a loss of hydrogen ions (acid), a gain in HCO_3^-, or both.
○ A partial arterial pressure of carbon dioxide ($Paco_2$) greater than 45 mm Hg indicates that the lungs are compensating for the alkalosis.
○ Renal compensation is more effective, but it takes longer.
○ Metabolic alkalosis commonly is accompanied by hypokalemia in which the kidneys conserve potassium and excrete hydrogen ions.

Causes
○ Cushing's disease
○ Drugs that contain sodium bicarbonate (such as corticosteroids and antacids)
○ Drugs
  – Antacids (sodium bicarbonate, calcium bicarbonate)
  – Corticosteroids
  – Thiazide and loop diuretics
○ Excessive acid loss from the gastrointestinal tract (as from vomiting, nasogastric suctioning)

 AGE AWARE Children who have pyloric stenosis are at risk for metabolic alkalosis.

○ Kidney disease
○ Multiple transfusions
○ Thiazide and loop diuretics

Prevalence
○ Depends on the underlying cause

Complications
○ Arrhythmias
○ Coma
○ Death

Assessment

History
○ Headache
○ Irritability
○ Lethargy
○ Muscle twitching and weakness
○ Nausea
○ Palpitations
○ Vomiting

Physical assessment
○ Confusion
○ Hyperactive deep tendon reflexes
○ Hypotension
○ Hypoxemia
○ Slow, shallow respirations

Test results
Laboratory
○ pH above 7.45
○ HCO_3^- level above 26 mEq/L (normal HCO_3^- level if the underlying cause is excessive acid loss)
○ $Paco_2$ level above 45 mm Hg in respiratory compensation is present
○ Hypokalemia
○ Hypocalcemia
○ Hypochloremia
Diagnostic tests
○ Electrocardiography reveals a low T wave that merges with the P wave and may reveal atrial tachycardia.

Nursing diagnoses

○ Acute confusion
○ Decreased cardiac output
○ Ineffective breathing pattern
○ Nausea

Key outcomes
The patient will:
○ maintain a normal pH on arterial blood gas analysis
○ maintain hemodynamic stability
○ describe the condition, its treatment, and its effects
○ maintain respiratory stability.

Interventions

General
○ Correction of acid-base imbalance
○ Seizure precautions
○ Treatment for hypoxemia
○ Stopping of nasogastric (NG) suctioning, if possible

Nursing
○ Irrigate NG tubes with normal saline solution instead of tap water to prevent loss of gastric electrolytes.
○ Maintain patient safety.
○ Assist patient with activities as needed.
○ Give prescribed drugs.

Drug therapy
○ Acetazolamide (Diamox)
○ Ammonium chloride I.V.

◢ **ALERT** *Infusing 0.9% ammonium chloride at more than 1 L over 4 hours may cause hemolysis of red blood cells. Excessive amounts may cause acidosis. Ammonium chloride is contraindicated in patients with liver or kidney failure.*

○ Antiemetics
○ No thiazide diuretics, if possible
○ Oxygen

Monitoring

○ Arterial blood gas analysis
○ Deep tendon reflexes and muscle strength
○ Intake and output
○ Level of consciousness
○ Respirations
○ Serum electrolytes
○ Vital signs

Patient teaching

Be sure to cover:
○ the disorder, diagnosis, and treatment
○ the need to avoid overuse of alkaline agents and diuretics
○ prescribed drugs, especially adverse effects of potassium-wasting diuretics or potassium chloride supplements
○ warning signs and symptoms and when to report them.

Discharge planning

○ Refer the patient to a nutritionist or social services, if needed.

Multiple myeloma

Overview

Description
- A disseminated neoplasm of marrow plasma cells
- Prognosis usually poor because diagnosis usually comes after infiltration of vertebrae, pelvis, skull, ribs, clavicles, and sternum
- Without treatment, causes vertebral collapse
- Fatal in 52% of patients within 3 months of diagnosis; 90% within 2 years
- Life commonly prolonged 3 to 5 years with early diagnosis and treatment
- Also called malignant plasmacytoma, plasma cell myeloma, and myelomatosis

Pathophysiology
- Infiltration of the bone produces osteolytic lesions throughout the skeleton.
- In late stages, the malignant plasma cells infiltrate into the lymph nodes, liver, spleen, and kidneys.

Risk factors
- Genetic predisposition
- Occupational exposure to radiation

Causes
- Exact cause unknown

Prevalence
- Strikes about 13,800 people yearly

 AGE AWARE Multiple myeloma is most common among men older than age 40.

Complications
- Dehydration
- Fractures
- Hematologic imbalance
- Hypercalcemia
- Hyperuricemia
- Infections (such as pneumonia)
- Pyelonephritis, renal calculi, and renal failure

Assessment

History
- Arthritic symptoms
- History of neoplastic fractures
- History of pneumonia
- Malaise
- Peripheral paresthesia and neuropathy
- Progressive weakness
- Severe, constant pain in back, ribs, or both that may increase with exercise and worsen at night
- Weight loss

Physical assessment
- Fever
- Joint swelling
- Noticeable thoracic deformities
- Reduction in body height of 5″ (12.7 cm)

Test results
Laboratory
- Moderate or severe anemia
- In differential, 40% to 50% lymphocytes but seldom more than 3% plasma cells
- Rouleau formation, which is often the first clue
- Elevation of the erythrocyte sedimentation rate
- Protein urea
- Bence Jones protein in urine (Absence doesn't rule out multiple myeloma, but presence almost always confirms it.)
- Hypercalciuria
- Elevated globulin spike in serum electrophoresis that's electrophoretically and immunologically abnormal

Imaging
- X-rays during the early stages may reveal diffuse osteoporosis. Eventually, they show characteristic lesions of multiple myeloma: multiple, sharply circumscribed osteolytic, or punched out, lesions, particularly on the skull, pelvis, and spine.

Diagnostic procedures
- Bone marrow aspiration reveals myelomatous cells and an abnormal number of immature plasma cells (10% to 95% instead of the normal 3% to 5%).

Nursing diagnoses

- Anticipatory grieving
- Chronic pain
- Death anxiety
- Disturbed body image
- Excess fluid volume
- Ineffective coping
- Risk for injury

Key outcomes
The patient will:
- express feelings about the illness
- maintain adequate ventilation
- express feelings of increased comfort and decreased pain
- demonstrate effective coping skills
- maintain fluid volume balance.

Interventions

General
- Activity, as tolerated
- Adjuvant local radiation
- Dialysis (if renal complications develop)
- Laminectomy for spinal cord compression

- Peripheral-blood stem-cell transplantation
- Plasmapheresis to remove protein from the blood and return the cells to the patient (temporary effect)
- Well-balanced diet

Nursing

- Encourage fluid intake of 3 to 4 qt (3 to 4 L) daily.
- Give prescribed drugs.
- Encourage mobilization.
- Assist with ambulation.

Drug therapy

- Analgesics
- Bisphosphonates
- Chemotherapeutic drugs
- Immunotherapy
- Interferon
- Possible use of thalidomide

Monitoring

- Complications of treatment
- Intake and output
- Pain control
- Proper positioning (alignment)
- Signs and symptoms of infection
- Signs and symptoms of severe anemia and fractures

Patient teaching

Be sure to cover:
- the disorder, diagnosis, and treatment
- importance of deep breathing and changing position every 2 hours after surgery
- appropriate dress for weather conditions (because the patient may be sensitive to cold)
- avoidance of crowds and people with infections
- prescribed drugs, dosages, administration, and possible adverse effects
- measuring daily intake and output
- use of assistive devices
- signs and symptoms of infection
- appropriate physical activity and exercises.

Discharge planning

- Refer the patient to community resources for additional support.
- Refer the patient to a physical therapist.

Myasthenia gravis

Overview

Description

- An acquired autoimmune disorder characterized by abnormal fatigability of striated (skeletal) muscles
- Sporadic but progressive weakness
- Muscle weakness worsened by exercise and repetitive movement
- Initial symptoms related to cranial nerves
- With respiratory system involvement, may be life-threatening
- Spontaneous remissions in about 25% of patients

Pathophysiology

- Blood cells and the thymus gland produce antibodies that block, destroy, or weaken neuroreceptors (which transmit nerve impulses).
- The result is failure of the transmission of nerve impulses at the neuromuscular junction.

Causes

- Autoimmune disorder related to the thymus gland
- Other immune and thyroid disorders

Prevalence

- Occurs at any age

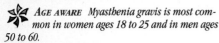 AGE AWARE *Myasthenia gravis is most common in women ages 18 to 25 and in men ages 50 to 60.*

- Three times more common in women than men
- Transient myasthenia in about 20% of infants born to myasthenic mothers

Complications

- Aspiration
- Pneumonia
- Respiratory distress

Assessment

History

- Difficulty chewing and swallowing
- Extreme muscle weakness and fatigue (cardinal symptoms)
- Head bobbing
- Jaw hanging open (especially when tired)
- Progressive muscle weakness (strongest in the morning, weakening during the day)
- Ptosis and diplopia (most common)
- Symptoms milder on awakening; worse as the day progresses

- Symptoms that become more intense during menses, after emotional stress, after prolonged exposure to sunlight or cold, and with infections
- Temporarily restored muscle function after a short rest
- Varying assessment findings

Physical assessment

- Decreased breath sounds
- Decreased tidal volume
- Drooping jaw
- Ptosis
- Respiratory distress and myasthenic crisis
- Sleepy, masklike expression

Test results

Imaging

- Chest X-ray or computed tomography scan shows thymoma.

Diagnostic procedures

- Positive Tensilon test shows temporarily improved muscle function and confirms the diagnosis.
- Electrodiagnostic tests show a rapid decline of more than 10% in the amplitude of evoked responses.

Nursing diagnoses

- Bathing or hygiene self-care deficit
- Disturbed body image
- Ineffective breathing pattern
- Ineffective coping
- Risk for aspiration
- Risk for imbalanced fluid volume
- Risk for injury
- Risk for urge urinary incontinence

Key outcomes

The patient will:

- maintain a patent airway and adequate ventilation
- maintain respiratory rate within 5 breaths/minute of baseline
- perform activities of daily living
- maintain range of motion and joint mobility
- express positive feelings about self
- demonstrate the ability to tolerate diet without aspiration
- have fewer episodes of incontinence
- mantain adequate fluid volume.

Interventions

General

- Activity, as tolerated (Exercise may worsen symptoms; planned rest periods may retard symptoms.)
- Diet, as tolerated
- Emergency airway and ventilation management

> ◢ **ALERT** *A patient with myasthenic crisis requires immediate hospitalization and vigorous respiratory support.*

○ Plasmapheresis
○ Relief of symptoms
○ Thymectomy, if needed

Nursing

○ Provide psychological support.
○ Provide frequent rest periods.
○ Plan activities to make the most of energy peaks.
○ Maintain the nutritional management program.
○ Maintain social activity.
○ Give prescribed drugs.
○ Allow the patient to participate in his care.
○ Promote soft, solid foods.

Drug therapy

○ Anticholinesterase drugs
○ Corticosteroids
○ I.V. immune globulin

Monitoring

○ Ability to tolerate diet
○ Neurologic and respiratory function (tidal volume and vital capacity)
○ Response to drugs
○ Signs of impending crisis

> ◢ **ALERT** *Signs of impending myasthenic crisis include increased muscle weakness, respiratory distress, and difficulty talking or chewing.*

Patient teaching

Be sure to cover:
○ the disorder, diagnosis, and treatment
○ surgery (preoperative and postoperative teaching)
○ energy conservation techniques
○ prescribed drugs, dosages, and possible adverse effects
○ avoidance of strenuous exercise, stress, infection, needless exposure to the sun or cold weather
○ activity planning
○ nutritional management program
○ swallowing therapy program.

Discharge planning

○ Refer the patient to the Myasthenia Gravis Foundation.
○ Refer the patient to a physical therapist, chest physiotherapist, and nutritionist, if needed.

Near drowning

Overview

Description
○ Victim survives physiologic effects of submersion
○ Primary problems: hypoxemia and acidosis
○ "Dry" near drowning
  – Fluid not aspirated
  – Respiratory obstruction or asphyxia
○ "Wet" near drowning
  – Fluid aspirated
  – Asphyxia or secondary changes from fluid aspiration
○ "Secondary" near drowning: recurrence of respiratory distress

Pathophysiology
○ Immersion stimulates hyperventilation.
○ Voluntary apnea occurs.
○ Laryngospasm develops.
○ Hypoxemia develops and can lead to brain damage and cardiac arrest.

Causes
○ Blow to the head while in the water
○ Boating accident
○ Dangerous water conditions
○ Decompression sickness from deep-water diving
○ Excessive alcohol consumption before swimming
○ Inability to swim
○ Panic
○ Sudden acute illness
○ Suicide attempt
○ Venomous stings from aquatic animals

Prevalence

▼ **ALERT** *Near drowning is the most common cause of injury and death in children ages 1 month to 14 years.*

○ More common in males

Complications
○ Bacterial aspiration
○ Cardiac complications
○ Neurologic impairment
○ Pulmonary complications
○ Pulmonary edema
○ Renal damage
○ Seizure disorder

Assessment

History
○ Victim found in water

Physical assessment
○ Abdominal distention
○ Altered level of consciousness
○ Cardiopulmonary arrest
○ Crackles, rhonchi, wheezing, or apnea
○ Cyanosis; pink, frothy sputum; or both
○ Fever or hypothermia
○ Hypoxia
○ Irregular heartbeat
○ Rapid, slow, or absent pulse
○ Seizures
○ Shallow, gasping, or absent respirations
○ Tachycardia

Test results
Laboratory
○ Arterial blood gas (ABG) level showing degree of hypoxia, intrapulmonary shunt, and acid-base balance
○ Possible hyperkalemia caused by acidosis or hemolysis of red blood cells
○ Hemolysis in complete blood count
○ Increased white blood cell (WBC) count caused by alveolar inflammation; decreased WBC count if patient is hypothermic
○ Increased blood urea nitrogen and creatinine levels, revealing impaired renal function
○ Signs of impaired renal function in urinalysis
Imaging
○ Cervical spine X-ray may show evidence of fracture.
○ Serial chest X-rays may show pulmonary edema.
Diagnostic procedures
○ Electrocardiography may show myocardial ischemia or infarct or cardiac arrhythmias.

Nursing diagnoses
○ Acute confusion
○ Anticipatory grieving
○ Death anxiety
○ Decreased cardiac output
○ Hyperthermia
○ Hypothermia
○ Ineffective airway clearance
○ Ineffective breathing pattern
○ Risk for post-trauma syndrome

Key outcomes
The patient will:
○ maintain adequate cardiac output
○ maintain adequate ventilation
○ maintain a patent airway
○ maintain a normal body temperature
○ develop effective coping mechanisms.

Interventions

General

- Activity based on extent of injury and success of resuscitation
- Airway and ventilation
- Correction of abnormal laboratory values
- Neck stabilization
- Nothing by mouth until swallowing ability has returned
- Warming measures, if hypothermic

Nursing

- Perform cardiopulmonary resuscitation if needed.
- For mild hypothermia (93.2° to 96.8° F [34° to 36° C]), provide active external rewarming and passive rewarming measures.
- For moderate hypothermia (86° F to 93.2° F [30° to 34° C]), provide active external rewarming of truncal areas only and passive rewarming measures.
- For severe hypothermia (less than 86° F [30° C]), provide active internal rewarming measures.
- Protect the cervical spine.
- Give prescribed drugs.
- Provide emotional support.

Drug therapy

- Bronchodilators
- Cardiac drug therapy if appropriate

Monitoring

- Cardiac rhythm
- Core body temperature
- Electrolyte and ABG measurement results
- Neurologic status
- Psychological state
- Respiratory status
- Vital signs, including oxygen saturation

Patient teaching

Be sure to cover:
- the injury, diagnosis, and treatment
- the need to avoid using alcohol or drugs before swimming
- water safety measures (such as the buddy system).

Discharge planning

- Recommend a water safety course given by the Red Cross, YMCA, or YWCA.
- Refer the patient or family for psychological counseling if appropriate.
- Refer the patient or family to resource and support services.

Nephrotic syndrome

Overview

Description

- Kidney disorder characterized by marked proteinuria, hypoalbuminemia, hyperlipidemia, increased coagulation, and edema
- Results from a glomerular defect that affects permeability, indicating renal damage
- Prognosis highly variable, depending on underlying cause
- In some forms, progression to end-stage renal failure

Pathophysiology

- Glomerular protein permeability increases.
- Urinary excretion of protein, especially albumin, increases.
- Hypoalbuminemia develops and decreases colloidal oncotic pressure.
- Leakage of fluid into interstitial spaces leads to acute, generalized edema.
- Loss of vascular volume leads to increased blood viscosity and coagulation disorders.
- The renin-angiotensin system is triggered, causing tubular reabsorption of sodium and water and contributing to edema. (See *What happens in nephrotic syndrome*.)

Risk factors

- Allergic reactions
- Hereditary nephritis
- Infection
- Long-term analgesic abuse
- Nephrotoxins
- Pregnancy

Causes

- Primary (idiopathic) glomerulonephritis (about 75% of cases)
- Lipid nephrosis (main cause in children younger than age 8)
- Membranous glomerulonephritis (most common lesion in adult idiopathic nephrotic syndrome)
- Focal glomerulosclerosis
  - May develop spontaneously at any age
  - May occur after kidney transplantation
  - May result from heroin injection
  - Develops in about 10% of childhood cases and up to 20% of adult cases
- Membranoproliferative glomerulonephritis
  - May occur after infection, particularly streptococcal infection
  - Occurs mainly in children and young adults
- Metabolic diseases
- Collagen-vascular disorders
- Circulatory diseases
- Certain neoplastic diseases, such as multiple myeloma

Prevalence

- In children, 1 in 50,000 yearly
- In adults, 1 or 2 in 50,000 yearly

 AGE AWARE *In children, nephrotic syndrome arises most often between ages 2 and 3.*

- Slightly more common in males than in females

Complications

- Accelerated atherosclerosis
- Acute renal failure
- Coagulation disorders
- Infection, including peritonitis
- Malnutrition
- Respiratory difficulty
- Thromboembolic vascular occlusion

Assessment

History

- Ankle, sacral, or periorbital swelling
- Anorexia
- Decreased urination
- Depression

What happens in nephrotic syndrome

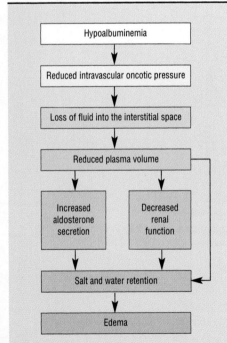

○ Lethargy
○ Presence of risk factor
○ Underlying cause

Physical assessment

○ Ascites
○ Mild to severe dependent edema
○ Orthostatic hypotension
○ Pallor
○ Periorbital edema
○ Signs of pleural effusion
○ Swollen external genitalia

Test results

Laboratory

○ Increased number of hyaline, granular, waxy, fatty casts and oval fat bodies in urinalysis
○ Consistent, heavy proteinuria (levels higher than 3.5 mg/dl for 24 hours)
○ Increased serum cholesterol, phospholipid, and triglyceride levels
○ Decreased serum albumin levels

Diagnostic procedures

○ Renal biopsy allows histologic identification of the lesion.

Nursing diagnoses

○ Decreased cardiac output
○ Disturbed body image
○ Excess fluid volume
○ Risk for infection

Key outcomes

The patient will:
○ avoid or have minimal complications
○ maintain fluid balance
○ identify risk factors that worsen tissue perfusion and modify lifestyle appropriately
○ maintain hemodynamic stability
○ express feelings about altered body image.

Interventions

General

○ Correction of the underlying cause if possible
○ Diet consisting of 0.6 g of protein per kg of body weight
○ Restricted sodium intake
○ Frequent rest between periods of activity

Nursing

○ Offer the patient reassurance and support, especially during the acute phase, when severe edema changes body image.
○ Provide information about dietary restrictions and fluid restriction.

○ Provide skin care.
○ Provide antiembolism stockings.
○ Encourage activity and periods of rest.

Drug therapy

○ Antibiotics for infection
○ Diuretics
○ Glucocorticoids
○ Possibly alkylating drugs
○ Possibly cytotoxic drugs

Monitoring

○ Bleeding and shock after kidney biopsy
○ Intake and output
○ Daily weight
○ Edema
○ Plasma albumin and transferrin levels
○ Urine for protein
○ Vital signs

Patient teaching

Be sure to cover:
○ the disorder, diagnosis, and treatments
○ signs of infection that should be reported
○ adherence to diet
○ prescribed drugs, dosages, administration, and possible adverse effects.

Discharge planning

○ Refer the patient to support services and psychological services, if needed.

Pancreatitis

Overview

Description
- Inflammation of the pancreas
- Acute and chronic forms
- In acute form, 10% mortality
- In chronic form, permanent tissue damage and tendency to progress to significant loss of pancreatic function
- May be idiopathic
- Sometimes related to biliary tract disease, alcoholism, trauma, and certain drugs

Pathophysiology
- Enzymes normally excreted into the duodenum by the pancreas are activated in the pancreas or its ducts and start to autodigest pancreatic tissue.
- Consequent inflammation causes intense pain, third spacing of large fluid volumes, pancreatic fat necrosis with consumption of serum calcium, and, occasionally, hemorrhage.

Risk factors
- Emotional factors
- Endoscopic retrograde cholangiopancreatography (ERCP)
- Heredity
- Kidney transplantation
- Neurogenic factors
- Renal failure
- Use of glucocorticoids, sulfonamides, thiazides, or hormonal contraceptives

Causes
- Alcoholism
- Abnormal organ structure
- Biliary tract disease
- Metabolic or endocrine disorders
- Pancreatic cancers
- Pancreatic cysts or tumors
- Penetrating peptic ulcers
- Penetrating trauma
- Viral or bacterial infection

Prevalence
- Acute form: 2 of every 10,000 people
- Chronic form: 2 of every 25,000 people
- Affects more men than women
- Affects Blacks four times more often than Whites

Complications
- Acute respiratory distress syndrome
- Atelectasis and pleural effusion
- Diabetic acidosis
- Diabetes mellitus
- Gastrointestinal bleeding
- Massive hemorrhage
- Pancreatic abscess and cancer
- Paralytic ileus
- Pneumonia
- Pseudocysts
- Shock and coma

Assessment

History
- Foul smelling, foamy stools
- Intense epigastric pain centered close to the umbilicus and radiating to the back, between the 10th thoracic and 6th lumbar vertebrae
- Malaise and restlessness
- Pain aggravated by fatty foods, alcohol consumption, or recumbent position
- Predisposing factor
- Weight loss with nausea and vomiting

Physical assessment
- Abdominal tenderness, rigidity, and guarding
- Crackles
- Cullen's sign (bluish periumbilical discoloration)
- Diminished bowel sounds
- Dyspnea, orthopnea
- Fever
- Generalized jaundice
- Hypotension
- Steatorrhea (with chronic pancreatitis)
- Tachycardia
- Turner's sign (bluish flank discoloration)

Test results
Laboratory
- Increased serum amylase, lipase, and bilirubin levels
- Increased white blood cell count
- Decreased serum calcium level
- Transient hyperglycemia and glycosuria
- Increased urinary amylase level
- In chronic pancreatitis: increased serum alkaline phosphatase, amylase, and bilirubin levels; transient increase in serum glucose level; and increased lipid and trypsin levels in stool

Imaging
- Abdominal and chest X-rays differentiate pancreatitis from other diseases that cause similar symptoms; they also detect pleural effusions.
- Computed tomography scans and ultrasonography show increased pancreatic diameter, pancreatic cysts, and pseudocysts.

Diagnostic procedures
- ERCP shows pancreatic anatomy, displays ductal system abnormalities, and allows pancreatitis to be differentiated from other disorders.

Nursing diagnoses

○ Acute pain
○ Dysfunctional family process: alcoholism
○ Excess fluid volume
○ Imbalanced nutrition: less than body requirements
○ Nausea
○ Noncompliance with needed lifestyle changes

Key outcomes

The patient will:
○ maintain normal fluid volume
○ maintain a patent airway
○ verbalize feelings of increased comfort
○ avoid complications
○ maintain skin integrity
○ initiate lifestyle changes.

Interventions

General

Crisis stage
○ Blood transfusions (for hemorrhage)
○ Emergency treatment of shock, as needed
○ I.V. replacement of fluid, electrolytes, and proteins

▶ **ALERT** *Acute pancreatitis is a life-threatening emergency; the patient will need vigorous supportive care and continuous monitoring of vital systems.*

○ Nasogastric suctioning
○ Nothing by mouth

Post-crisis stage
○ Activity, as tolerated
○ Alcohol and caffeine abstention
○ Oral low-fat, low-protein feedings implemented gradually
○ Surgery
   – For chronic pancreatitis: sphincterotomy
   – Pancreaticojejunostomy

Nursing

○ Give prescribed drugs and I.V. therapy.
○ Encourage the patient to express his feelings.
○ Offer emotional support.
○ Provide mouth and nose care.

Drug therapy

○ Albumin
○ Analgesics
○ Antacids
○ Antibiotics
○ Anticholinergics
○ Electrolyte replacement
○ Histamine antagonists
○ Insulin
○ Pancreatic enzymes
○ Total parenteral nutrition

Monitoring

○ Acid-base balance
○ Adverse reactions to antibiotics
○ Daily weight
○ Fluid and electrolyte balance
○ Nasogastric tube function and drainage
○ Nutritional status and metabolic requirements
○ Pain control
○ Respiratory status
○ Serum glucose level
○ Vital signs and electrocardiogram

Patient teaching

Be sure to cover:
○ the disorder, diagnosis, and treatment
○ identification and avoidance of acute pancreatitis triggers
○ dietary needs
○ prescribed drugs, dosages, administration, and possible adverse effects.

Discharge planning

○ Refer the patient to community resource and support services, as needed.
○ Refer the patient to Alcoholics Anonymous if pancreatitis is alcohol related.

Pericarditis

Overview

Description

○ Inflammation of the pericardium—the fibroserous sac that envelops, supports, and protects the heart
○ Acute form
  – May be fibrinous or effusive
  – Characterized by serous, purulent, or hemorrhagic exudate
○ Chronic form
  – Characterized by dense fibrous pericardial thickening
  – Also called constrictive pericarditis

Pathophysiology

○ Pericardial tissue is damaged by bacteria or another substance that releases chemical mediators of inflammation into surrounding tissue.
○ Friction results from inflamed layers rubbing against each other.
○ Chemical mediators dilate blood vessels and increase vessel permeability.
○ Vessel walls leak fluids and proteins, causing extracellular edema.

Causes

○ Aortic aneurysm with pericardial leakage
○ Bacterial, fungal, or viral infection (in infectious pericarditis)
○ Cardiac surgery
○ Chest trauma
○ Drugs, such as hydralazine or procainamide
○ High-dose chest radiation
○ Hypersensitivity or autoimmune disease
○ Idiopathic factors
○ Myocardial infarction (MI)
○ Myxedema with cholesterol deposits in pericardium
○ Neoplasms (primary or metastatic)
○ Radiation
○ Rheumatologic conditions
○ Tuberculosis
○ Uremia

Prevalence

○ Affects males more than females

 AGE AWARE Pericarditis is most common in men ages 20 to 50.

Complications

○ Cardiac tamponade
○ Pericardial effusion

Assessment

History

○ Chest pain (may mimic MI pain)
○ Dyspnea
○ Pleuritic pain, increasing with deep inspiration and decreasing when the patient sits up and leans forward
○ Predisposing factor
○ Sharp, sudden pain, usually starting over the sternum and radiating to the neck, shoulders, back, and arms

Physical assessment

○ Diminished or muffled apical impulse
○ Fluid retention, ascites, hepatomegaly (resembling chronic right-sided heart failure)
○ Pericardial friction rub
○ With cardiac tamponade: clammy skin, dyspnea, hypotension, jugular vein distention, pallor, and pulsus paradoxus
○ With pericardial effusion: tachycardia

Test results

Laboratory
○ Increased white blood cell count (especially in infectious pericarditis)
○ Elevated erythrocyte sedimentation rate
○ Slightly increased serum creatinine kinase-MB levels (with myocarditis)
○ Possible causative organism in pericardial fluid culture (bacterial or fungal pericarditis)
○ Increased blood urea nitrogen level in uremia
○ Increased antistreptolysin-O titers (may indicate rheumatic fever)
○ Positive reaction in purified protein derivative skin test; indicates tuberculosis

Imaging
○ Echocardiography shows an echo-free space between the ventricular wall and the pericardium that indicates pericardial effusion.
○ High-resolution computed tomography and magnetic resonance imaging reveals pericardial thickness.

Diagnostic procedures
○ Electrocardiography shows initial ST-segment elevation across the precordium.

Nursing diagnoses

○ Acute pain
○ Decreased cardiac output
○ Excess fluid volume
○ Ineffective breathing pattern

Key outcomes

The patient will:
○ maintain hemodynamic stability and adequate cardiac output

- avoid arrhythmias
- maintain adequate ventilation
- verbalize feelings of increased comfort and decreased pain.

Interventions

General

- Bed rest as long as fever and pain persist
- Dietary restrictions based on underlying disorder
- Management of rheumatic fever, uremia, tuberculosis, or other underlying disorder
- Relief of symptoms
- Surgery
  - Partial pericardectomy (for recurrent pericarditis)
  - Pericardiocentesis
  - Surgical drainage
  - Total pericardectomy (for constrictive pericarditis)

▼ **ALERT** *Place a pericardiocentesis tray at the patient's bedside whenever you suspect pericardial effusion.*

Nursing

- Give prescribed analgesics, antibiotics, and oxygen.
- Stress the importance of bed rest. Provide a bedside commode.
- Place the patient upright to relieve dyspnea and chest pain.
- Encourage the patient to express concerns about the effects of activity restrictions on responsibilities and routines.
- Review the patient's allergy history.
- Provide appropriate postoperative care.

Drug therapy

- Antibiotics
- Corticosteroids
- Diuretics
- Nonsteroidal anti-inflammatory drugs

▼ **ALERT** *Post–MI patients should avoid nonsteroidal anti-inflammatory drugs and corticosteroids because these drugs may interfere with myocardial scar formation.*

Monitoring

- Heart rhythm
- Heart sounds
- Hemodynamic values
- Pain
- Vital signs including central venous pressure

Patient teaching

Be sure to cover:
- the disorder, diagnosis, and treatment
- how to perform deep-breathing and coughing exercises
- the need to resume daily activities slowly and to schedule rest periods in daily routine, as instructed by the doctor.

Discharge planning

- Refer the patient to a physical therapist or chest physiotherapist if needed.

Peritonitis

Overview

Description

- Inflammation of the peritoneum
- May extend throughout the peritoneum or localize as an abscess
- Commonly decreases intestinal motility and causes intestinal distention with gas
- Fatal in 10% of cases, with bowel obstruction the usual cause of death
- May be acute or chronic

Pathophysiology

- The peritoneum is the membrane that lines the abdominal cavity and covers the visceral organs.
- Bacteria invade the peritoneum after inflammation and perforation of the gastrointestinal (GI) tract.
- Fluid containing protein and electrolytes accumulates in the peritoneal cavity; normally transparent, the peritoneum becomes opaque, red, inflamed, and edematous.
- Infection may localize as an abscess rather than disseminate as a generalized infection.

Causes

- Bacterial or chemical inflammation
- GI tract perforation (from appendicitis, diverticulitis, peptic ulcer, or ulcerative colitis)
- Ruptured ectopic pregnancy

Prevalence

- More common in men

Complications

- Abscess
- Bowel obstruction
- Respiratory compromise
- Septicemia
- Shock

Assessment

History

Early phase
- Vague, generalized abdominal pain
- If localized: pain over a specific area (usually the inflammation site)
- If generalized: diffuse pain over the abdomen

With progression
- Anorexia, nausea, and vomiting
- Hiccups
- Inability to pass stools and flatus
- Increasingly severe and constant abdominal pain that increases with movement and breathing
- Possible referral of pain to shoulder or thoracic area

Physical assessment

- Abdominal rigidity
- Fever
- General abdominal tenderness
- Hypotension
- Positive bowel sounds (early); absent bowel sounds (later)
- Rebound tenderness
- Shallow breathing
- Signs of dehydration
- Tachycardia
- Typical patient positioning: lying very still with knees flexed

Test results

Laboratory
- Leukocytosis in complete blood count

Imaging
- Abdominal X-rays show edematous and gaseous distention of the small and large bowel. With perforation of a visceral organ, X-rays show air in the abdominal cavity.
- Chest X-rays may reveal elevation of the diaphragm.
- Computed tomography reveals fluid and inflammation.

Diagnostic procedures
- Paracentesis shows the exudate's nature and permits bacterial culture testing.

Nursing diagnoses

- Acute pain
- Constipation
- Decreased cardiac output
- Imbalanced nutrition: less than body requirements
- Ineffective tissue perfusion: GI
- Nausea
- Risk for infection

Key outcomes

The patient will:
- regain normal vital signs
- express feelings of increased comfort
- maintain normal fluid volume
- show no signs or symptoms of infection
- maintain adequate ventilation.

Interventions

General

- Bed rest until condition improves
- Gradual increase in diet
- I.V. fluids
- Nasogastric (NG) intubation and, possibly, rectal tube
- Nothing by mouth until bowel function returns
- Parenteral nutrition, if necessary
- Semi-Fowler's position

- ○ Surgery: the treatment of choice; procedure varies with the cause of peritonitis
- ○ After surgery: avoidance of lifting for at least 6 weeks

Nursing

- ○ Give prescribed drugs.
- ○ Encourage early postoperative ambulation.
- ○ Allow the patient to express his feelings.
- ○ Offer emotional support.
- ○ Provide mouth and nose care.

Drug therapy

- ○ Analgesics
- ○ Antibiotics, based on infecting organism
- ○ Electrolyte replacement

Monitoring

- ○ Bowel function
- ○ Fluid and nutritional status
- ○ NG tube and rectal tube function and drainage
- ○ Pain control
- ○ Signs and symptoms of dehiscence
- ○ Vital signs
- ○ Wound site

▼ **ALERT** *Monitor the patient for signs and symptoms of abscess formation, including persistent abdominal tenderness and fever.*

Patient teaching

Be sure to cover:
- ○ the disorder, diagnosis, and treatment
- ○ preoperatively, coughing and deep-breathing techniques
- ○ postoperative care procedures
- ○ signs and symptoms of infection
- ○ proper wound care
- ○ prescribed drugs, dosages, administration, and possible adverse effects
- ○ dietary and activity limitations (depending on type of surgery).

Discharge planning

- ○ Refer the patient to a nutritionist, if needed.

Pheochromocytoma

Overview

Description

○ Catecholamine-producing tumor
  – Typically benign
  – Usually derived from adrenal medullary cells
○ Most common cause of adrenal medullary hyper-secretion
  – Usually produces norepinephrine
  – May secrete both epinephrine and norepinephrine if tumor is large
○ Potentially fatal, but good prognosis with treatment
○ Also known as chromaffin tumor

Pathophysiology

○ Pheochromocytoma causes excessive catecholamine production from autonomous tumor functioning.
○ The tumor stems from a chromaffin cell tumor of the adrenal medulla or sympathetic ganglia (more often in the right adrenal gland than in the left).
○ Extra-adrenal pheochromocytomas may occur in the abdomen, thorax, urinary bladder, neck, or vicinity of the 9th and 10th cranial nerves.

Causes

○ May be inherited as an autosomal dominant trait

Prevalence

○ Rare
○ Seen in about 0.5% of newly diagnosed hypertensive patients
○ Affects all races
○ Affects both sexes equally
○ Typically familial

 AGE AWARE Pheochromocytoma is most common in patients ages 30 to 50.

Complications

○ Acute pulmonary edema
○ Cardiac arrhythmias
○ Cerebrovascular accident
○ Cholelithiasis
○ Heart failure
○ Irreversible kidney damage
○ Retinopathy

ALERT Pheochromocytoma may become evident during pregnancy when uterine pressure on the tumor causes more frequent hypertensive crises. These crises carry a high risk for spontaneous abortion and can be fatal for both mother and fetus.

Assessment

History

○ Hypertension that responds poorly to conventional treatment
○ Hypotension or shock after surgery or diagnostic procedures
○ Paroxysmal symptoms suggesting a seizure disorder or anxiety attack
○ Unpredictable episodes of hypertensive crisis

During paroxysms or crisis

○ Blurred vision
○ Dizziness or light-headedness when moving to an upright position
○ Feelings of impending doom
○ Moderate weight loss
○ Nausea and vomiting
○ Palpitations
○ Precordial or abdominal pain
○ Severe diaphoresis
○ Throbbing headache

Physical assessment

During paroxysms or crisis

○ Hypertension
○ Pallor or flushing
○ Profuse sweating
○ Seizures
○ Tachycardia
○ Tachypnea
○ Tremor

Test results

Laboratory

○ Increased levels of vanillylmandelic acid and metanephrine in 24-hour urine specimen
○ Total plasma catecholamine levels 10 to 50 times higher than normal on direct assay

Imaging

○ Computed tomography (CT) scan or magnetic resonance imaging of adrenal glands may show intra-adrenal lesions.
○ CT scan, chest X-rays, or abdominal aortography may reveal extra-adrenal pheochromocytoma.

Nursing diagnoses

○ Acute pain
○ Anxiety
○ Decreased cardiac output
○ Deficient fluid volume
○ Ineffective breathing pattern
○ Nausea
○ Risk for injury

Key outcomes

The patient will:
○ maintain stable vital signs

○ maintain fluid balance
○ maintain normal cardiac output
○ express feelings of increased comfort.

Interventions

General

○ Avoidance of complications
○ High-protein diet with adequate calories
○ Rest during acute attacks
○ Surgical removal of pheochromocytoma

Nursing

○ Take orthostatic blood pressures.
○ Give prescribed drugs.
○ Ensure the reliability of urine catecholamine measurements.
○ Provide comfort measures.
○ Consult a dietitian, as needed.
○ Tell the patient to report symptoms of an acute attack.
○ Encourage the patient to express his feelings.
○ Help the patient develop effective coping strategies.

Drug therapy

○ Alpha blockers
○ Beta blockers
○ Calcium channel blockers
○ Catecholamine-synthesis antagonists
○ I.V. phentolamine or nitroprusside during paroxysms or crises

▼ **ALERT** *Because severe and occasionally fatal paroxysms have been induced by opioids, histamines, and other drugs, all drugs should be considered carefully and given cautiously to patients with known or suspected pheochromocytoma.*

Monitoring

○ Adverse reactions to drugs
○ Cardiovascular status
○ Daily weight
○ Neurologic status
○ Renal function
○ Serum glucose level
○ Vital signs, especially blood pressure
After adrenalectomy
○ Bowel sounds
○ Incision
○ Pain
○ Signs and symptoms of hemorrhage
○ Vital signs
○ Wound dressings

▼ **ALERT** *Hypertension is common after adrenalectomy because the stress of surgery and adrenal gland manipulation stimulates catecholamine secretion.*

Patient teaching

Be sure to cover:
○ the disorder, diagnosis, and treatment
○ prescribed drugs, dosages, administration, and possible adverse effects
○ when to contact a doctor
○ how to prevent paroxysmal attacks
○ signs and symptoms of adrenal insufficiency
○ importance of wearing medical identification jewelry
○ how to monitor blood pressure.

Discharge planning

○ Refer family members for genetic counseling if autosomal dominant transmission of pheochromocytoma is suspected.

Pleural effusion and empyema

Overview

Description

- Fluid accumulation in the pleural space
- Variable fluid type
  - Bilious fluid
  - Blood in hemothorax
  - Chyle in chylothorax
  - Extracellular
  - Pus in empyema
- Effusion may be transudative or exudative

Pathophysiology

- Typically, fluid and other blood components migrate through the walls of intact capillaries bordering the pleura.
- In transudative effusion, fluid is watery and diffuses out of the capillaries if hydrostatic pressure increases or capillary oncotic pressure decreases.
- In exudative effusion, inflammatory processes increase capillary permeability. Fluid is less watery and contains high levels of white blood cells and plasma proteins.
- Empyema occurs when pulmonary lymphatics become blocked and contaminated lymphatic fluid pours into the pleural space.

Causes

Transudative pleural effusion
- Cardiovascular disease
- Hepatic disease with ascites
- Hypoproteinemia
- Renal disease

Exudative pleural effusion
- Chest trauma
- Pancreatitis
- Pleural infection
- Pleural inflammation
- Pleural malignancy

Empyema
- Infected wound
- Intra-abdominal infection
- Lung abscess
- Pulmonary infection
- Thoracic surgery

Prevalence

- May occur at any age
- Affects both sexes equally

Complications

- Atelectasis
- Hypoxemia
- Infection

Assessment

History

- Chest pain
- Malaise
- Nonproductive cough
- Shortness of breath
- Underlying pulmonary disease

Physical assessment

- Bronchial breath sounds
- Diminished or absent breath sounds
- Dullness and decreased tactile fremitus over the effusion
- Fever
- Foul-smelling sputum in empyema
- Pleural friction rub
- Trachea deviated away from the affected side

Test results

Laboratory
- In transudative effusion: specific gravity lower than 1.015; less than 3 g/dl of protein
- In exudative effusion: 0.5 or higher ratio of protein in pleural fluid to protein in serum; lactate dehydrogenase (LDH) level of 200 international units/L or higher; 0.6 or higher ratio of LDH in pleural fluid to LDH in serum
- In empyema: microorganisms present, increased white blood cell count, decreased glucose level
- In esophageal rupture or pancreatitis: pleural fluid amylase levels exceeding serum amylase levels

Imaging
- Chest X-rays may show pleural effusions; lateral decubitus films may show loculated pleural effusions or small pleural effusions not visible on standard chest X-rays.
- Computed tomography scan of the thorax shows small pleural effusions.

Diagnostic procedures
- Thoracentesis is used to obtain pleural fluid specimens for analysis.
- Tuberculin skin test may be positive for tuberculosis.
- Pleural biopsy may be positive for carcinoma.

Nursing diagnoses

- Chronic pain
- Impaired nutrition: less than body requirements
- Ineffective airway clearance
- Ineffective breathing pattern
- Risk for imbalanced fluid volume
- Risk for infection

Key outcomes

The patient will:
- maintain adequate ventilation
- remain free from infection

- consume the specified number of calories daily
- maintain adequate fluid volume
- express an understanding of the illness
- demonstrate effective coping mechanisms.

- Refer the patient to a chest physiotherapist, if needed.

Interventions

General

- Activity, as tolerated
- High-calorie diet
- Possible chemical pleurodesis
- Possible chest-tube insertion
- Surgery to remove thick coating over lung (decortication) or rib resection
- Thoracentesis to remove fluid

Nursing

- Give prescribed drugs and oxygen.
- Assist during thoracentesis.
- Encourage the patient to use incentive spirometry.
- Encourage deep-breathing exercises.
- Provide meticulous chest-tube care.
- Ensure chest-tube patency.
- Keep petroleum gauze and a hemostat at the bedside.

Drug therapy

- Antibiotics
- Oxygen
- Sclerosing agent

Monitoring

- Chest tube drainage
- Intake and output
- Pulse oximetry
- Respiratory status
- Signs and symptoms of pneumothorax
- Vital signs

Patient teaching

Be sure to cover:
- the disorder, diagnosis, and treatment
- prescribed drugs, dosages, administration, and possible adverse effects
- prethoracentesis and post-thoracentesis procedures
- chest tube insertion and drainage
- signs and symptoms of infection
- signs and symptoms of pleural fluid reaccumulation
- when to contact a doctor
- deep breathing and incentive spirometry.

Discharge planning

- Provide a home health referral for follow-up care.
- Refer the patient to a smoking-cessation program, if needed.

Poisoning

Overview

Description
- Contact with a harmful substance via inhalation, ingestion, injection, or skin contact
- Prognosis varies with the amount of poison absorbed, its toxicity, and the time between poisoning and treatment

Pathophysiology
- Varies with the type of poison

Risk factors
- Employment in a chemical plant
- Inappropriate labeling of drugs or chemicals
- Inappropriate storage of drugs or chemicals

Causes
- Accidental drug ingestion
- Homicide attempt
- Improper cooking, canning, or storage of food
- Suicide attempt

Prevalence
- Affects 1 million people annually; fatal in about 800 cases

 AGE AWARE *Poisoning is the fourth most common cause of death in children.*

Complications
- Cardiac arrhythmias
- Cardiovascular collapse
- Coma and death
- Neurogenic shock
- Seizures

Assessment

History
- Drug overdose
- Poison exposure

Physical assessment
- Acute renal failure
- Cardiac arrhythmias
- Cardiovascular depression
- Cardiovascular excitation
- Central nervous system depression or excitability
- Liver failure
- Respiratory depression
- Varies with type of poison

Test results

Laboratory
- Increased or decreased lactate level
- Increased serum calcium and magnesium levels
- Poison identified in the patient's mouth, vomitus, urine, feces, or blood or on the patient's hands or clothing
- Hypoxemia or metabolic abnormalities in arterial blood gas analysis
- Imbalanced serum electrolyte levels such as hypokalemia; possibly anion-gap metabolic acidosis

Imaging
- Chest X-rays may show pulmonary infiltrates or edema in inhalation poisoning; they may show aspiration pneumonia in petroleum distillate inhalation.
- Abdominal X-rays may reveal iron pills or other radiopaque substances.

Diagnostic procedures
- Electrocardiography may show arrhythmias or QRS-complex and QT-interval prolongation.

Nursing diagnoses
- Acute confusion
- Acute pain
- Anxiety
- Ineffective airway clearance
- Ineffective breathing pattern
- Ineffective tissue perfusion (renal)
- Risk for suicide

Key outcomes
The patient will:
- maintain adequate ventilation
- maintain a patent airway
- maintain orientation to time, place, and person
- express feelings of increased comfort and pain relief
- identify factors that increase the risk for injury
- maintain adequate tissue perfusion.

Interventions

General
- Airway and ventilation maintenance
- Emergency resuscitation, as needed
- Hyperthermia blanket, as needed
- Nasogastric tube
- Nothing by mouth until the episode resolves
- Oxygen administration
- Peritoneal dialysis or hemodialysis
- Recommendations of local poison control center
- Safety measures
- Symptomatic care

Nursing
- Perform cardiopulmonary resuscitation, if needed.
- Induce emesis, if recommended.

○ Perform gastric lavage and give a cathartic, as prescribed.
○ Provide supplemental oxygen as ordered and needed.
○ Send vomitus and aspirate for analysis.
○ In severe poisoning, provide peritoneal dialysis or hemodialysis.
○ Ensure patient safety (suicide precautions).

Drug therapy
○ Activated charcoal, if appropriate
○ I.V. hydration
○ Specific antidote, if available
○ Syrup of ipecac, if appropriate

▼ **ALERT** *Never induce vomiting if you suspect corrosive acid poisoning, the patient is unconscious, or the gag reflex is impaired.*

Monitoring
○ Level of consciousness
○ Respiratory status
○ Serum toxin levels
○ Suicidal ideations, if indicated
○ Vital signs

Patient teaching

Be sure to cover:
○ importance of reading all labels before taking drugs
○ proper drug and chemical storage
○ dangers of taking drugs prescribed for someone else
○ dangers of transferring drugs or chemicals from their original container
○ dangers of telling children that medication is "candy"
○ importance of keeping ipecac syrup available at home
○ use of childproof caps on drug containers.

Discharge planning

○ Refer the patient for psychological counseling in case of suicide attempt.
○ Refer the patient to the proper authorities in case of deliberate poisoning.
○ Refer the patient to a poison control center, the local police, and the local fire department for guidelines on how to keep his environment as safe as possible.

Poliomyelitis

Overview

Description

- An acute communicable disease caused by the polio virus
- Ranges in severity from subclinical infection to fatal paralytic illness (mortality 5% to 10%)
- Prognosis excellent if central nervous system (CNS) is spared
- Also called polio or infantile paralysis

Pathophysiology

- The poliovirus has three antigenically distinct serotypes (types I, II, and III) that cause poliomyelitis.
- The incubation period ranges from 5 to 35 days (7 to 14 days on average).
- The virus usually enters the body through the alimentary tract, multiplies in the oropharynx and lower intestinal tract, and then spreads to regional lymph nodes and the blood.
- Factors that increase the risk of paralysis include pregnancy; old age; localized trauma, such as a recent tonsillectomy, tooth extraction, or inoculation; and unusual physical exertion at or just before the clinical onset of poliomyelitis.

Causes

- Contraction of the virus from direct contact with infected oropharyngeal secretions or feces

Prevalence

- Minor polio outbreaks, usually among nonimmunized groups
- Onset during the summer and fall
- Mostly occurs in people older than age 15
- Adults and girls at greater risk for infection; boys, for paralysis

Complications

- Atelectasis
- Cor pulmonale
- Death
- Hypertension
- Myocarditis
- Paralytic ileus
- Paralysis
- Pneumonia
- Skeletal and soft-tissue deformities
- Urinary tract infection
- Urolithiasis

Assessment

History

- Exposure to polio virus
- Fever

Physical assessment

- Muscle weakness
- Patient "tripods" (extend his arms behind him for support) when sitting up
- Patient's head falls back when supine and shoulders are elevated (Hoyne's sign)
- Inability to raise legs 90 degrees when in a supine position
- Kernig's and Brudzinski's signs (paralytic poliomyelitis)

Abortive infection

- Headache
- Inflamed pharynx
- Malaise
- Slight fever
- Sore throat
- Vomiting

Major poliomyelitis, nonparalytic

- Headache
- Irritability
- Lethargy
- Moderate fever
- Muscle tenderness, weakness, and spasms in the extensors of the neck and back and sometimes in the hamstring and other muscles
- Pains in neck, back, arms, legs, and abdomen
- Vomiting

Major poliomyelitis, paralytic

- Abdominal distention
- Asymmetrical weakness of various muscles
- Constipation
- Hypersensitivity to touch
- Loss of superficial and deep reflexes
- Paresthesia
- Symptoms similar to those of nonparalytic poliomyelitis
- Urine retention

Bulbar paralytic

- Difficulty chewing
- Diplopia
- Dysphasia
- Dyspnea
- Facial weakness
- Inability to swallow or expel saliva
- Regurgitation of food through the nasal passages
- Respiratory paralysis
- Symptoms of encephalitis

Test results

Laboratory

- Polio virus isolated from throat washings early in the disease, from stools throughout the disease, and from cerebrospinal fluid cultures in CNS infection

- Convalescent serum antibody titers four times greater than acute titers
- Coxsackievirus and echovirus infections ruled out

Nursing diagnoses

- Acute pain
- Bathing or hygiene self-care deficit
- Hyperthermia
- Ineffective breathing pattern
- Ineffective coping
- Risk for aspiration
- Risk for imbalanced fluid volume
- Risk for injury

Key outcomes

The patient will:
- report feelings of increased comfort
- maintain adequate ventilation
- demonstrate effective coping mechanisms
- use available support systems
- continue to perform activities of daily living
- maintain adequate fluid volume.

Interventions

General

- Activity, as tolerated
- Airway patency, using a tracheostomy if needed
- Assistive devices
- Moist heat application
- Physical therapy
- Supportive care
- Well-balanced diet

Nursing

- Provide emotional support.
- Provide good skin care, reposition the patient often, and keep the bed dry.
- Encourage mild activity as the patient tolerates it.
- Maintain contact isolation.
- Encourage oral intake, and give intravenous fluids as prescribed to ensure an adequate daily output of low–specific-gravity urine (1.5 to 2 L daily for adults).

Drug therapy

- Analgesics
- Antipyretics

▼ **ALERT** *Morphine is contraindicated because of the danger of additional respiratory suppression.*

Monitoring

- Nutritional status
- Respiratory status

- Signs of impaction
- Signs of neurologic damage
- Signs of paralysis
- Vital signs

Patient teaching

Be sure to cover:
- physical therapy
- avoiding complications of limited mobility
- proper hand-washing and contact isolation techniques.

Discharge planning

- Refer the patient to support services and physical rehabilitation services, as appropriate.

Polycystic kidney disease

Overview

Description
- Growth of multiple, bilateral, grapelike clusters of fluid-filled cysts in the kidneys (See *Polycystic kidney.*)
- May progress slowly even after renal insufficiency symptoms appear
- Two forms
  - Infantile form, which causes stillbirth or early neonatal death
  - Adult form, which has insidious onset but usually becomes obvious between ages 30 and 50
- Usually fatal within 4 years of uremic symptom onset, unless dialysis begins
- Widely varying prognosis in adults
- Also known as PKD

Pathophysiology
- Cysts enlarge the kidneys, compressing and eventually replacing functioning renal tissue.
- Renal deterioration results, a process that's more gradual in adults than in infants.
- The condition progresses to fatal uremia.

Causes
- Familial
- Infantile form: inherited as an autosomal recessive trait
- Adult form: inherited as an autosomal dominant trait

Prevalence
- Affects both sexes equally
- Infantile form: 1 in 6,000 to 40,000 infants
- Adult form: 1 in 50 to 1,000 adults

Polycystic kidney

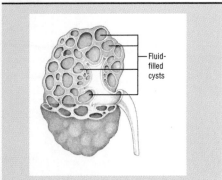

Fluid-filled cysts

Complications
- Heart failure
- Hepatic failure
- Life-threatening retroperitoneal bleeding
- Proteinuria
- Recurrent hematuria
- Renal failure
- Respiratory failure

Assessment

History
Adult form
- Abdominal pain, usually worsened on exertion and eased by lying down
- Family history
- Gross hematuria
- Headaches
- Pain in back or flank area
- Polyuria
- Urinary tract infections

Physical assessment
Infantile form
- Floppy, low set ears (Potter facies)
- Pronounced bilateral, symmetrical flank masses that are tense and can't be transilluminated
- Pronounced epicanthal folds
- Pointed nose
- Signs of portal hypertension (bleeding varices)
- Signs of respiratory distress, heart failure and, eventually, uremia and renal failure
- Small chin

Adult form
- Grossly enlarged kidneys (advanced stages)
- Hypertension
- Signs of an enlarging kidney mass

Test results
Laboratory
- Possible blood, bacteria, or protein in urine
- Possible renal insufficiency or failure in creatinine clearance test
- Possible sodium loss or retention

Imaging
- Excretory or retrograde urography reveals enlarged kidneys with pelvic elongation, flattening of the calyces, and indentations caused by cysts. In a neonate, excretory urography shows poor excretion of contrast medium.
- Ultrasonography, tomography, and radioisotopic scans show kidney enlargement and cysts.
- Tomography, computed tomography scan, and magnetic resonance imaging show multiple areas of cystic damage.

Nursing diagnoses

○ Acute pain
○ Death anxiety
○ Decreased cardiac output
○ Excess fluid volume
○ Ineffective tissue perfusion: renal
○ Risk for infection

Key outcomes

The patient will:
○ maintain fluid balance
○ maintain urine specific gravity within designated limits
○ maintain hemodynamic stability
○ report feelings of increased comfort
○ identify risk factors that further decrease tissue perfusion, and modify lifestyle appropriately.

Interventions

General

○ Avoidance of contact sports
○ Dialysis
○ Drainage of cystic abscess or retroperitoneal bleeding
○ Fluid restriction (in renal failure)
○ Low-protein and, possibly, low-sodium diet
○ Monitoring of renal function
○ Prevention of infections
○ Rarely, kidney transplantation

Nursing

○ Give prescribed drugs.
○ Provide supportive care to minimize symptoms.
○ Individualize patient care accordingly.

Drug therapy

○ Analgesics
○ Antibiotics for urinary tract infection
○ Antihypertensives for hypertension

Monitoring

○ Access site for dialysis
○ Electrolytes
○ Intake and output
○ Urine (for blood, cloudiness, calculi, granules, culture, and creatinine clearance)
○ Vital signs

Patient teaching

Be sure to cover:
○ the disorder, diagnosis, and treatment
○ prescribed drugs, dosages, administration, and possible adverse effects

○ follow-up with the doctor for severe or recurring headaches
○ signs and symptoms of urinary tract infection and the need to notify the doctor promptly
○ importance of blood pressure control
○ possible need for dialysis or transplantation.

Discharge planning

○ Refer a young adult patient or the parents of an infant with polycystic kidney disease for genetic counseling.

Pregnancy-induced hypertension

Overview

Description
○ High blood pressure, typically after the 20th week of gestation in a nulliparous woman
○ Carries a high risk for fetal mortality because of the increased risk of premature delivery
○ Among the most common causes of maternal death in developed countries (especially when complications occur)
○ Nonconvulsive form
  – Also called preeclampsia
  – Occurs after the 20th week of gestation
  – May be mild or severe
○ Convulsive form
  – Also called eclampsia
  – Occurs between the 24th week of gestation and the end of the first postpartum week

Pathophysiology
○ Generalized arteriolar vasoconstriction probably decreases blood flow through the placenta and maternal organs.
○ This leads to intrauterine growth retardation or restriction, placental infarcts, and abruptio placentae.

Causes
○ Unknown
○ Contributing factors: geographic, ethnic, racial, nutritional, immunologic, and familial factors; vascular disease; maternal age; autolysis of placental infarcts; autointoxication; uremia; maternal sensitization to total proteins; pyelonephritis; and diabetes

 AGE AWARE *Adolescents and primiparas older than age 35 are at higher risk for preeclampsia.*

Prevalence
○ Occurs in about 7% of pregnancies; more common in women from lower socioeconomic groups
○ Progresses to eclampsia in about 5% of preeclampsia cases
○ Fatal in about 15% of patients with eclampsia, from pregnancy-induced hypertension itself or from complications

Complications
○ Abruptio placentae
○ Coagulopathy
○ Coma
○ HELLP syndrome: hemolysis, elevated liver enzyme levels, low platelet count
○ Maternal hepatic damage
○ Premature labor
○ Renal failure
○ Seizures
○ Stillbirth

Assessment

History
○ Blurred vision
○ Emotional tension
○ Epigastric pain or heartburn
○ Irritability
○ Sudden weight gain: more than 3 lb weekly during the second trimester or 1 lb during the third trimester
○ Severe frontal headache

Physical assessment
○ Generalized edema, especially of the face
○ Hyperreflexia
○ Hypertension
  – Preeclampsia: blood pressure of 160/110 mm Hg or higher
  – Eclampsia: systolic blood pressure of 180 or 200 mm Hg or higher
○ Oliguria
○ Pitting edema of the legs and feet
○ Seizures

Test results
Laboratory
○ Proteinuria
  – In preeclampsia: more than 300 mg/24 hours [1+]
  – In severe eclampsia: 5 g/24 hours [5+] or more
○ In HELLP syndrome: hemolysis, elevated liver enzymes, and low platelet count
Imaging
○ Ultrasonography aids evaluation of fetal well-being.
Diagnostic procedures
○ Stress and nonstress tests and biophysical profiles help evaluate fetal well-being.
○ Vascular spasm, papilledema, retinal edema or detachment, and arteriovenous nicking or hemorrhage may be seen using ophthalmoscopy.

Nursing diagnoses
○ Acute confusion
○ Anticipatory grieving
○ Anxiety
○ Compromised family coping
○ Death anxiety
○ Decreased cardiac output
○ Excess fluid volume
○ Risk for impaired parent/infant attachment

Key outcomes

The patient will:
○ maintain normal vital signs
○ maintain adequate fluid volume
○ avoid complications
○ remain oriented to the environment.

Interventions

General

○ Adequate nutrition
○ Complete bed rest
○ Left lateral lying position
○ Limited caffeine
○ Low-sodium diet, if indicated
○ Measures to halt progression of the disorder and ensure fetal survival
○ Possible cesarean delivery
○ Prompt labor induction, especially if the patient is near term (advocated by some clinicians)

Nursing

○ Give prescribed drugs.
○ Elevate edematous arms or legs.
○ Eliminate constricting hose, slippers, and bed linens.
○ Assist with or insert an indwelling urinary catheter, if needed.
○ Provide a quiet, darkened room.
○ Enforce absolute bed rest.
○ Provide emotional support.
○ Encourage the patient to express her feelings.
○ Help the patient develop effective coping strategies.

Drug therapy

○ Antihypertensives

 ALERT *Diuretics aren't appropriate during pregnancy.*

○ Magnesium sulfate
○ Oxygen
○ Oxytocin

Monitoring

○ Complications
○ Daily weight
○ Deep tendon reflexes
○ Edema
○ Fetal heart rate
○ Headache unrelieved by medication
○ Intake and output
○ Vision
○ Vital signs
○ Level of consciousness

Patient teaching

Be sure to cover:
○ the disorder, diagnosis, and treatment
○ signs and symptoms of preeclampsia and eclampsia
○ importance of bed rest in the left lateral position, as ordered
○ adequate nutrition and a low-sodium diet
○ good prenatal care
○ control of hypertension
○ early recognition and prompt treatment of preeclampsia
○ likelihood that the neonate will be small for gestational age, with the probability that he'll do better than other premature babies of the same weight.

Discharge planning

○ Refer the patient for professional counseling, as indicated.

Protein-losing enteropathy

Overview

Description
- An abnormal loss of protein from the digestive tract or the inability of the gastrointestinal (GI) tract to absorb proteins
- Normally, 10% to 20% of albumin turnover in the GI tract

Pathophysiology
- Disease processes that cause protein-losing enteropathy are grouped into two major categories.
  - Lymphatic obstruction increases pressure in the lymphatic system of the GI tract, causing stasis of lymph and loss of albumin and protein-rich lymphatic fluid into the lumen of the GI tract. When albumin loss exceeds the rate of synthesis, hypoalbuminemia and edema occur.
  - Mucosal erosion or ulceration prevents protein absorption along the GI tract.

Causes
Lymphatic obstruction
- Idiopathic intestinal lymphangiectasia
- Lymphoma
- Tumor

GI mucosal ulceration
- Celiac sprue
- Crohn's disease
- Fistulae
- Gastric cancer
- Gastric ulcer
- Irritable bowel syndrome
- Ulcerative colitis

Other
- Heart failure

Prevalence
- Unknown
- No prevalence patterns related to race, sex, or age

Complications
- Heart failure
- Infection
- Respiratory insufficiency

Assessment

History
- Predisposing condition
- Swelling

Physical assessment
- Abdominal tenderness
- Diarrhea
- Edema
- Hypertension
- Jugular vein distention

Test results
Laboratory
- Decreased serum albumin levels
- Confirmation of intestinal tract as site of protein loss via alpha$_1$-antitrypsin stool clearance test, which involves 24-hour stool and blood collection

Nursing diagnoses
- Decreased cardiac output
- Diarrhea
- Excess fluid volume
- Impaired nutrition: less than body requirements

Key outcomes
The patient will:
- maintain adequate fluid and electrolyte balance
- maintain normal serum albumin levels
- maintain stable vital signs
- maintain adequate cardiac output
- express an understanding of the disorder and treatment.

Interventions

General
- Treatment for underlying cause
- Adequate intake of dietary protein
- Maintenance of fluid balance

Nursing
- Give prescribed drugs.
- Provide comfort measures.
- Elevate limbs to prevent or treat edema.
- Encourage activity and ambulation as tolerated.

Drug therapy
- Albumin replacement
- Diuretics
- Electrolyte supplementation, if indicated
- Fat-soluble vitamin supplementation
- Histamine$_2$ blockers

Monitoring
- Daily weight
- Intake and output
- Serum albumin levels
- Stool for occult blood
- Vital signs

Patient teaching

Be sure to cover:
○ the diagnosis, prognosis, and treatment
○ prescribed drugs, dosages, administration, and possible adverse effects
○ importance and components of a high-protein diet
○ importance of daily weight monitoring and when to call the doctor
○ importance of abstaining from alcohol.

Discharge planning

○ Refer the patient to a nutritionist, as indicated.

Psychogenic polydipsia

Overview

Description
○ A disorder that causes excessive water-drinking in the absence of a physiologic stimulus to drink

Pathophysiology
○ Psychogenic polydipsia is a psychiatric condition.
○ There's no apparent reason for excessive thirst or intake.
○ The condition is well tolerated if water intoxication and hyponatremia don't occur.

Causes
○ Unknown

Prevalence
○ Uncommon
○ Most common among long-term psychiatric patients, especially schizophrenics

 AGE AWARE In children, this disorder may reflect emotional difficulties.

Complications
○ Coma
○ Seizures

Assessment

History
○ Excessive intake of water or other fluid
○ Excessive thirst
○ Frequent and copious urination
Water intoxication
○ Confusion
○ Headache
○ Irritability
○ Weight gain

Physical assessment
○ Intake of about 4 or more gallons of fluid daily, usually water
○ Urine output up to 5 L daily
○ Pale or colorless urine
○ No signs or symptoms of dehydration (no dry mucous membranes or poor skin turgor)
Water intoxication
○ Mental status changes
○ Seizures

Test results
Laboratory
○ Decreased serum sodium level and hematocrit
○ Urine specific gravity less than 1.005
○ Urine protein less than 2 mg/dl
○ Urine osmolality less than 100 mOsm/kg
Diagnostic procedures
○ The water deprivation test measures serum and urine osmolality after drastically decreasing fluid intake over a number of hours. It illustrates that drinking less does not cause the patient to become ill and that the patient will produce less urine with less fluid intake.

Nursing diagnoses

○ Acute confusion
○ Excess fluid volume
○ Ineffective coping

Key outcomes
The patient will:
○ maintain hemodynamic stability
○ maintain an adequate fluid balance
○ have normal serum sodium levels
○ experience no mental status changes
○ verbalize an understanding of the disorder and its consequences.

Interventions

General
○ Fluid restriction
○ No treatment unless hyponatremia or water intoxication occurs

Nursing
○ Give prescribed drugs.
○ Offer emotional support.
○ Provide safety measures.

Drug therapy
○ Clozapine
Hyponatremia
○ Demeclocycline or lithium
○ Hypertonic (3% or 5%) saline solutions (if serum sodium level is less than 110 mEq/L)
○ Normal saline solution
○ Oral sodium supplements

ALERT Monitor the patient carefully when giving hypertonic saline solutions. They can cause water to shift out of the cells, which may lead to intravascular volume overload and serious brain damage.

Monitoring
○ Intake and output
○ Serum sodium and serum and urine osmolality
○ Signs and symptoms of cerebral edema
○ Vital signs

Patient teaching

Be sure to cover:
- the diagnosis, prognosis, and treatment
- prescribed drugs, dosages, administration, and possible adverse reactions
- how to monitor intake and output
- signs and symptoms of cerebral edema and hyponatremia and when to contact the doctor
- fluid restrictions, if needed
- foods high in sodium, if needed.

Discharge planning

- Refer the patient to a psychiatrist or psychologist.
- Refer the patient to a nutritionist.

Pulmonary edema

Overview

Description
○ Accumulation of fluid in the extravascular spaces of the lung
○ Common complication of cardiovascular disorders
○ May be chronic or acute
○ Can become fatal rapidly

Pathophysiology
○ Pulmonary edema results from either increased pulmonary capillary hydrostatic pressure or decreased colloid osmotic pressure. Normally, the two pressures are in balance.
○ If pulmonary capillary hydrostatic pressure increases, the compromised left ventricle needs higher filling pressures to maintain adequate output; these pressures are transmitted to the left atrium, pulmonary veins, and pulmonary capillary bed. Fluids and solutes are then forced from the intravascular compartment into the lung interstitium. With fluid overloading the interstitium, some fluid floods peripheral alveoli and impairs gas exchange.
○ If colloid osmotic pressure decreases, the pulling force that contains intravascular fluids is lost, and nothing opposes the hydrostatic force. Fluid flows freely into the interstitium and alveoli, causing pulmonary edema.

Causes
○ Acute myocardial ischemia and infarction
○ Arrhythmias
○ Barbiturate or opioid poisoning
○ Diastolic dysfunction
○ Fluid overload
○ Impaired pulmonary lymphatic drainage
○ Inhalation of irritating gases
○ Left atrial myxoma
○ Left-sided heart failure
○ Pneumonia
○ Pulmonary veno-occlusive disease
○ Valvular heart disease

Prevalence
○ More common in middle-age and elderly people
○ Affects both sexes equally

Complications
○ Cardiac or respiratory arrest
○ Death
○ Respiratory and metabolic acidosis

Assessment

History
○ Dyspnea on exertion
○ Orthopnea
○ Paroxysmal nocturnal dyspnea
○ Persistent cough
○ Predisposing factor

Physical assessment
○ Crackles
○ Diastolic S_3 gallop
○ Frothy, bloody sputum
○ Hepatomegaly
○ Hypotension
○ Intense, productive cough
○ Jugular vein distention
○ Mental status changes
○ Peripheral edema
○ Rapid, labored breathing
○ Restlessness and anxiety
○ Sweaty, cold, clammy skin
○ Tachycardia
○ Thready pulse
○ Wheezing

Test results
Laboratory
○ Hypoxemia, hypercapnia, or acidosis in arterial blood gas analysis
Imaging
○ Chest X-rays show diffuse haziness of the lung fields, cardiomegaly, and pleural effusion.
Diagnostic procedures
○ Pulse oximetry may show decreased oxygen saturation.
○ Pulmonary artery catheterization may reveal increased pulmonary artery wedge pressures.
○ Electrocardiography may show valvular disease and left ventricular hypokinesis or akinesis.

Nursing diagnoses

○ Anxiety
○ Decreased cardiac output
○ Excess fluid volume
○ Fatigue
○ Fear
○ Ineffective breathing pattern
○ Ineffective coping

Key outcomes
The patient will:
○ maintain adequate ventilation
○ maintain fluid balance
○ maintain adequate cardiac output
○ verbalize decreased anxiety and fear
○ demonstrate adequate coping mechanisms.

Interventions

General

- Fluid overload reduction
- Improved gas exchange and myocardial function
- Correction of underlying disease
- Sodium-restricted diet
- Fluid restriction
- Activity, as tolerated
- Valve repair or replacement or myocardial revascularization, if appropriate, to correct the underlying cause

Nursing

- Give prescribed drugs and oxygen.
- Place the patient in high Fowler's position.
- Restrict fluids and sodium intake.
- Promote rest and relaxation.
- Provide emotional support.

Drug therapy

- Afterload-reducing drugs
- Antiarrhythmics
- Bronchodilators
- Diuretics
- Morphine

▼ *ALERT Morphine may further compromise respiration in a patient with respiratory distress. Keep resuscitation equipment nearby in case the patient stops breathing.*

- Positive inotropic drugs
- Preload-reducing drugs
- Supplemental oxygen
- Vasopressors

Monitoring

- Arterial blood gas values
- Complications
- Daily weight
- Heart rhythm
- Hemodynamic values
- Intake and output
- Pulse oximetry values
- Respiratory status
- Response to treatment
- Vital signs

Patient teaching

Be sure to cover:
- the disorder, diagnosis, and treatment
- prescribed drugs, dosages, administration, and possible adverse reactions
- fluid and sodium restrictions
- daily weight
- signs and symptoms of fluid overload
- energy conservation strategies
- avoidance of alcohol
- when to contact the doctor.

Discharge planning

- Refer the patient to a cardiac rehabilitation program, if indicated.
- Refer the patient to a smoking-cessation program, if needed.

Pulmonary embolism

Overview

Description

O Obstruction of the pulmonary arterial bed when a mass lodges in the main pulmonary artery or branch, partially or completely blocking it
O Blockage usually from a thrombus dislodged from a deep leg vein
O May be asymptomatic
O May be rapidly fatal from pulmonary infarction

Pathophysiology

O Thrombus formation results from vascular wall damage, venous stasis, or blood hypercoagulability.
O Trauma, clot dissolution, sudden muscle spasm, intravascular pressure changes, or peripheral blood flow changes can cause the thrombus to loosen or fragmentize.
O The thrombus (now an embolus) floats through the right side of the heart and enters the lung through the pulmonary artery. There, the embolus may dissolve, fragment, or grow.
O By occluding the pulmonary artery, the embolus prevents alveoli from producing enough surfactant to maintain alveolar integrity. Alveoli collapse, and atelectasis develops.
O If the embolus enlarges, it may occlude most or all of the pulmonary vessels and cause death.

Causes

O Atrial fibrillation
O Deep vein thrombosis
O Pelvic, renal, and hepatic vein thrombosis
O Rarely, other types of emboli, such as bone, air, fat, amniotic fluid, tumor cells, or a foreign body
O Right heart thrombus
O Upper extremity thrombosis
O Valvular heart disease

Prevalence

O The most common pulmonary complication in hospitalized patients
O 600,000 to 700,000 cases annually
O Affects both sexes equally
O More common with advancing age

Complications

O Acute respiratory distress syndrome
O Death
O Embolic extension
O Hepatic congestion and necrosis
O Massive atelectasis
O Pulmonary abscess
O Pulmonary hypertension
O Pulmonary infarction
O Right-sided heart failure

Assessment

History

O Pleuritic pain or angina
O Predisposing factor
O Shortness of breath for no apparent reason

Physical assessment

O Crackles
O Hypotension
O Low-grade fever
O Productive cough, possibly with blood-tinged sputum
O Restlessness
O S_3 and S_4 sounds, with increased intensity of the pulmonic component of S_2
O Tachycardia
O Transient pleural friction rub
O Warmth, tenderness, and edema of the lower leg
O Weak, rapid pulse
O With a large embolus: cyanosis, distended jugular veins, syncope

Test results

Laboratory
O Hypoxemia on arterial blood gas analysis
O Elevated D-dimer level
Imaging
O Lung ventilation perfusion scan shows a ventilation-perfusion mismatch.
O Pulmonary angiography shows a pulmonary vessel filling defect or an abrupt vessel ending and reveals the location and extent of pulmonary embolism.
O Chest X-rays may show a small infiltrate or effusion.
O Spiral chest computed tomography scan may show central pulmonary emboli.
Diagnostic procedures
O Electrocardiography may reveal right axis deviation and right bundle-branch block; it also may show atrial fibrillation.

Nursing diagnoses

O Acute pain
O Anxiety
O Decreased cardiac output
O Deficient fluid volume
O Impaired gas exchange
O Ineffective breathing pattern
O Ineffective coping

Key outcomes

The patient will:
O maintain adequate ventilation
O maintain adequate cardiac output
O maintain a patent airway

- verbalize feelings of increased comfort
- demonstrate effective coping mechanisms
- maintain fluid volume balance.

Interventions

General

- Bed rest during the acute phase
- Maintenance of adequate cardiovascular and pulmonary function
- Mechanical ventilation, if indicated
- Possible fluid restriction
- Surgery
  - Vena caval interruption
  - Vena caval filter placement
  - Pulmonary embolectomy

Nursing

- Give prescribed drugs.
- Avoid I.M. injections.
- Encourage active and passive range-of-motion exercises, unless contraindicated.
- Avoid massaging the lower legs.
- Apply antiembolism stockings.
- Provide adequate nutrition.
- Assist with ambulation as soon as the patient is stable.
- Encourage use of incentive spirometry.

Drug therapy

- Antiarrhythmics
- Antibiotics (for septic embolus)
- Anticoagulation
- Corticosteroids (controversial)
- Diuretics
- Oxygen
- Thrombolytics
- Vasopressors (for hypotension)

Monitoring

- Abnormal bleeding
- Arterial blood gas values
- Coagulation study results
- Complications
- Intake and output
- Pulse oximetry
- Respiratory status
- Signs of deep vein thrombosis
- Stools for occult blood
- Vital signs

Patient teaching

Be sure to cover:
- the disease, diagnosis, and treatment
- prescribed drugs, dosages, administration, and possible adverse effects

- ways to prevent deep vein thrombosis and pulmonary embolism
- signs and symptoms of abnormal bleeding
- prevention of abnormal bleeding
- how to monitor anticoagulant effects
- the need for follow-up blood work
- dietary sources of vitamin K
- when to notify the doctor.

Discharge planning

- Refer the patient to a weight-management program, if indicated.
- Refer the patient to a nutritionist, if needed.

Radiation exposure

Overview

Description
○ Exposure to excessive tissue-damaging radiation
○ Variable damage based on amount of body area exposed, length of exposure, dosage absorbed, distance from the source, and presence of protective shielding
○ May result from cancer radiotherapy, working in a radiation facility, or other exposure to radioactive materials
○ May be acute or chronic

Pathophysiology
○ Ionization occurs in the molecules of living cells.
○ Electrons are removed from atoms. Charged atoms or ions form and react with other atoms to cause cell damage.
○ Rapidly dividing cells are the most susceptible to radiation damage. Highly differentiated cells are more resistant to radiation.

Risk factors
○ Cancer
○ Employment in a facility that contains or uses radiation

Causes
○ Exposure to radiation through inhalation, ingestion, or direct contact

Prevalence
○ Unknown

Complications
○ Anemia
○ Bone necrosis and fractures
○ Decreased fertility
○ Fetal growth retardation or genetic defects in offspring (from exposure during childbearing years)
○ Leukemia
○ Malignant neoplasms
○ Shortened life span
○ Thyroid cancer

Assessment

History
Acute hematopoietic radiation toxicity
○ Bleeding from the skin, genitourinary tract, and gastrointestinal (GI) tract
○ Hemorrhage
○ Increased susceptibility to infection
○ Nosebleeds

GI radiation toxicity
○ Intractable nausea, vomiting, and diarrhea
Cerebral radiation toxicity
○ Nausea, vomiting, and diarrhea
○ Lethargy
Cardiovascular radiation toxicity
○ Hypotension, shock, and cardiac arrhythmias

Physical assessment
Acute hematopoietic radiation toxicity
○ Oropharyngeal abscesses
○ Pallor
○ Petechiae
○ Weakness
GI radiation toxicity
○ Circulatory collapse and death
○ Mouth and throat ulcers and infection
Cerebral radiation toxicity
○ Coma and death
○ Confusion
○ Seizures
○ Tremors
Generalized radiation exposure
○ Alopecia
○ Brittle nails
○ Cataracts
○ Signs of hypothyroidism
○ Skin dryness, erythema, atrophy, and malignant lesions

Test results
Laboratory
○ Decreased white blood cell, platelet, and lymphocyte counts
○ Decreased serum potassium and chloride levels
Imaging
○ X-rays may reveal bone necrosis.
Diagnostic procedures
○ Bone marrow studies may show blood dyscrasia.
○ A Geiger counter helps determine if radioactive material was ingested or inhaled and allows evaluation of the amount of radiation in open wounds.

Nursing diagnoses

○ Fatigue
○ Deficient fluid volume
○ Imbalanced nutrition: less than body requirements
○ Impaired oral mucous membrane
○ Impaired skin integrity
○ Risk for infection

Key outcomes
The patient will:
○ maintain an acceptable weight
○ maintain normal fluid volume
○ remain free from signs and symptoms of infection.

Interventions

General

- Activity as tolerated
- High-protein, high-calorie diet
- Management of life-threatening injuries
- Symptomatic and supportive treatment based on the type and extent of radiation injury

Nursing

- Implement appropriate respiratory and cardiac support measures.
- Give prescribed I.V. fluids and electrolytes.
- For skin contamination, wash the patient's body thoroughly with mild soap and water.
- Debride and irrigate open wounds, as ordered.
- For ingested radioactive material, perform gastric lavage and whole-bowel irrigation, and give activated charcoal, as ordered.
- Dispose of contaminated clothing properly.
- Dispose of contaminated excrement and body fluids according to facility policy.
- Use strict sterile technique.

Drug therapy

- Aluminum phosphate gel
- Antiemetics
- Barium sulfate
- Chelating drugs
- Potassium iodide

Monitoring

- Fluid and electrolyte balance
- Intake and output
- Nutritional status
- Signs and symptoms of hemorrhage
- Vital signs

Patient teaching

Be sure to cover:
- the injury process, diagnosis, and treatment
- effects of radiation exposure
- how to prevent a recurrence
- skin care
- wound care
- need for follow-up care.

Discharge planning

- Refer the patient to resource and support services.
- If the patient was exposed to significant amounts of radiation, provide a referral to genetic counseling resources.

Rapidly progressing glomerulonephritis

Overview

Description
○ A form of kidney disease
○ Involves the glomeruli: portions of the internal kidney structures where the blood flows through very small capillaries and is filtered through membranes to form urine
○ Includes any type of glomerulonephritis (inflammation of the glomerulus) in which progressive loss of kidney function occurs over weeks to months

Pathophysiology
○ Rapidly progressing glomerulonephritis causes damage to the internal structures of the kidneys.
○ The kidneys quickly lose function.
○ The condition may develop as acute nephritic syndrome or unexplained renal failure.

Causes
○ Abscess of any internal organ
○ Anti-glomerular basement membrane antibody
○ Goodpasture's syndrome
○ Immunoglobulin A nephropathy
○ Lupus nephritis
○ Lymphatic system disorders
○ Malignant tumors or blood
○ Membranoproliferative glomerulonephritis
○ Polyarteritis
○ Vasculitis

Prevalence

�֎ AGE AWARE *Rapidly progressing glomerulonephritis is most common in people ages 40 to 60. It's rare in preschool-age children and slightly more common in later childhood.*

○ Slightly more common in men

Complications
○ Acute or chronic renal failure and end-stage renal disease
○ Heart failure
○ Infection
○ Pulmonary edema

Assessment

History
○ Abdominal pain
○ Anorexia
○ Cough
○ Diarrhea
○ Malaise
○ Muscle and joint aches
○ Predisposing condition
○ Shortness of breath

Physical assessment
○ Arrhythmias
○ Crackles
○ Dark urine
○ Dyspnea
○ Edema
○ Fever
○ Hypertension
○ Jugular vein distention
○ Oliguria

Test results
Laboratory
○ Hematuria
○ Proteinuria
○ White blood cells and casts in urine
○ Decreased 24-hour creatinine clearance
○ Increased serum blood urea nitrogen, creatinine, and potassium levels
○ Possible positive anti-glomerular basement membrane antibody test
Diagnostic procedures
○ The diagnosis is confirmed when 50% or more glomeruli reveal crescents on kidney biopsy.
○ Electrocardiography may show arrhythmias caused by hyperkalemia.

Nursing diagnoses

○ Acute pain
○ Decreased cardiac output
○ Diarrhea
○ Excess fluid volume
○ Imbalanced nutrition: less than body requirements
○ Impaired urinary elimination
○ Ineffective breathing pattern
○ Risk for infection

Key outcomes
The patient will:
○ maintain hemodynamic stability
○ remain free of signs and symptoms of infection
○ maintain respiratory sufficiency
○ produce adequate urine output
○ verbalize increased comfort.

Interventions

General
○ Dialysis
○ Kidney transplant
○ Plasmapheresis
○ Treatment for causative disorder

Nursing

- ○ Give prescribed drugs.
- ○ Provide comfort measures.
- ○ Promote activity and ambulation as tolerated.
- ○ Elevate limbs to prevent or treat edema.

Drug therapy

- ○ Antibiotics
- ○ Corticosteroids
- ○ Immunosuppressants
- ○ Oxygen

Monitoring

- ○ Daily weight
- ○ Electrocardiogram
- ○ Intake and output
- ○ Pain level
- ○ Respiratory status
- ○ Serum blood urea nitrogen, creatinine, and electrolytes
- ○ Vital signs

Patient teaching

Be sure to cover:
- ○ the diagnosis, prognosis, and treatment
- ○ the importance of daily weights
- ○ prescribed drugs, dosages, administration, and possible adverse effects
- ○ how to measure intake and output, and when to call the doctor
- ○ signs and symptoms of infection.

Discharge planning

- ○ Refer the patient to an outpatient dialysis center, if appropriate.
- ○ Refer the patient to support services and a nutritionist, as indicated.

Renal calculi

Overview

Description
- Formation of calculi (commonly called stones) anywhere in the urinary tract
- Most common in the renal pelvis or calyces
- Variable size and quantity
- Warrant hospitalization in about 1 of every 1,000 Americans

Pathophysiology
- Calculi form when substances normally dissolved in the urine, such as calcium oxalate and calcium phosphate, precipitate.
- Large, rough calculi may occlude the opening to the ureteropelvic junction.
- The frequency and force of peristaltic contractions increase, causing pain.

Risk factors
- Dehydration
- Immobilization
- Infection
- Metabolic factors
- Urinary tract obstruction
- Urine pH changes

Causes
- Unknown

Prevalence
- Occur in 1 in 1,000 Americans
- Affect more men than women
- Rare in Blacks and children

Complications
- Complete ureteral obstruction
- Hydronephrosis
- Renal cell necrosis
- Renal parenchymal damage

Assessment

History
- Anuria (rare)
- Classic renal colic pain: severe pain that travels from the costovertebral angle to the flank and then to the suprapubic region and external genitalia
- Fever, chills
- Nausea, vomiting
- Pain of fluctuating intensity; may be excruciating at its peak
- With calculi in the renal pelvis and calyces: relatively constant, dull pain

Physical assessment
- Abdominal distention
- Hematuria

Test results
Laboratory
- Calcium oxalate, phosphorus, and uric acid in 24-hour urine collection
- Increased urine specific gravity
- Hematuria and pyuria
- Crystals and casts in urine
- Mineral content of calculi available through analysis

Imaging
- Kidney-ureter-bladder (KUB) X-rays reveal most renal calculi.
- Excretory urography helps confirm the diagnosis and determines calculi size and location.
- Kidney ultrasonography can detect obstructive changes and radiolucent calculi not seen on KUB films.
- Computed tomography scan is highly sensitive for identifying hydronephrosis and detecting small renal and urethral calculi.

Nursing diagnoses
- Acute pain
- Impaired urinary elimination
- Nausea
- Readiness for enhanced knowledge related to prevention of renal calculi
- Risk for imbalanced fluid volume

Key outcomes
The patient will:
- maintain fluid balance
- report increased comfort
- identify risk factors that increase calculus formation and modify lifestyle accordingly
- demonstrate the ability to manage urinary elimination problems.

Interventions

General
- Dietary restrictions based on composition of calculi
- Extracorporeal shock wave lithotripsy
- Percutaneous ultrasonic lithotripsy
- Surgery
  - Cystoscopy
  - Parathyroidectomy for hyperparathyroidism
- Vigorous hydration (more than 3 qt [3 L] daily)

Nursing
- Provide I.V. fluids, as ordered; force fluids as needed.
- Strain all urine and save solid material for analysis.

○ Encourage ambulation to aid spontaneous calculus passage.

Drug therapy
○ Allopurinol (for uric acid calculi)
○ Analgesics
○ Antibiotics
○ Ascorbic acid
○ Diuretics
○ Methenamine mandelate

Monitoring
○ Catheter function and drainage
○ Daily weight
○ Intake and output
○ Pain control
○ Signs and symptoms of infection

Patient teaching

Be sure to cover:
○ the disorder, diagnosis, and treatment
○ prescribed diet and importance of compliance
○ prescribed drugs, dosages, administration, and possible adverse effects
○ ways to prevent recurrences
○ how to strain urine for stones
○ immediate return visit to hospital for fever, uncontrolled pain, or vomiting.

Discharge planning

○ Patients who don't meet admission criteria should arrange for a follow-up with a urologist in 2 to 3 days.
○ Refer the patient to a nutritionist, if needed.

Renal failure, acute

Overview

Description

○ Sudden interruption of renal function caused by obstruction, reduced circulation, or renal parenchymal disease
○ Classified as prerenal failure, intrarenal failure (also called intrinsic or parenchymal failure), or postrenal failure
○ Usually reversible with treatment
○ Untreated, may progress to end-stage renal disease, uremia, and death
○ Normally occurs in three phases: oliguric, diuretic, and recovery

Prerenal failure
○ Prerenal failure is caused by impaired blood flow.
○ Decrease in filtration pressure causes decline in glomerular filtration rate.
○ Failure to restore blood volume or blood pressure may cause acute tubular necrosis or acute cortical necrosis. (See *Preventing acute tubular necrosis.*)

Intrarenal failure
○ Intrarenal failure results from damage to the kidneys themselves.

Postrenal failure
○ Postrenal failure usually occurs with urinary tract obstruction that affects both kidneys, such as prostatic hyperplasia.

Pathophysiology

Oliguric phase
○ This phase may last a few days or several weeks.
○ Urine output drops below 400 ml daily.
○ Fluid volume excess, azotemia, and electrolyte imbalance develop.
○ Local mediators are released, causing intrarenal vasoconstriction.
○ Medullary hypoxia causes cellular swelling and adherence of neutrophils to capillaries and venules.
○ Hypoperfusion develops, and cells are injured or die.
○ Reperfusion causes reactive oxygen species to form, leading to further cellular injury.

Diuretic phase
○ Renal function is recovered.
○ Urine output gradually increases.
○ Glomerular filtration rate improves, although tubular transport systems remain abnormal.

Recovery phase
○ This phase may last 3 to 12 months, possibly longer.
○ The patient gradually returns to normal or near normal renal function.

Causes

Prerenal failure
○ Hemorrhagic blood loss
○ Hypotension or hypoperfusion
○ Hypovolemia
○ Loss of plasma volume
○ Water and electrolyte losses

Intrarenal failure
○ Acute tubular necrosis
○ Coagulation defects
○ Glomerulopathies
○ Malignant hypertension

Postrenal failure
○ Bladder neck obstruction
○ Obstructive uropathies, usually bilateral
○ Ureteral destruction

Prevalence

○ Seen in 5% of hospitalized patients

Complications

○ Acute pulmonary edema
○ Electrolyte imbalance
○ Hypertensive crisis
○ Infection
○ Metabolic acidosis
○ Renal shutdown

Assessment

History

○ Predisposing disorder
○ Recent fever, chills, or central nervous system problem
○ Recent gastrointestinal problem

Physical assessment

○ Altered level of consciousness
○ Bibasilar crackles
○ Bleeding abnormalities
○ Dry mucous membranes
○ Dry, pruritic skin
○ Irritability, drowsiness, or confusion
○ Uremic breath odor

Test results

Laboratory
○ Increased blood urea nitrogen, serum creatinine, and potassium levels
○ Decreased blood pH, bicarbonate, and hemoglobin levels
○ Decreased hematocrit
○ Casts and cellular debris in urine
○ Decreased urine specific gravity
○ In glomerular disease: proteinuria and urine osmolality close to serum osmolality level
○ Urine sodium level less than 20 mEq/L, caused by decreased perfusion in oliguria
○ Urine sodium level above 40 mEq/L from an intrarenal problem in oliguria

○ Glomerular filtration rate and number of remaining functioning nephrons measured by urine creatinine clearance

Imaging

The following imaging tests may show the cause of renal failure:

○ computed tomography scan
○ excretory urography renal scan
○ kidney ultrasonography
○ kidney-ureter-bladder radiography
○ nephrotomography
○ retrograde pyelography.

Diagnostic procedures

○ If the patient has hyperkalemia, electrocardiography will show tall, peaked T waves; a widening QRS complex; and disappearing P waves.

Nursing diagnoses

○ Acute pain
○ Excess fluid volume
○ Impaired urinary elimination
○ Ineffective tissue perfusion: renal
○ Readiness for enhanced knowledge related to dietary and fluid restrictions and treatment protocols
○ Risk for impaired skin integrity
○ Risk for infection

Key outcomes

The patient will:

○ avoid complications
○ maintain fluid balance
○ maintain hemodynamic stability
○ verbalize risk factors for decreased tissue perfusion and modify lifestyle appropriately
○ demonstrate the ability to manage urinary elimination problems
○ verbalize increased comfort.

Interventions

General

○ Fluid restriction
○ Hemodialysis or peritoneal dialysis, as appropriate
○ High-calorie, low-protein, low-potassium, low-sodium diet
○ Rest periods when fatigued
○ Surgery to create vascular access for hemodialysis

Nursing

○ Give prescribed drugs.
○ Encourage the patient to express feelings.
○ Provide emotional support.
○ Identify patients at risk for and take steps to prevent acute tubular necrosis.
○ Use sterile technique.
○ Ensure patient safety.

Preventing acute tubular necrosis

Acute tubular necrosis may develop after aminoglycoside therapy or exposure to industrial chemicals, heavy metals, and contrast media. It occurs mainly in elderly hospitalized patients.

To prevent acute tubular necrosis, make sure every patient is well hydrated before and after surgery or imaging procedures that use a contrast agent. For high-risk patients, give mannitol, as ordered, before and during these procedures. If the patient is receiving a blood transfusion, monitor him carefully, and stop the transfusion immediately if signs of transfusion reaction occur (such as fever, rash, and chills).

All patients at risk for acute tubular necrosis need adequate hydration; monitor their urine output closely.

Drug therapy

○ Diuretics
○ Supplemental vitamins
○ In hyperkalemia: hypertonic glucose-and-insulin infusions, sodium bicarbonate, sodium polystyrene sulfonate

Monitoring

○ Daily weight
○ Dialysis access site
○ Effects of excess fluid volume
○ Electrolyte levels
○ Intake and output
○ Renal function studies
○ Vital signs

Patient teaching

Be sure to cover:

○ the disorder, diagnosis, and treatment
○ prescribed drugs, dosages, administration, and possible adverse effects
○ recommended fluid allowance
○ compliance with diet and drug regimen
○ daily weight and importance of immediately reporting changes of 3 lb or more
○ signs and symptoms of edema and importance of reporting them to the doctor.

Discharge planning

○ Encourage follow-up care with nephrologist.
○ Refer the patient to a nutritionist, if needed.

Renal failure, chronic

Overview

Description

- The end result of gradually progressive loss of renal function
- Occasionally, the result of a rapidly progressive disease of sudden onset
- Symptoms sparse until more than 75% of glomerular filtration lost, worsening as renal function declines
- Fatal unless treated
- May require maintenance dialysis or kidney transplantation

Pathophysiology

- Nephron destruction eventually causes irreversible renal damage.
- Disease may progress through the following stages: reduced renal reserve, renal insufficiency, renal failure, and end-stage renal disease.

Causes

- Chronic glomerular disease
- Chronic infections such as chronic pyelonephritis
- Collagen diseases such as systemic lupus erythematosus
- Congenital anomalies such as polycystic kidney disease
- Endocrine disease
- Nephrotoxic agents
- Obstructive processes such as calculi
- Vascular diseases

Prevalence

- Affects about 2 of every 100,000 people
- May occur at all ages, but more common in adults
- Affects more men than women
- Affects more Blacks than Whites

Complications

- Anemia
- Electrolyte imbalances
- Lipid disorders
- Peripheral neuropathy
- Platelet dysfunction
- Pulmonary edema
- Sexual dysfunction

Assessment

History

- Amenorrhea
- Dry mouth
- Fasciculations, twitching
- Fatigue
- Hiccups
- Impotence
- Infertility, decreased libido
- Muscle cramps
- Nausea
- Pathologic fractures
- Predisposing factor

Physical assessment

- Abdominal pain on palpation
- Altered level of consciousness
- Bibasilar crackles
- Cardiac arrhythmias
- Decreased urine output
- Growth retardation (in children)
- Gum ulceration and bleeding
- Hypotension or hypertension
- Pale, yellowish bronze skin color
- Peripheral edema
- Pleural friction rub
- Poor skin turgor
- Thin, brittle fingernails and dry, brittle hair
- Uremic fetor

Test results

Laboratory

- Increased blood urea nitrogen, serum creatinine, sodium, and potassium levels
- Decreased arterial pH and bicarbonate levels (metabolic acidosis)
- Decreased hemoglobin level and hematocrit
- Decreased red blood cell survival time
- Mild thrombocytopenia and platelet defects
- Increased aldosterone secretion
- Hyperglycemia
- Hypertriglyceridemia
- Decreased high-density lipoprotein levels
- Urine specific gravity 1.010 and fixed
- Proteinuria
- Glycosuria
- Red blood cells, leukocytes, casts, and crystals in urine

Imaging

- Kidney-ureter-bladder X-rays, excretory urography, nephrotomography, renal scan, and renal arteriography show reduced kidney size.

Diagnostic procedures

- Renal biopsy allows histologic identification of the underlying pathology.
- Electroencephalography shows changes suggesting metabolic encephalopathy.

Nursing diagnoses

- Chronic pain
- Decreased cardiac output
- Excess fluid volume
- Fatigue

- Impaired mucous membranes
- Impaired skin integrity
- Impaired urinary elimination
- Nausea
- Risk for infection

Key outcomes

The patient will:
- avoid complications
- maintain fluid balance
- report feelings of increased comfort
- maintain hemodynamic stability
- demonstrate the ability to manage urinary elimination problems
- perform activities of daily living within the confines of the disease
- remain free from infection.

Interventions

General

- Fluid restriction
- Hemodialysis or peritoneal dialysis

✳ *AGE AWARE Children need more dialysis in relation to their body weight than adults because their metabolic rates and, therefore, food intake are relatively higher.*

- Low-protein (with peritoneal dialysis, high-protein), high-calorie, low-sodium, low-phosphorus, and low-potassium diet
- Rest periods when fatigued
- Surgery
  - Creation of vascular access for dialysis
  - Possible kidney transplant

Nursing

- Give prescribed drugs.
- Perform meticulous skin care and oral hygiene.
- Encourage the patient to express feelings.
- Provide emotional support.
- Maintain sterile technique.

Drug therapy

- Antiemetics
- Antihypertensives
- Antipruritics
- Cardiac glycosides
- Erythropoietin
- Iron and folate supplements
- Loop diuretics
- Supplementary vitamins and essential amino acids

Monitoring

- Daily weight
- Electrocardiogram
- Electrolyte levels
- Intake and output

- Renal function studies
- Signs and symptoms of bleeding
- Signs and symptoms of fluid overload
- Vital signs

Patient teaching

Be sure to cover:
- the disorder, diagnosis, and treatment
- dietary changes
- fluid restrictions
- dialysis site care, as appropriate
- importance of wearing or carrying medical identification.

Discharge planning

- Refer the patient to resource and support services.
- Refer the patient to a nutritionist, if needed.

Renal tubular acidosis

Overview

Description
- A syndrome of persistent dehydration, hyperchloremia, hypokalemia, metabolic acidosis, and nephrocalcinosis
- Occurs as distal (type I, or classic) or proximal (type II) types
- Usually a good prognosis, but depends on the severity of renal damage before treatment

Pathophysiology
- Metabolic acidosis results from the kidneys' inability to conserve bicarbonate and adequately acidify urine.
- Distal renal tubular acidosis (primary and secondary) results from an inability of the distal tubules to secrete hydrogen ions against established gradients across the tubular membrane. This results in decreased excretion of titratable acids and ammonium, increased loss of potassium and bicarbonate in the urine, and systemic acidosis.
- Proximal renal tubular acidosis (primary and secondary) results from defective reabsorption of bicarbonate in the proximal tubules. This causes bicarbonate to flood the distal tubules, which normally secrete hydrogen ions, and leads to impaired formation of titratable acids and ammonium for excretion.

Causes
Primary distal form
- Unknown
- Hereditary defect

Secondary distal form
- Hepatic cirrhosis
- Malnutrition
- Several genetically transmitted disorders
- Starvation

Primary proximal form
- Idiopathic

Secondary proximal form
- Fanconi's syndrome

Prevalence
- Primary distal renal tubular acidosis: most common in females, older children, adolescents, and young adults

Complications
- Pyelonephritis
- Renal calculi
- Urinary tract infection

Assessment

History
- Anorexia
- Constipation
- Polyuria
- Vomiting

Physical assessment
- Apathy
- Dehydration
- Fever
- Growth retardation
- Muscle wasting
- Rickets

Test results
Laboratory
- Decreased serum bicarbonate, pH, potassium, and phosphorus levels
- Increased serum chloride and alkaline phosphatase levels
- Alkaline pH with low titratable acids and ammonium content
- Increased urinary bicarbonate and potassium levels
- Low urine specific gravity

Imaging
- In later stages, X-rays may show nephrocalcinosis.

Nursing diagnoses
- Constipation
- Deficient fluid volume
- Hyperthermia
- Impaired nutrition: less than body requirements
- Risk for delayed development
- Risk for infection

Key outcomes
The patient will:
- avoid complications
- maintain fluid balance
- remain free from infection.

Interventions

General
- Surgery for severe obstruction from renal calculi
- High-potassium diet

Nursing
- Give prescribed drugs.
- Strain urine for calculi.
- Provide comfort measures.
- Encourage activity, as tolerated.

Drug therapy
- Analgesics for renal calculi
- Antibiotics for pyelonephritis
- Bicarbonate replacement
- Potassium supplementation
- Vitamin D

Monitoring
- Daily weight
- Intake and output
- Laboratory values, especially potassium, for hypokalemia
- Urine pH

Patient teaching

Be sure to cover:
- relationship between prognosis, bone healing, and the adequacy of treatment
- diagnosis and treatment of rickets if it develops
- signs and symptoms of calculi and the need to report them immediately.

Discharge planning

- Because renal tubular acidosis may be caused by a genetic defect, encourage family members to seek genetic counseling or screening for this disorder.

Renal vein thrombosis

Overview

Description
○ Clotting in the renal vein
○ Thrombosis affecting one or both kidneys
○ May be acute or chronic
○ Poor prognosis in thrombosis affecting both kidneys

Pathophysiology
○ Thrombosis results in renal congestion, engorgement, and possibly infarction.
○ Chronic thrombosis usually impairs renal function, causing nephrotic syndrome.
○ Abrupt onset of thrombosis that causes extensive damage may precipitate rapidly fatal renal infarction.

Causes
○ Heart failure
○ Periarteritis
○ Thrombophlebitis of the inferior vena or blood vessels of the legs
○ Tumor obstructing the renal vein (usually hypernephroma)

 AGE AWARE *In infants, renal vein thrombosis usually follows diarrhea that causes severe dehydration.*

Prevalence
○ Unknown
○ Possibly more common in males, with no specific numbers available as proof
○ Most common between ages 40 and 60

Complications
○ Acute or chronic renal failure
○ Urinary tract infection

Assessment

History
○ Clotting disorder
○ Fever
○ Severe lumbar pain
○ Tenderness in the epigastric region and costovertebral angle
○ Weight gain

Physical assessment
○ Enlarged and easily palpated kidneys
○ Hematuria
○ Hypertension (rare)
○ Oliguria and uremia with bilateral obstruction
○ Pallor
○ Peripheral edema

Test results

Laboratory
○ Gross or microscopic hematuria
○ Proteinuria
○ Casts in urine
○ Oliguria
○ Serum leukocytosis, hypoalbuminemia, and hyperlipidemia

Imaging
○ Computed tomography with contrast reveals enlargement and distention of the affected renal vein and clots inside the vein.
○ Excretory urography differentiates acute from chronic thrombosis.

Diagnostic procedures
○ Renal arteriography and biopsy and venography confirm the diagnosis.

Nursing diagnoses

○ Acute pain
○ Excess fluid volume
○ Hyperthermia
○ Impaired urinary elimination
○ Ineffective tissue perfusion: renal
○ Risk for infection

Key outcomes
The patient will:
○ avoid complications
○ maintain fluid balance
○ remain free from infection
○ maintain an adequate comfort level.

Interventions

General
○ Hemodialysis
○ Potassium- and sodium-restricted diet
○ Surgery
  – Possible kidney transplant for nephrotic syndrome
  – Possible nephrectomy for intrarenal bleeding
  – Rarely, a thrombectomy, which must be performed within 24 hours of thrombosis

Nursing
○ Give prescribed drugs.
○ Provide comfort measures.
○ Enforce dietary restrictions.

Drug therapy
○ Analgesics
○ Anticoagulants
○ Diuretics
○ Thrombolytics

Monitoring
- Daily weight
- Electrolytes
- Intake and output
- Prothrombin time, international normalized ratio, and activated partial thromboplastin time
- Renal function via blood urea nitrogen and creatinine levels
- Signs and symptoms of bleeding
- Signs and symptoms of pulmonary emboli
- Vital signs

Patient teaching

Be sure to cover:
- the diagnosis and treatment
- how to maintain bleeding precautions
- avoiding foods high in vitamin K
- the importance of wearing medical identification when taking Coumadin
- the importance of follow-up blood work.

Discharge planning

- Refer the patient to resource and support services.
- Refer the patient to a nutritionist, if needed.

Respiratory acidosis

Overview

Description

- Acid-base disturbance characterized by reduced alveolar ventilation, as shown by partial pressure of arterial carbon dioxide ($Paco_2$) higher than 45 mm Hg (hypercapnia)
- Varying prognosis depending on the severity of the underlying disturbance and the patient's general clinical condition
- May be acute or chronic

Pathophysiology

- Depressed ventilation causes respiratory acidosis.
- Carbon dioxide is then retained, and hydrogen ion concentration increases.
- Respiratory acidosis results.

Causes

- Airway obstruction
- Asthma
- Central nervous system (CNS) trauma
- Chronic bronchitis
- Chronic metabolic alkalosis
- Chronic obstructive pulmonary disease
- CNS-depressant drugs
- Extensive pneumonia
- Large pneumothorax
- Neuromuscular disease
- Parenchymal lung disease
- Pulmonary edema
- Severe acute respiratory distress syndrome
- Ventilation therapy

Prevalence

- Affects males and females equally

Complications

- Cardiac arrest
- Respiratory arrest
- Shock

Arterial blood gas results in respiratory acidosis

This table shows typical arterial blood gas findings in uncompensated and compensated respiratory acidosis.

	Uncompensated	Compensated
pH	< 7.35	Normal
$Paco_2$ (mm Hg)	> 45	> 45
HCO_3^- (mEq/L)	Normal	> 26

Assessment

History

- Headache
- Nausea and vomiting
- Predisposing factor
- Shortness of breath

Physical assessment

- Asterixis (tremor)
- Bounding pulses
- Depressed deep tendon reflexes
- Diaphoresis
- Hypotension
- Mental status changes
- Papilledema
- Rapid, shallow respirations
- Tachycardia

Test results

Laboratory
- Hypercapnia, in which arterial blood pH is below 7.35, and $Paco_2$ is above 45 mm Hg (See *Arterial blood gas results in respiratory acidosis*.)

Nursing diagnoses

- Acute confusion
- Decreased cardiac output
- Ineffective breathing pattern
- Nausea
- Readiness for enhanced coping
- Risk for imbalanced fluid volume

Key outcomes

The patient will:
- maintain a patent airway
- maintain adequate ventilation
- maintain fluid balance
- maintain adequate cardiac output
- demonstrate effective coping strategies.

Interventions

General

- Activity as tolerated
- Bronchoscopy
- Correction of the condition causing alveolar hypoventilation
- Correction of metabolic alkalosis
- Possible mechanical ventilation
- Possible dialysis or charcoal

Nursing

- Give prescribed drugs and oxygen.
- Provide adequate fluids.
- Maintain a patent airway.

- Perform tracheal suctioning, as needed.
- Administer vigorous chest physiotherapy.
- Encourage turning, coughing, and deep breathing.

Drug therapy

- Antibiotics
- Bronchodilators
- Drug therapy for the underlying condition
- I.V. fluid
- Oxygen
- Parenteral nutrition
- Sodium bicarbonate

▼ **ALERT** *Dangerously low blood pH (less than 7.15) can produce profound CNS and cardiovascular deterioration; careful administration of I.V. sodium bicarbonate may be needed.*

Monitoring

- Arterial blood gas values
- Intake and output
- Mechanical ventilator settings
- Neurologic status
- Respiratory status

▼ **ALERT** *Pulse oximetry, used to monitor oxygen saturation, won't reveal increasing carbon dioxide levels.*

- Serum electrolyte values
- Vital signs

Patient teaching

Be sure to cover:
- the disorder, diagnosis, and treatment
- how to administer supplemental oxygen
- prescribed drugs and possible adverse effects
- how to perform coughing and deep-breathing exercises
- signs and symptoms of acid-base imbalance and when to notify the doctor.

Discharge planning

- Refer the patient for home oxygen therapy if indicated.
- Refer the patient to a chest physiotherapist if needed

Respiratory alkalosis

Overview

Description
- Acid-base disturbance characterized by a decrease in partial pressure of arterial carbon dioxide ($Paco_2$) to less than 35 mm Hg
- May be acute, resulting from a sudden increase in ventilation
- May be chronic and difficult to identify because of renal compensation

Pathophysiology
- Alveolar hyperventilation and hypocapnia result in respiratory alkalosis.
- Uncomplicated respiratory alkalosis leads to a decrease in hydrogen ion levels, which increases the blood pH level.
- Hypercapnia occurs when the elimination of CO_2 by the lungs exceeds the production of CO_2 at the cellular level.

Causes
- Acute asthma
- Anxiety
- Aspirin toxicity
- Central nervous system disease
- Fever
- Hepatic failure
- Interstitial lung disease
- Metabolic acidosis
- Pain
- Pneumonia
- Pregnancy
- Pulmonary vascular disease
- Sepsis
- Severe hypoxemia

Prevalence
- Unknown
- Depends on underlying condition

Arterial blood gas results in respiratory alkalosis

This table shows typical arterial blood gas findings in uncompensated and compensated respiratory alkalosis.

	Uncompensated	Compensated
pH	> 7.45	Normal
Paco$_2$ (mm Hg)	< 35	< 35
HCO$_3^-$ (mEq/L)	Normal	< 22

Complications
- Cardiac arrest
- Respiratory arrest
- Seizures

Assessment

History
- Difficulty breathing
- Dizziness
- Light-headedness
- Muscle weakness
- Restlessness

Physical assessment
- Altered level of consciousness
- Cardiac arrhythmias
- Carpopedal spasms
- Deep, rapid breathing, possibly exceeding 40 breaths/minute
- Hyperreflexia
- Twitching

Test results
Laboratory
- $Paco_2$ less than 35 mm Hg
- pH above 7.45
- HCO_3^- level normal in the acute stage, below normal in the chronic stage (See *Arterial blood gas results in respiratory alkalosis.*)
- Possible salicylate poisoning revealed in toxicology screening

Diagnostic procedures
- Electrocardiography may show arrhythmias or changes caused by hypokalemia or hypocalcemia.

Nursing diagnoses
- Acute confusion
- Decreased cardiac output
- Ineffective breathing pattern
- Readiness for enhanced coping
- Risk for imbalanced fluid volume
- Risk for injury

Key outcomes
The patient will:
- maintain a patent airway
- maintain adequate ventilation
- maintain fluid balance
- maintain adequate cardiac output
- demonstrate effective coping strategies.

Interventions

General

- Treatment of the underlying condition
- Mechanical ventilation, if indicated
- Undisturbed rest periods

Nursing

- Give prescribed drugs.
- Allay anxiety, and recommend activities that promote relaxation.
- Assist the patient with breathing into a paper bag, if indicated.
- Institute safety measures and seizure precautions.

Drug therapy

- Diamox
- Oxygen

Monitoring

- Arterial blood gas and serum electrolyte levels
- Cardiovascular status
- Deep tendon reflexes
- Neurologic status
- Ventilator settings
- Vital signs

Patient teaching

Be sure to cover:
- the disorder, diagnosis, and treatment
- how to administer supplemental oxygen
- prescribed drugs, dosages, and possible adverse effects
- how to hyperventilate into a paper bag
- signs and symptoms of acid-base imbalance
- when to contact a doctor.

Discharge planning

- Refer the patient to an outpatient oxygen delivery service, if indicated.

Respiratory distress syndrome

Overview

Description

- Respiratory disorder that involves widespread alveolar collapse
- Most common cause of neonatal death
- If mild, subsides slowly after about 3 days
- Also called RDS or hyaline membrane disease

Pathophysiology

- In neonates born before the 27th week of gestation, immaturity of alveoli and capillary blood supply lead to alveolar collapse from lack of surfactant (a lipoprotein normally present in alveoli and respiratory bronchioles).
- Surfactant deficiency causes widespread atelectasis, resulting in inadequate alveolar ventilation and shunting of blood through collapsed lung areas.
- Hypoxia and acidosis result.
- Compensatory grunting occurs, producing positive end-expiratory pressure (PEEP) that helps prevent further alveolar collapse.

Causes

- Surfactant deficiency stemming from preterm birth

Prevalence

AGE AWARE *Respiratory distress syndrome occurs almost exclusively in neonates born before the 27th gestational week; it affects about 60% of those born before the 28th week.*

- Most common among neonates who weigh 1,000 g to 1,500 g (about 2 to 3 lb)
- Most common in neonates of mothers with diabetes, neonates delivered by cesarean birth, and neonates delivered suddenly after antepartum hemorrhage

Complications

- Bronchopulmonary dysplasia
- Death
- Respiratory insufficiency
- Shock

Assessment

History

- Cesarean birth
- Maternal history of diabetes or antepartum hemorrhage
- Preterm birth

Physical assessment

- Audible expiratory grunting
- Diminished air entry and crackles
- Frothy sputum
- Intercostal, subcostal, or sternal retractions
- Low body temperature
- Nasal flaring
- Pallor
- Possible apnea, bradycardia, and cyanosis
- Possible hypotension, peripheral edema, and oliguria
- Rapid, shallow respirations

Test results

Laboratory

- Decreased partial pressure of arterial oxygen (Pao_2)
- Possibly normal, decreased, or increased partial pressure of arterial carbon dioxide
- Decreased arterial pH
- Prenatal lung development and risk of respiratory distress syndrome shown in lecithin:sphingomyelin ratio

Imaging

- Chest X-rays may show a fine reticulonodular pattern and dark streaks, indicating air-filled, dilated bronchioles.

Nursing diagnoses

- Caregiver role strain
- Decreased cardiac output
- Death anxiety
- Ineffective airway clearance
- Ineffective breathing pattern
- Ineffective infant feeding pattern
- Risk for imbalanced fluid volume
- Risk for impaired parent/infant attachment
- Risk for infection
- Risk for spiritual distress

Key outcomes

The patient will:

- maintain adequate ventilation
- maintain a patent airway
- remain free from infection
- maintain adequate fluid volume
- maintain intact skin integrity.

The patient's family will:

- identify factors that increase the risk of neonatal injury.

Interventions

General

- Aggressive management, assisted by mechanical ventilation with PEEP or continuous positive airway pressure (CPAP) administered by a tight-fitting face mask or, when needed, an endotracheal tube

- For a neonate who can't maintain adequate gas exchange, high-frequency oscillation ventilation
- Extracorporeal membrane oxygenation as a last resort for ventilation
- Radiant warmer or Isolette
- Warm, humidified, oxygen-enriched gases given by oxygen hood or mechanical ventilation
- Tube feedings or total parenteral nutrition
- Possible tracheostomy

Nursing

- Give prescribed drugs.
- Check the umbilical catheter for arterial or venous hypotension, as appropriate.
- Suction, as needed.
- Change the transcutaneous Pao_2 monitor lead placement site every 2 to 4 hours.
- Adjust PEEP or CPAP settings as indicated by arterial blood gas (ABG) values.

▼ **ALERT** *In a neonate on a mechanical ventilator, watch carefully for signs of barotrauma and accidental disconnection from the ventilator. Check the ventilator settings often. Be alert for signs of complications of PEEP or CPAP therapy, such as decreased cardiac output, pneumothorax, and pneumomediastinum.*

- Implement measures to prevent infection.
- Provide mouth care every 2 hours.
- Encourage parents to participate in the infant's care.
- Encourage parents to ask questions and to express their fears and concerns.
- Advise parents that full recovery may take up to 12 months.
- Offer emotional support.

Drug therapy

- Antenatal corticosteroids
- Diuretics
- I.V. fluids and sodium bicarbonate
- Oxygen therapy
- Pancuronium bromide
- Prophylactic antibiotics
- Surfactant replacement therapy
- Total parenteral nutrition
- Vitamin E

▼ **ALERT** *Watch for evidence of complications from oxygen therapy: lung capillary damage, decreased mucus flow, impaired ciliary functioning, and widespread atelectasis. Also be alert for signs of patent ductus arteriosus, heart failure, retinopathy, pulmonary hypertension, necrotizing enterocolitis, and neurologic abnormalities.*

Monitoring

- ABG values
- Central venous pressure
- Daily weight
- Decreased peripheral circulation
- Intake and output
- Mechanical ventilator settings
- Pulse oximetry
- Respiratory status
- Signs and symptoms of infection
- Skin color
- Skin integrity
- Thrombosis
- Vital signs

Patient teaching

Be sure to cover (with parents):
- the disorder, diagnosis, and treatment
- prescribed drugs, dosages, administration, and possible adverse effects
- explanations of respiratory equipment, alarm sounds, and mechanical noise
- potential complications
- when to contact the doctor.

Discharge planning

- Refer the patient for follow-up care with a neonatal ophthalmologist, as indicated.
- When prognosis is poor, refer the patient's family to pastoral care and social services to help prepare them for the infant's impending death.

Respiratory syncytial virus infection

Overview

Description

○ Virus that's the leading cause of lower respiratory tract infection in infants and young children and upper respiratory infections in adults
○ Suspected cause of fatal respiratory diseases in infants
○ Can cause serious illness in immunocompromised adults, institutionalized elderly people, and patients with underlying cardiopulmonary disease
○ Also known as RSV

Pathophysiology

○ The virus attaches to cells, eventually resulting in necrosis of the bronchiolar epithelium; in severe infection, lymphocytes and mononuclear cells infiltrate the bronchioles.
○ As a result, alveoli thicken, and alveolar spaces fill with fluid.
○ Narrowing of the airway passages on expiration prevents air from leaving the lungs, causing progressive overinflation.

Causes

○ Respiratory syncytial virus, a subgroup of myxoviruses resembling paramyxovirus
○ Transmitted by respiratory secretions
○ Probably spread to infants and young children by school-age children, adolescents, and young adults with mild reinfections

Prevalence

✳ AGE AWARE *Respiratory syncytial virus almost exclusively affects infants and young children, especially those in daycare settings. It's most common among infants ages 1 to 6 months, peaking between ages 2 and 3 months.*

○ Annual epidemics during winter and spring

Complications

○ Bronchiolitis
○ Croup
○ Otitis media
○ Pneumonia and progressive pneumonia
○ Residual lung damage
○ Respiratory failure
○ Sudden infant death syndrome

Assessment

History

○ Coughing
○ Dyspnea
○ Earache
○ Fever
○ Malaise
○ Nasal congestion
○ Sore throat
○ Wheezing

Physical assessment

○ Nasal and pharyngeal inflammation
○ Otitis media
○ Severe respiratory distress (nasal flaring, retraction, cyanosis, and tachypnea)
○ Wheezes, rhonchi, and crackles

Test results

Laboratory
○ Respiratory syncytial virus present in cultures of nasal and pharyngeal secretions
○ Elevated serum respiratory syncytial virus antibody titers
○ Hypoxemia
○ Respiratory acidosis
○ Increased blood urea nitrogen levels if the patient is dehydrated
Imaging
○ Chest X-rays help detect pneumonia.

Nursing diagnoses

○ Acute pain
○ Fatigue
○ Impaired gas exchange
○ Ineffective airway clearance
○ Ineffective breathing pattern
○ Risk for imbalanced fluid volume

Key outcomes

The patient will:
○ maintain a respiratory rate within 5 breaths/minute of baseline
○ express or indicate feelings of increased comfort while maintaining adequate air exchange
○ cough effectively
○ maintain adequate fluid volume.

Interventions

General

○ Respiratory support
○ Adequate nutrition
○ Avoidance of overhydration

○ Rest periods when fatigued
○ Possible tracheostomy

Nursing

○ Institute contact isolation.
○ Perform percussion, drainage, and suction when needed.
○ Give prescribed oxygen.
○ Use a croup tent, as needed.
○ Place the patient in semi-Fowler's position.
○ Watch for signs and symptoms of dehydration, and give I.V. fluids accordingly.
○ Promote bed rest.
○ Offer diversional activities tailored to the patient's condition and age.
○ Promote bonding between infants and parents.

Drug therapy

○ I.V. fluids
○ Ribavirin in aerosol form

Monitoring

○ Arterial blood gas levels
○ Fluid and electrolyte status
○ Respiratory status
○ Vital signs including oxygen saturation

Patient teaching

Be sure to cover (with parents):
○ the disorder, diagnosis, and treatment
○ how the infection spreads
○ preventive measures (administration of immune globulin)
○ prescribed drugs, dosages, administration, and possible adverse effects
○ importance of a nonsmoking environment in the home
○ follow-up care.

Discharge planning

○ Refer the patient to a chest physiotherapist, if indicated.
○ Refer the patient for home oxygen and nebulizer treatment services, if indicated.

Rhabdomyolysis

Overview

Description
- Breakdown of muscle fibers and release of muscle fiber contents into the circulation

Pathophysiology
- Myoglobin, the oxygen-binding protein pigment in skeletal muscle, is released into the bloodstream after skeletal muscles sustain damage.
- The kidneys filter myoglobin from the bloodstream.
- Myoglobin may occlude kidney structures, causing damage.

Measuring limb circumference

To ensure accurate and consistent limb circumference measurements, use a consistent reference point each time and measure with the limb in full extension. The drawing below shows correct reference points for arm and leg measurements.

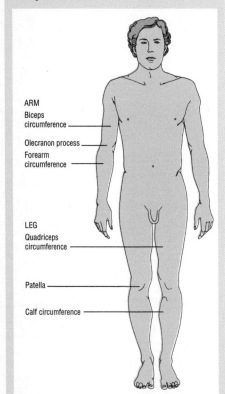

ARM
Biceps
circumference

Olecranon process
Forearm
circumference

LEG
Quadriceps
circumference

Patella

Calf circumference

Causes
- Alcoholism
- Burns
- Drugs (cocaine, amphetamines, statins, heroin, or PCP)
- Heatstroke
- Hereditary disorders
- Hyperthermia or hypothermia
- Ischemia
- Necrosis
- Physical exertion
- Seizures
- Trauma

Prevalence
- About 26,000 cases reported annually in the United States
- Accounts for about 8% to 15% of acute renal failure cases
- Overall mortality rate about 5%; varies with specific cause
- Affects males more than females

✳ *AGE AWARE Rhabdomyolysis may occur in infants, toddlers, and adolescents who have inherited enzyme deficiencies of carbohydrate or lipid metabolism or myopathies.*

Complications
- Compartment syndrome
- Death
- Disseminated intravascular coagulation
- Heart failure
- Infection
- Renal failure

Assessment

History
- Fatigue
- Joint pain
- Muscle stiffness and aching
- Precipitating factor
- Weakness
- Weight gain

Physical assessment
- Arrhythmias
- Dark urine
- Tender or damaged skeletal muscles

Test results
Laboratory
- Casts in urine
- Hemoglobin but no red blood cells in urine
- Myoglobin present in urine and serum
- Increased creatinine kinase (decreasing by 40% daily after the initial insult) and serum potassium levels

Diagnostic procedures
○ Electrocardiography may reveal changes similar to those of acute hyperkalemia (peaked T waves, prolonged PR and QRS intervals, and absence of P wave).

Nursing diagnoses

○ Acute pain
○ Decreased cardiac output
○ Excess fluid volume
○ Fatigue
○ Impaired urinary elimination
○ Ineffective tissue perfusion: renal

Key outcomes

The patient will:
○ maintain adequate fluid and electrolyte balance
○ maintain hemodynamic stability
○ exhibit respiratory sufficiency
○ verbalize comfort
○ perform activities of daily living
○ maintain adequate urine output.

Interventions

General
○ Dialysis
○ Fasciotomy for compartment syndrome
○ Fresh frozen plasma, cryoprecipitate, and platelets for disseminated intravascular coagulation
○ Hydration to flush myoglobin from the kidneys
○ Low-potassium diet

Nursing
○ Give prescribed drugs.
○ Provide comfort measures.
○ Promote activity and ambulation as tolerated.
○ Warm or cool a hypothermic or hyperthermic patient, respectively, according to facility policy.

Drug therapy
○ Analgesics
○ Diuretics
○ Insulin and 50% dextrose or Kayexalate for elevated potassium levels
○ Isotonic crystalloids
○ I.V. sodium bicarbonate
○ Oxygen

▼ **ALERT** *Hyperkalemia is the most dangerous electrolyte disorder and can lead to serious cardiac arrhythmias and cardiac arrest. Report increased potassium levels immediately.*

Monitoring
○ Daily weight
○ Intake and output
○ Limb circumference to check for compartment syndrome (See *Measuring limb circumference.*)
○ Pain level
○ Prothrombin time, activated partial thromboplastin time, and other signs and symptoms of disseminated intravascular coagulation
○ Serum levels of blood urea nitrogen, creatinine, creatine kinase, and electrolytes
○ Respiratory status
○ Vital signs

Patient teaching

Be sure to cover:
○ the diagnosis, prognosis, and treatment
○ dietary restrictions
○ importance of daily weights
○ monitoring intake and output
○ prescribed drugs, dosages, administration, and possible adverse effects
○ ways to prevent skeletal muscle damage, if appropriate
○ signs and symptoms of worsening renal failure and when to contact the doctor
○ importance of follow-up care and blood work.

Discharge planning

○ Refer the patient to a physical therapist, nutritionist, and outpatient hemodialysis center, as appropriate.
○ Refer the patient to a drug rehabilitation facility or Alcoholics Anonymous, as appropriate.

Salmonella infection

Overview

Description
- One of the most common intestinal infections in the United States
- Occurs as typhoid fever, paratyphoid fever, enterocolitis, bacteremia, or localized infection
- Typhoid fever
  - Most severe form
  - Usually lasts 1 to 4 weeks
  - Confers lifelong immunity
  - May cause carrier state
- Nontyphoid forms
  - Usually mild to moderate illness
  - Low risk of death
- Enterocolitis and bacteremia
  - Especially common (and more virulent) among infants, elderly people, and those already weakened by other infections, especially human immunodeficiency virus infection

Pathophysiology
- Bacteria move across the mucosa of the small intestine, altering the plasma membrane and entering the lamina propria.
- Invasion activates cell-signaling pathways, which alter electrolyte transport, and may cause diarrhea.
- Some salmonella produce a molecule that increases electrolyte and fluid secretion.

Causes
- Gram-negative bacilli of the genus *Salmonella* (a member of the Enterobacteriaceae family)
  - Typhoid fever: *S. typhi*
  - Enterocolitis: *S. enteritidis*
  - Bacteremia: *S. choleresis*
- Contact with infected person or animal
- Ingestion of contaminated dry milk, chocolate bars, or pharmaceuticals of animal origin
- Nontyphoidal infection — usually, ingestion of contaminated water or food or inadequately processed food, especially eggs, chicken, turkey, and duck
- Typhoid fever — usually, drinking water contaminated by excretions of a carrier

AGE AWARE Salmonella infection may occur in children younger than age 5 and from fecal-oral spread.

Prevalence
- Increasing in the United States because of travel to endemic areas, especially the borders of Mexico

AGE AWARE Most typhoid patients are younger than age 30; most carriers are women older than age 50.

- Lifelong immunity after initial attack of typhoid fever, but patient may become a carrier
- Paratyphoid fever rare in the United States

Complications
- Abscess formation
- Dehydration
- Hypovolemic shock
- Sepsis
- Toxic megacolon

Assessment

History
- With enterocolitis, possible report of contaminated food eaten 6 to 48 hours before onset of symptoms
- With bacteremia, patient usually reveals immunocompromised condition, especially acquired immunodeficiency syndrome
- With typhoid fever, possible ingestion of contaminated food or water, typically 1 to 2 weeks before symptoms develop

Physical assessment
- Abdominal pain
- Fever
- With enterocolitis, severe diarrhea
- With typhoidal infection, headache, increasing fever, and constipation

Test results
Laboratory
- Causative organism and bacteremia usually in blood culture in typhoid or paratyphoid fever
- Causative organism in stool culture in typhoid or paratyphoid fever and enterocolitis
- Causative organism in other culture specimens (urine, bone marrow, pus, and vomitus)
- Presence of *S. typhi* in stools 1 year or more after treatment in about 3% of patients (carrier state)
- Fourfold increase in titer in Widal's test, an agglutination reaction against somatic and flagellar antigens, which suggests typhoid fever
- Transient leukocytosis during the first week of typhoidal salmonella infection
- Leukopenia during the third week of typhoidal salmonella infection
- Leukocytosis with local infection

Nursing diagnoses
- Acute pain
- Deficient fluid volume
- Fatigue
- Impaired urinary elimination

Key outcomes

The patient will:
- regain and maintain fluid and electrolyte balance
- return to a normal elimination pattern
- conserve energy while carrying out daily activities
- report adequate pain relief
- experience no further weight loss
- undergo further testing to determine if he's a carrier.

Interventions

General
- Usually no treatment
- Activity as tolerated
- Bed rest
- Fluid and electrolyte replacement
- High-calorie fluids
- Possible hospitalization for severe diarrhea
- Surgical drainage of localized abscesses

Nursing
- Follow enteric precautions until three consecutive stool cultures are negative — the first one 48 hours after antibiotic treatment ends, followed by two more at 24-hour intervals.
- Watch closely for signs of bowel perforation.
- Maintain adequate I.V. fluid and electrolyte therapy, as ordered.
- Provide skin and mouth care.
- Apply mild heat to relieve abdominal cramps.
- Report salmonella cases to public health officials.

Drug therapy
- Antidiarrheals
- Antimicrobials
- Electrolyte supplements
- I.V. fluids

▼ **ALERT** *Don't give antipyretics. They may mask fever and lead to hypothermia. Instead, promote heat loss by applying tepid, wet towels to the patient's groin and axillae.*

Monitoring
- Calorie count
- Daily weight
- Fluid and electrolyte status
- Intake and output
- Vital signs

Patient teaching

Be sure to cover:
- the disorder, diagnosis, and treatment
- the need for close contacts to obtain a medical examination and treatment if cultures are positive

Preventing salmonella infection

To prevent salmonella infection, follow these teaching guidelines:
- Explain the causes of salmonella infection.
- Show the patient how to wash his hands by wetting them under running water, lathering with soap, scrubbing, rinsing under running water with his fingers pointing down, and drying with a clean cloth or paper towel.
- Tell the patient to wash his hands after using the bathroom and before eating.
- Tell him to cook foods thoroughly—especially eggs and chicken—and to refrigerate them at once.
- Teach him how to avoid cross-contaminating foods by cleaning preparation surfaces with hot, soapy water and drying them thoroughly after use; cleaning surfaces between foods when preparing more than one food; and washing his hands before and after handling each food.
- Tell a patient with a positive stool culture to avoid handling food and to use a separate bathroom or clean the bathroom after each use.
- Tell the patient to report dehydration, bleeding, or recurrence of signs of salmonella infection.

- ways to prevent salmonella infections (See *Preventing salmonella infection.*)
- the need to be vaccinated (for those at high risk for contracting typhoid fever, such as laboratory workers and travelers)
- the importance of proper hand-washing
- the need to avoid preparing food or pouring water for others until salmonella infection is eliminated.

Discharge planning

- Arrange for follow-up with an infectious disease specialist or a gastroenterologist as needed.

Sarcoidosis

Overview

Description

○ A multisystem, granulomatous disorder that typically produces lymphadenopathy, pulmonary infiltration, and skeletal, liver, eye, or skin lesions
○ May be acute (usually resolves within 2 years) or chronic
○ Chronic, progressive sarcoidosis (uncommon) includes pulmonary fibrosis and progressive pulmonary disability

Pathophysiology

○ An excessive inflammatory process begins in the alveoli, bronchioles, and pulmonary blood vessels.
○ Monocyte-macrophages accumulate in the target tissue, where they induce the inflammatory process.
○ CD4+ T-lymphocytes and sensitized immune cells form a ring around the inflamed area.
○ Fibroblasts, mast cells, collagen fibers, and proteoglycans encase the inflammatory and immune cells, causing granuloma formation.

Causes

○ Exact cause unknown
○ Possible causes:
  – Chemicals
  – Hypersensitivity response to atypical mycobacteria, fungi, and pine pollen
  – Lymphokine production abnormalities
  – T-cell abnormalities

Prevalence

 AGE AWARE *Sarcoidosis is most common in people ages 20 to 40.*

○ Predominant among Blacks in the United States
○ Affects twice as many women as men
○ Slightly more common among families, suggesting genetic predisposition

Complications

○ Cor pulmonale
○ Pulmonary fibrosis
○ Pulmonary hypertension

Assessment

History

○ Dyspnea
○ General fatigue and malaise
○ Nonproductive cough
○ Pain in the wrists, ankles, and elbows
○ Substernal pain
○ Unexplained weight loss

Physical assessment

○ Anterior uveitis
○ Arrhythmias
○ Bilateral hilar and paratracheal lymphadenopathy
○ Cranial or peripheral nerve palsies
○ Erythema nodosum
○ Extensive nasal mucosal lesions
○ Glaucoma and blindness occasionally in advanced disease
○ Irregular pulse
○ Muscle weakness
○ Polyarthralgia
○ Punched out lesions on the fingers and toes
○ Splenomegaly

Test results

Laboratory
○ Decreased partial pressure of arterial oxygen
○ Increased carbon dioxide levels
○ Hypercalcemia in urinalysis

Imaging
○ Chest X-rays show bilateral hilar and right paratracheal adenopathy, with or without diffuse interstitial infiltrates.

Diagnostic procedures
○ Electrocardiography shows arrhythmias with:
  – Premature beats
  – Bundle-branch or complete heart block.
○ Kveim-Siltzbach skin test shows granuloma development at the injection site in 2 to 4 weeks when positive.
○ Lymph node, skin, or lung biopsy shows noncaseating granulomas with negative cultures for mycobacteria and fungi.
○ Pulmonary function tests show decreased total lung capacity and compliance and reduced diffusing capacity.

Nursing diagnoses

○ Activity intolerance
○ Decreased cardiac output
○ Deficient knowledge: disease process
○ Ineffective breathing pattern
○ Ineffective individual coping
○ Risk for imbalanced fluid volume
○ Risk for infection

Key outcomes

The patient will:
○ maintain adequate ventilation
○ demonstrate effective coping mechanisms
○ express an understanding of the illness
○ perform activities of daily living within the confines of the illness
○ remain free from signs and symptoms of infection
○ verbalize increased comfort
○ maintain adequate cardiac output
○ maintain adequate fluid volume.

Interventions

General

- ○ None needed for asymptomatic sarcoidosis
- ○ Protection from sunlight
- ○ Low-calcium diet for hypercalcemia
- ○ Reduced-sodium, high-calorie diet
- ○ Adequate fluids
- ○ Activity as tolerated

Nursing

- ○ Give prescribed drugs.
- ○ Give supplemental oxygen.
- ○ Provide a nutritious, high-calorie diet.
- ○ Encourage oral fluid intake.
- ○ Provide a low-calcium diet for hypercalcemia.
- ○ Provide emotional support.
- ○ Provide comfort measures.
- ○ Include the patient in care decisions whenever possible.

Drug therapy

- ○ Analgesics
- ○ Corticosteroids
- ○ Oxygen therapy

Monitoring

- ○ Arterial blood gas results
- ○ Cardiac rhythm
- ○ Chest X-ray results
- ○ Daily weight
- ○ Fingerstick tests of glucose level
- ○ Intake and output
- ○ Respiratory status
- ○ Sputum production
- ○ Vital signs

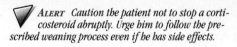 **ALERT** *Because corticosteroids may induce or worsen diabetes mellitus, test the patient's blood by fingerstick for glucose and acetone levels at least every 12 hours at the start of corticosteroid therapy. Also, watch for other adverse effects, such as fluid retention, electrolyte imbalance (especially hypokalemia), moon face, hypertension, and personality changes.*

Patient teaching

Be sure to cover:
- ○ the disorder, diagnosis, and treatment
- ○ prescribed drugs, dosages, administration, and possible adverse effects
- ○ when to consult a doctor
- ○ corticosteroid therapy
- ○ the need for regular follow-up examinations
- ○ the importance of wearing a medical identification bracelet
- ○ infection prevention.

ALERT *Caution the patient not to stop a corticosteroid abruptly. Urge him to follow the prescribed weaning process even if he has side effects.*

Discharge planning

- ○ Refer a patient with failing vision to community support and resource groups such as the American Foundation for the Blind, if needed.

Sheehan's syndrome

Overview

Description
○ Postpartum necrosis of the pituitary gland
○ Usually involves the anterior pituitary gland

Pathophysiology
○ The pituitary gland is normally hypertrophic during pregnancy.
○ Metabolic requirements are increased and so is pressure in the sella turcica.
○ The pituitary becomes susceptible to decreased blood pressure from problems during delivery, such as hemorrhage.
○ Damage to the anterior pituitary gland causes hypopituitarism and partial or complete loss of thyroid, adrenocortical, and gonadal function.
○ In the chronic form, symptoms may take years to develop after the initial damage. In the rare acute form symptoms are evident immediately after delivery.

Risk factors
○ Multiple pregnancies
○ Placental abnormalities

Causes
○ Obstetric hemorrhage
○ Obstetric shock

Prevalence
○ A rare disorder because of widespread access to obstetric care
○ Occurs in 1 in 10,000 pregnancies
○ The most common cause of ischemic necrosis of the anterior pituitary gland

Complications
○ Infection
○ Death

Assessment

History
○ Failure of lactation
○ Failure of menstruation
○ Fatigue
○ Postpartum

Physical assessment
○ Hypotension
○ Lack of pubic or axillary hair growth
○ Symptoms of thyroid and adrenocortical failure

Test results
Laboratory
○ Decreased serum thyroid and adrenal hormone levels
Imaging
○ A computed tomography scan of the head rules out other abnormalities of the pituitary gland, such as a tumor.

Nursing diagnoses

○ Decreased cardiac output
○ Deficient fluid volume
○ Ineffective breast-feeding
○ Risk for deficient parenting
○ Situational low self-esteem

Key outcomes
The patient will:
○ maintain adequate cardiac output
○ maintain stable vital signs
○ maintain balanced fluid status
○ breast-feed her newborn, if appropriate
○ maintain hematocrit within normal limits
○ verbalize her feelings related to the diagnosis
○ express positive feelings about self
○ bond with her newborn.

Interventions

General
○ Administration of blood products
○ Prevention of hypotension during delivery
○ Prevention of postpartum hemorrhage

Nursing
○ Give prescribed drugs.
○ Assist the patient in feeding her newborn, either breast-feeding, if appropriate, or bottle feeding.
○ Encourage the patient to bond with her newborn or child.
○ Encourage periods of rest to cope with fatigue.
○ Provide emotional support, especially related to the patient's verbalizations about altered body image.

Drug therapy
○ Lifelong hormone replacement therapy
  – Adrenal hormones
  – Estrogen
  – Progesterone
  – Thyroid hormones
○ I.V. fluids

Monitoring
○ Lactation
○ Menstrual cycles
○ Serum hormone levels

○ Serum thyroid function tests
○ Vital signs

Patient teaching

Be sure to cover:
○ the diagnosis, prognosis, and treatment
○ the importance of regular prenatal, postnatal, and obstetric care
○ the importance of follow-up blood work
○ how to keep a calendar of her menstrual cycles and when to notify the doctor
○ breast and bottle feeding
○ the importance of adequate rest and balanced diet
○ signs and symptoms of infection
○ ways to prevent infection.

Discharge planning

○ Refer the patient to community support groups.
○ Refer the patient to a lactation consultant, if appropriate.
○ Refer the patient to an endocrinologist for follow-up care.

Shock, cardiogenic

Overview

Description
○ A condition of diminished cardiac output that severely impairs tissue perfusion
○ The most lethal form of shock
○ Sometimes called pump failure

Pathophysiology
○ Left ventricular dysfunction starts a series of compensatory mechanisms to increase cardiac output.
○ As cardiac output decreases, aortic and carotid baroreceptors activate sympathetic nervous responses.
○ Responses increase heart rate, left ventricular filling pressure, and peripheral resistance to flow to enhance venous return to the heart.
○ This action initially stabilizes the patient but later causes deterioration with increasing oxygen demands on the already compromised myocardium.
○ These events create a cycle of low cardiac output, sympathetic compensation, myocardial ischemia, and even lower cardiac output.

Causes
○ Acute mitral or aortic insufficiency
○ End-stage cardiomyopathy
○ Myocardial infarction (MI, the most common)
○ Myocardial ischemia
○ Myocarditis
○ Papillary muscle dysfunction
○ Ventricular aneurysm
○ Ventricular septal defect

Prevalence
○ Typically affects patients in whom an area of MI involves 40% or more of the left ventricular muscle mass (a group in which mortality may exceed 85%)

Complications
○ Multiple organ dysfunction
○ Death

▽ *ALERT Most patients with cardiogenic shock die within 24 hours. Those who survive have a poor prognosis.*

Assessment

History
○ Anginal pain
○ Disorder that decreases left ventricular function
○ Disorder, such as an MI or cardiomyopathy, that severely decreases left ventricular function

Physical assessment
○ Cyanosis
○ Decreased level of consciousness (LOC)
○ Decreased sensorium
○ Gallop rhythm, faint heart sounds, and, possibly, a holosystolic murmur
○ Jugular vein distention
○ Mean arterial pressure of less than 60 mm Hg in adults
○ Pale, cold, clammy skin
○ Pulmonary crackles
○ Rapid, shallow respirations
○ Rapid, thready pulse
○ Severe anxiety
○ Urine output less than 20 ml/hour

Test results
Laboratory
○ Increased serum levels of creatine kinase, lactate dehydrogenase, aspartate aminotransferase, and alanine aminotransferase
○ Increased troponin levels
○ Metabolic and respiratory acidosis and hypoxia in arterial blood gas (ABG) analysis
Diagnostic procedures
○ Cardiac catheterization and echocardiography may reveal conditions that can lead to pump dysfunction and failure, such as cardiac tamponade, papillary muscle infarct or rupture, ventricular septal rupture, pulmonary emboli, venous pooling, and hypovolemia.
○ Pulmonary artery pressure monitoring reveals increased pulmonary artery pressure and pulmonary artery wedge pressure, reflecting an increase in left ventricular end-diastolic pressure (preload) and heightened resistance to left ventricular emptying (afterload) caused by ineffective pumping and increased peripheral vascular resistance.
○ Invasive arterial pressure monitoring shows systolic arterial pressure less than 80 mm Hg caused by impaired ventricular ejection.
○ Electrocardiography demonstrates possible evidence of acute MI, ischemia, or ventricular aneurysm.

Nursing diagnoses

○ Acute pain
○ Decreased cardiac output
○ Excessive fluid volume
○ Impaired spontaneous ventilation
○ Ineffective individual coping

Key outcomes
The patient will:
○ maintain adequate cardiac output and hemodynamic stability
○ develop no complications of fluid volume excess

- maintain adequate ventilation
- express feelings and develop adequate coping mechanisms
- remain free from chest pain.

Interventions

General

- Bed rest
- Intra-aortic balloon pump (IABP)
- Percutaneous transluminal coronary angioplasty, stents, or bypass grafting to increase myocardial perfusion
- Possible parenteral nutrition or tube feedings
- Possible ventricular assist device
- Possible heart transplant

Nursing

- Administer oxygen therapy.
- Follow IABP protocols and policies.

> **ALERT** *When a patient is on an IABP, move him as little as possible. Never place the patient in a sitting position higher than 45 degrees (including for chest X-rays) because the balloon may tear through the aorta and cause immediate death. Assess pedal pulses and skin temperature and color. Check the dressing on the insertion site frequently for bleeding, and change it according to facility protocol. Also check the site for hematoma or signs of infection, and culture any drainage.*

- Monitor the patient for cardiac arrhythmias.
- Plan your care to allow frequent rest periods, and provide as much privacy as possible.
- Provide explanations and reassurance for the patient and his family as appropriate.
- Prepare the patient and his family for a possibly fatal outcome, and help them find coping strategies.

Drug therapy

- Analgesics
- Inotropics
- Osmotic diuretics
- Oxygen
- Sedatives
- Vasoconstrictors
- Vasodilators
- Vasopressors

Monitoring

- ABG levels (acid-base balance) and pulse oximetry
- Cardiac status and rhythm
- Complete blood count and electrolyte levels
- Hemodynamics
- Intake and output
- LOC
- Pulmonary artery and wedge pressures
- Respiratory status
- Vital signs and peripheral pulses

Patient teaching

Be sure to cover:
- the disorder, diagnosis, and treatment
- explanations and reassurance for the patient and the family
- the possibly fatal outcome.

Discharge planning

- Refer the patient to community support servics.
- Refer the patient and family to pastoral care to discuss feelings of grief.
- Refer the patient for hospice care, as appropriate.

Shock, hypovolemic

Overview

Description
○ Reduced intravascular blood volume causing circulatory dysfunction and inadequate tissue perfusion resulting from loss of blood, plasma, or fluids
○ Potentially life-threatening

Pathophysiology
○ When fluid is lost from the intravascular space, venous return to the heart is reduced.
○ This decreases ventricular filling, which decreases stroke volume.
○ Cardiac output falls, causing reduced perfusion to tissues and organs.
○ Tissue anoxia prompts a shift in cellular metabolism from aerobic to anaerobic pathways.
○ Lactic acid accumulates, resulting in metabolic acidosis.

Causes
○ Acute blood loss (about one-fifth of total volume)
○ Acute pancreatitis
○ Ascites
○ Burns
○ Dehydration, as from excessive perspiration, severe diarrhea, protracted vomiting, diabetes insipidus, diuresis, or inadequate fluid intake
○ Diuretic abuse
○ Intestinal obstruction
○ Peritonitis

Prevalence
○ Affects all ages
○ Affects males and females equally
○ Depends on cause
○ More frequent and less tolerated in elderly patients

Complications
○ Acute respiratory distress syndrome
○ Acute tubular necrosis and renal failure
○ Cardiac arrest
○ Disseminated intravascular coagulation
○ Multiple organ dysfunction
○ Permanent cerebral damage

Assessment

History
○ Disorders or conditions that reduce blood volume, such as gastrointestinal hemorrhage, trauma, and severe diarrhea and vomiting
○ With cardiac disease, possible anginal pain from of decreased myocardial perfusion and oxygenation

Physical assessment
○ Altered level of consciousness
○ Decreased sensorium
○ Mean arterial pressure less than 60 mm Hg in adults (in chronic hypotension, mean pressure may fall below 50 mm Hg before signs of shock)
○ Narrowing pulse pressure
○ Orthostatic vital signs and tilt test results consistent with hypovolemic shock (See *What happens in hypovolemic shock.*)
○ Pale, cool, clammy skin
○ Pallor, tachycardia, hypotension
○ Rapid, shallow respirations
○ Rapid, thready pulse
○ Urine output usually less than 20 ml/hour

Test results
Laboratory
○ Decreased hematocrit
○ Decreased red blood cell and platelet counts
○ Decreased hemoglobin levels
○ Increased serum potassium, sodium, lactate dehydrogenase, creatinine, and blood urea nitrogen levels
○ Increased urine specific gravity (greater than 1.020) and urine osmolality
○ Decreased pH and partial pressure of arterial oxygen
○ Increased partial pressure of arterial carbon dioxide
○ Aspiration of gastric contents through a nasogastric tube identifies internal bleeding
○ Positive result in guaiac testing of nasogastric tube aspirate
○ Positive result in occult blood tests
○ Coagulopathy from disseminated intravascular coagulation
Imaging
○ X-rays (chest or abdominal) help to identify internal bleeding sites.
Diagnostic procedures
○ Gastroscopy helps to identify internal bleeding sites.
○ Invasive hemodynamic monitoring shows reduced central venous pressure, right atrial pressure, pulmonary artery pressure, pulmonary artery wedge pressure, and cardiac output.

Nursing diagnoses
○ Decreased cardiac output
○ Deficient fluid volume
○ Impaired spontaneous ventilation
○ Ineffective individual coping

Key outcomes
The patient will:
○ maintain adequate cardiac output
○ maintain hemodynamic stability
○ maintain adequate ventilation
○ express feelings and develop adequate coping mechanisms
○ regain adequate fluid volume.

Interventions

General

▶ **ALERT** *Emergency treatment must include prompt blood and fluid replacement to restore intravascular volume and raise blood pressure.*

- ○ In severe cases, intra-aortic balloon pump, ventricular assist device, or pneumatic antishock garment
- ○ Oxygen administration
- ○ Bleeding control by direct application of pressure and related measures
- ○ Possible parenteral nutrition or tube feedings
- ○ Bed rest
- ○ Possible surgery to correct underlying problem

Nursing

- ○ Check for a patent airway and adequate circulation. If blood pressure and heart rate are absent, start cardiopulmonary resuscitation.
- ○ Obtain type and crossmatch, as ordered.
- ○ Give I.V. solutions, blood products, and drugs.
- ○ Insert an indwelling urinary catheter.
- ○ Give prescribed oxygen.
- ○ Explain all treatments and procedures.
- ○ Provide emotional support to the patient and family.

▶ **ALERT** *Don't start an I.V. line in the legs of a patient in shock after abdominal trauma because infused fluid may escape through ruptured vessels into the abdomen.*

Drug therapy

- ○ Oxygen
- ○ Plasma proteins or other plasma expanders
- ○ Positive inotropes
- ○ Possibly diuretics
- ○ Prompt and vigorous blood and fluid replacement

Monitoring

- ○ Airway patency
- ○ Arterial blood gas levels
- ○ Cardiac rhythm
- ○ Coagulation studies for impending coagulopathy
- ○ Complete blood count and electrolyte measurements
- ○ Hemodynamics
- ○ Intake and output
- ○ Peripheral pulses
- ○ Signs of fluid overload
- ○ Vital signs

▶ **ALERT** *If blood pressure drops below 80 mm Hg, increase the oxygen flow rate and notify the doctor right away.*

Patient teaching

Be sure to cover:
- ○ the disorder, diagnosis, and treatment
- ○ all procedures and their purposes

What happens in hypovolemic shock

In hypovolemic shock, loss of vascular volume causes extreme tissue hypoperfusion. Internal fluid loss can result from hemorrhage or third-space fluid shifting. External fluid loss can result from severe bleeding or severe diarrhea, diuresis, or vomiting. Inadequate vascular volume decreases venous return and cardiac output. The resulting drop in arterial blood pressure activates the body's compensatory mechanisms in an attempt to increase vascular volume. If compensation is unsuccessful, decompensation and death may occur.

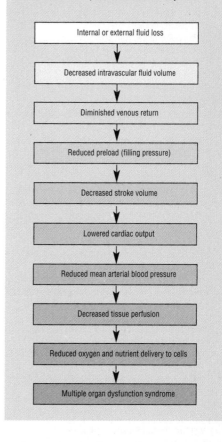

- ○ the risks of blood transfusions
- ○ the purpose of all equipment
- ○ dietary restrictions
- ○ prescribed drugs, dosages, administration, and possible adverse effects.

Discharge planning

- ○ Refer the patient to a nutritionist to determine the patient's daily fluid needs, if appropriate.
- ○ Refer the patient to a diabetes educator, or arrange a gastrointestinal follow-up, if appropriate.

Shock, septic

Overview

Description
○ Low systemic vascular resistance and an elevated cardiac output
○ Probably a response to infections that release microbes or an immune mediator
○ Second to cardiogenic shock as the leading cause of shock-related death
○ Leading cause of death in acute care units in the United States

Pathophysiology
○ Initially, the body's defenses activate chemical mediators in response to the invading organisms.
○ The release of these mediators results in low systemic vascular resistance and increased cardiac output.
○ Blood flow is unevenly distributed in the microcirculation, and plasma leaking from capillaries causes functional hypovolemia.
○ Diffuse increase in capillary permeability occurs.
○ Eventually, cardiac output decreases, and poor tissue perfusion and hypotension cause multisystem dysfunction syndrome and death.

Causes
○ Any pathogenic organism
○ Gram-negative bacteria, such as *Escherichia coli*, *Klebsiella pneumoniae*, *Serratia*, *Enterobacter*, and *Pseudomonas*, are most common causes (up to 70% of cases)
○ Translocation of bacteria from other areas of the body (surgery, I.V. therapy, catheters)

Prevalence
○ Possible in any person with impaired immunity

 AGE AWARE Neonates and elderly people are at greatest risk for septic shock.

○ About two-thirds of cases in hospitalized patients (most have underlying diseases)

Complications
○ Abnormal liver function
○ Disseminated intravascular coagulation
○ Gastrointestinal ulcers
○ Heart failure
○ Renal failure
○ Shock in about 25% of patients with gram-positive bacteremia
○ Death

Assessment

History
○ Possible disorder or treatment that can cause immunosuppression
○ Possible previous invasive tests or treatments, surgery, or trauma
○ Possible fever and chills (although 20% of patients possibly hypothermic)

Physical assessment
Hyperdynamic or warm phase
○ Altered level of consciousness (LOC) reflected in agitation, anxiety, irritability, and shortened attention span
○ Blood pressure normal or slightly elevated
○ Peripheral vasodilation
○ Rapid, full, bounding pulse
○ Respirations rapid and shallow
○ Skin possibly pink and flushed or warm and dry
○ Urine output below normal
Hypodynamic or cold phase
○ Cold, clammy skin
○ Crackles or rhonchi if pulmonary congestion is present
○ Decreased LOC; possible obtundation and coma
○ Hypotension
○ Irregular pulse if arrhythmias are present
○ Pale skin and possible cyanosis
○ Peripheral vasoconstriction and inadequate tissue perfusion
○ Rapid, weak, thready pulse
○ Respirations possibly rapid and shallow
○ Urine output possibly less than 25 ml/hour or absent

Test results
Laboratory
○ Causative organism in blood cultures
○ Presence or absence of anemia and leukopenia, severe or absent neutropenia, and usually the presence of thrombocytopenia
○ Increased blood urea nitrogen and creatinine levels
○ Decreased creatinine clearance
○ Abnormal prothrombin time and partial thromboplastin time
○ Elevated serum lactate dehydrogenase levels, with metabolic acidosis
○ Increased urine specific gravity (more than 1.020), increased osmolality
○ Decreased sodium levels
○ Increased blood pH and partial pressure of arterial oxygen and decreased partial pressure of arterial carbon dioxide with respiratory alkalosis in early stages
Diagnostic procedures
○ Electrocardiography shows ST-segment depression, inverted T waves, and arrhythmias resembling a myocardial infarction.

○ Invasive hemodynamic monitoring shows:
  – increased cardiac output and decreased systemic vascular resistance in warm phase
  – decreased cardiac output and increased systemic vascular resistance in cold phase.

Nursing diagnoses

○ Decreased cardiac output
○ Deficient fluid volume
○ Ineffective individual coping
○ Ineffective spontaneous ventilation
○ Risk for infection

Key outcomes
The patient will:
○ maintain adequate cardiac output
○ maintain hemodynamic stability
○ maintain adequate ventilation
○ show no signs of infection
○ express feelings and develop adequate coping mechanisms
○ maintain adequate fluid volume.

Interventions

General

○ Administration of whole blood or plasma
○ Bed rest
○ Fluid volume replacement
○ In patients immunosuppressed from drug therapy, drugs reduced or stopped, if possible
○ Mechanical ventilation if respiratory failure occurs
○ Possible parenteral nutrition or tube feedings
○ Removal of I.V., intra-arterial, or urinary drainage catheters whenever possible
○ Surgery and debridement to drain and excise abscesses

Nursing

○ Remove any I.V., intra-arterial, or urinary drainage catheters, and send them to the laboratory to culture for the presence of the causative organism.
○ Give prescribed I.V. fluids and blood products.

▷ **ALERT** *A progressive drop in blood pressure accompanied by a thready pulse typically signals inadequate cardiac output from reduced intravascular volume. Notify a doctor immediately and increase the infusion rate.*

○ Give appropriate antimicrobial I.V. drugs.
○ Notify a doctor if urine output is less than 30 ml/hour.
○ Give prescribed oxygen.
○ Provide emotional support to the patient and his family.
○ Document the occurrence of a nosocomial infection, and report it to the infection-control practitioner.

Drug therapy
○ Antimicrobial
○ Antipyretics
○ Colloid or crystalloid infusions
○ Corticosteroids
○ Diuretics
○ Granulocyte transfusions
○ I.V. bicarbonate
○ Oxygen
○ Vasopressors

Monitoring
○ Arterial blood gas levels and pulse oximetry
○ Cardiac rhythm
○ Complete blood count
○ Daily weight
○ Heart and breath sounds
○ Hemodynamics
○ Intake and output
○ Mental status
○ Serum antibiotic levels
○ Vital signs and peripheral pulses

Patient teaching

Be sure to cover:
○ the disorder, diagnosis, and treatment
○ all procedures and their purposes, to ease the patient's anxiety
○ risks of blood transfusions
○ all equipment and purposes
○ drugs and possible adverse effects
○ possible complications
○ infection-control precautions and the importance of hand-washing.

Discharge planning

○ Refer the patient for outpatient I.V. infusion services if prolonged I.V. antibiotics are needed.

Sickle cell anemia

Overview

Description
○ A congenital hemolytic anemia

Pathophysiology
○ An inherited defective hemoglobin molecule (hemoglobin S) causes red blood cells (RBCs) to roughen and become sickle-cell shaped.
○ Defective RBCs become insoluble whenever hypoxia occurs. As a result, they become rigid, rough, and elongated into a crescent or sickle shape.

▼ *ALERT Infection, stress, dehydration, strenuous exercise, high altitude, unpressurized aircraft, cold, and vasoconstrictive drugs are conditions that may provoke hypoxia and periodic crises.*

○ Sickling can cause hemolysis and RBCs to pile up, resulting in more viscous blood and impaired circulation.
○ A painful (vasoocclusive or infarctive) crisis results from blood vessel obstruction by tangled sickle cells, which causes tissue anoxia and possible necrosis.

✳ *AGE AWARE A painful crisis, the hallmark of the disease, usually appears periodically after age 5.*

○ Autosplenectomy, which happens with long-term disease, occurs when the splenic damage and scarring is so extensive that the spleen shrinks and becomes impalpable.

▼ *ALERT Autosplenectomy can lead to increased susceptibility to Streptococcus pneumoniae sepsis, which can be fatal without prompt treatment.*

○ Anaplastic (megaloblastic) crisis results from bone marrow depression and is associated with infection, usually viral.
○ Acute sequestration crisis may cause sudden massive entrapment of RBCs in the spleen and liver.

✳ *AGE AWARE Acute sequestration crisis occurs in infants between ages 8 months and 2 years. If untreated, it commonly progresses to hypovolemic shock and death.*

○ Hemolytic crisis rarely occurs in patients with glucose-6-phosphate dehydrogenase deficiency.

Causes
○ Homozygous inheritance of the gene that produces hemoglobin S.

Prevalence
○ Occurs mainly but not only in Blacks; most common in tropical Africans and in persons of African descent.
○ Overall, 1 in 400 to 600 Black children has sickle cell anemia; about 1 in 10 American Blacks carries the abnormal gene.
○ Also occurs in people of Mediterranean or East Indian ancestry.
○ Half of patients with sickle cell anemia die by their early twenties; few live to middle age.

Complications
○ Chronic ill health
○ Infection
○ Periodic crises
○ Premature death
○ Organ infarction

Assessment

History

✳ *AGE AWARE Symptoms usually don't develop until after age 6 months because large amounts of fetal hemoglobin protect infants for the first few months after birth.*

✳ *AGE AWARE Children with sickle cell anemia tend to be small for their age with delayed puberty. Adults tend to have a spiderlike body build with narrow shoulders and hips, long limbs, curved spine, barrel chest, and elongated skull.*

○ Aching bones
○ Chest pains
○ Difficulty awakening
○ Dyspnea or dyspnea on exertion
○ Family history or the sickle cell trait
○ Fatigue, listlessness
○ Fever over 104° F (40° C) or fever of 100° F (37.8° C) that persists for 2 days
○ Increased susceptibility to infection
○ Irritability
○ Pain
○ Sudden, painful episodes of priapism in adolescent or adult males
Painful crisis
○ Dark urine
○ Severe abdominal pain
○ Thoracic, muscular, and bone pain
Autosplenectomy
○ Lethargy
Anaplastic crisis
○ Dyspnea
○ Lethargy
Acute sequestration crisis
○ Lethargy

Physical assessment
○ Hepatomegaly
○ Ischemic leg ulcers
○ Jaundice
○ Joint swelling
○ Pallor (lips, tongue, palms, nail beds)

○ Systolic and diastolic murmurs
○ Tachycardia
Painful crisis
○ Low-grade fever
○ Worsening jaundice
Autosplenectomy
○ Apathy
○ Fever
Anaplastic crisis
○ Pallor
○ Possible coma
Acute sequestration crisis
○ Decreased level of consciousness
○ Dehydration
○ Hypotension
Hemolytic crisis
○ Hepatomegaly
○ Worsening and chronic jaundice

Test results
Laboratory
○ Hemoglobin S or other hemoglobinopathies in electrophoresis
○ Electrophoresis on umbilical cord blood at birth for all at-risk newborns
○ Decreased RBC count, erythrocyte sedimentation rate, and RBC survival
○ Increased white blood cell and platelet counts and serum iron level
○ Reticulocytosis
○ Possibly low or normal hemoglobin

Nursing diagnoses

○ Acute pain
○ Deficient fluid volume
○ Ineffective spontaneous ventilation

Key outcomes
The patient will:
○ maintain hemodynamic stability
○ not exhibit signs of dehydration or crisis
○ maintain adequate respirations and prevent hypoxia
○ verbalize comfort
○ remain alert and oriented.

Interventions

General
○ Prevention of crisis
○ Supportive measures during crisis
○ Prevention of dehydration
Crisis
○ Infusion of packed RBCs
○ Bed rest

Nursing
○ Provide comfort measures.

○ Encourage adequate fluid intake.
○ Provide support to the patient and family.
○ Encourage normal mental and social development in children.
Crisis
○ Apply warm compresses to painful areas.

▼ **ALERT** *Never use cold compresses because they aggravate the condition.*

○ Cover the patient with a blanket.

Drug therapy
○ Prophylactic penicillin starting before age 4 months
○ Sodium cyanate
Crisis
○ Analgesics
○ Antipyretic
○ I.V. fluids
○ Sedation

Monitoring
○ Intake and output
○ Laboratory values
○ Mental status
○ Pain score
○ Respiratory status
○ Signs and symptoms of crisis
○ Vital signs

Patient teaching

Be sure to cover:
○ avoiding tight clothing that restricts circulation
○ avoiding strenuous exercise, vasoconstricting drugs, cold temperatures, unpressurized aircraft, high altitude, and other conditions that provoke hypoxia
○ the importance of childhood immunizations, meticulous wound care, oral hygiene, regular dental checkups, and a balanced diet to prevent infection
○ the importance of wearing an alert bracelet and informing all health care providers about the disorder.

Discharge planning

○ Refer the parents of children with sickle cell anemia for genetic counseling and recommend screening of other family members to determine if they're heterozygous carriers.
○ Refer the parents of children with sickle cell anemia to psychological counseling to cope with feelings of guilt.
○ Refer the patient and family to a community support group.
○ Refer women to a qualified obstetrician or gynecologist because sickle cell anemia may increase obstetric risks; use of hormonal contraceptives may be risky as well.

Silicosis

Overview

Description
○ Progressive pneumoconiosis characterized by nodular lesions, commonly leading to fibrosis
○ Classified according to severity of pulmonary disease and rapidity of onset and progression
○ Usually a simple, asymptomatic illness
○ Considered an industrial disease
○ Prognosis good unless complications occur

Pathophysiology
○ Small particles of mineral dust are inhaled and deposited in the respiratory bronchioles, alveolar ducts, and alveoli.
○ The surface of these particles generates silicon-based radicals that lead to the production of hydroxy, hydrogen peroxide, and other oxygen radicals that damage cell membranes and inactivate essential cell proteins.
○ Alveolar macrophages ingest the particles, become activated, and release cytokines, such as tumor necrosis factor and others that attract other inflammatory cells.
○ The inflammation damages resident cells and the extracellular matrix.
○ Fibroblasts are stimulated to produce collagen, resulting in fibrosis.

Causes
○ Silica dust
  – Manufacture of ceramics (flint) and building materials (sandstone)
  – Mixed form in construction materials (cement)
  – Powder form (silica flour) in paints, porcelain, scouring soaps, and wood fillers
  – Mining of gold, lead, zinc, and iron

Prevalence
○ Most common in those who work around silica dust, such as foundry workers, boiler scalers, and stone cutters
○ Acute silicosis possible after 1 to 3 years in sand blasters, tunnel workers, and others exposed to high concentrations of respirable silica
○ Accelerated silicosis possible in those exposed to lower concentrations of free silica, usually after about 10 years of exposure

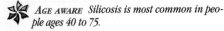 *AGE AWARE Silicosis is most common in people ages 40 to 75.*

○ More common in males than in females

Complications
○ Cardiac or respiratory failure
○ Cor pulmonale
○ Lung infection
○ Pneumothorax
○ Pulmonary fibrosis
○ Pulmonary tuberculosis

Assessment

History
○ Long-term exposure to silica dust
○ Dyspnea on exertion
○ Dry cough, especially in the morning

Physical assessment
○ Areas of increased and decreased resonance
○ Decreased chest expansion
○ Decreased mentation
○ Diminished breath sounds
○ Hemoptysis
○ Lethargy
○ Medium crackles, wheezing
○ Tachypnea

> *ALERT Assess the patient for an intensified ventricular gallop on inspiration, which is a hallmark of cor pulmonale.*

Test results
Laboratory
○ Normal partial pressure of oxygen in simple silicosis (may be significantly decreased in late stages or complicated disease)
○ Normal partial pressure of carbon dioxide in early stages of the disease (may decrease with hyperventilation; may increase if restrictive lung disease develops)
Imaging
○ Chest X-rays in simple silicosis show small, discrete, nodular lesions in both lung fields, although they typically concentrate in the upper lung.
○ Lung nodes may appear enlarged and show eggshell calcification.
○ Chest X-rays in complicated silicosis show one or more conglomerate masses of dense tissue.
Diagnostic procedures
○ Forced vital capacity (FVC) is reduced in complicated silicosis.
○ Forced expiratory volume in 1 second (FEV_1) is reduced with obstructive disease.
○ FEV_1 is reduced, with a normal or high ratio of FEV_1 to FVC, in complicated silicosis.
○ Diffusing capacity for carbon monoxide is reduced when fibrosis destroys alveolar walls and obliterates pulmonary capillaries or when it thickens the alveolocapillary membrane.
○ Pulmonary artery monitoring reveals pulmonary hypertension.

Nursing diagnoses

○ Deficient knowledge (disease process)
○ Fatigue
○ Imbalanced nutrition: less than body requirements
○ Ineffective individual coping
○ Ineffective spontaneous ventilation
○ Risk for deficient fluid volume

Key outcomes

The patient will:
○ maintain adequate ventilation
○ use energy conservation techniques
○ express an understanding of the illness
○ demonstrate effective coping mechanisms
○ maintain adequate caloric intake
○ maintain adequate fluid volume.

Interventions

General

○ Relief of respiratory symptoms
○ Management of hypoxia and cor pulmonale
○ Prevention of respiratory tract infections
○ Steam inhalation and chest physiotherapy
○ Increased fluid intake
○ High-calorie, high-protein diet
○ Regular exercise program, as tolerated
○ Surgery
 – Possible tracheostomy
 – Possible lung transplantation
 – Whole lung lavage

Nursing

○ Give prescribed drugs.
○ Perform chest physiotherapy.
○ Provide a high-calorie, high-protein diet.
○ Provide small, frequent meals.
○ Provide frequent mouth care.
○ Ensure adequate hydration (3 quarts [3 L] daily).
○ Encourage daily exercise as tolerated.
○ Provide diversional activities as appropriate.
○ Provide frequent rest periods.
○ Help with adjustment to the lifestyle changes demanded by a chronic illness.
○ Include the patient and family in care decisions whenever possible.
○ Perform tuberculosis testing if ordered.

Drug therapy

○ Antibiotics
○ Anti-inflammatories
○ Bronchodilators
○ I.V. fluids
○ Oxygen

Monitoring

○ Activity tolerance
○ Breath sounds
○ Changes in mentation
○ Complications
○ Daily weight
○ Intake and output
○ Respiratory status
○ Sputum production
○ Vital signs

Patient teaching

Be sure to cover:
○ the disorder, diagnosis, and treatment
○ prescribed drugs, dosages, administration, and possible adverse effects
○ when to consult a doctor
○ the need to avoid crowds and people with infections
○ home oxygen therapy, if needed
○ transtracheal catheter care, if needed
○ postural drainage and chest percussion
○ coughing and deep-breathing exercises
○ the need to consume a high-calorie, high-protein diet
○ adequate hydration
○ the risk of tuberculosis
○ energy conservation techniques
○ methods of preventing infection.

Discharge planning

○ Refer the patient for influenza and pneumococcus immunizations, as needed.
○ Refer the patient to a smoking-cessation program, if indicated.
○ Refer the patient for tuberculosis testing, if indicated.

Syndrome of inappropriate antidiuretic hormone secretion

Overview

Description

- Disease of the posterior pituitary marked by excessive release of antidiuretic hormone (ADH), also known as vasopressin
- Potentially life-threatening
- Prognosis depends on underlying disorder and response to treatment
- Also known as SIADH

Pathophysiology

- Excessive ADH secretion occurs in the absence of normal physiologic stimuli for its release.
- Excessive water reabsorption from the distal convoluted tubule and collecting ducts results in hyponatremia and normal to slightly increased extracellular fluid volume.

Causes

- Central nervous system disorders
- Drugs
- Myxedema
- Neoplastic diseases
- Oat cell carcinoma of the lung
- Psychosis
- Pulmonary disorders

Prevalence

- Common cause of hospital-acquired hyponatremia

Complications

- Cerebral edema
- Coma
- Heart failure
- Seizures
- Severe hyponatremia
- Water intoxication
- Death

Assessment

History

- Anorexia, nausea, vomiting
- Cancer
- Cerebrovascular disease
- Emotional and behavioral changes
- Headaches
- Lethargy
- Possible clue to the cause
- Pulmonary disease
- Recent head injury
- Weight gain

Physical assessment

- Disorientation
- Increased water retention
- Muscle weakness
- Seizures and coma
- Sluggish deep tendon reflexes
- Tachycardia

Test results

Laboratory

- Serum osmolality levels less than 280 mOsm/kg
- Serum sodium levels less than 123 mEq/L
- Urine sodium levels more than 20 mEq/L without diuretics
- Normal renal function tests

Nursing diagnoses

- Deficient fluid volume
- Deficient knowledge (disease process)
- Risk for injury

Key outcomes

The patient will:
- develop no complications
- remain alert and oriented to the environment
- verbalize an understanding of the disorder and treatment regimen
- maintain adequate fluid balance.

Interventions

General

- Based mainly on symptoms
- Correction of the underlying cause
- Restricted water intake (500 to 1,000 ml/day)
- High-salt, high-protein diet or urea supplements to enhance water excretion
- Activity as tolerated
- Surgery, with radiation or chemotherapy, to treat underlying cause such as cancer

Nursing

- Restrict fluids.
- Provide comfort measures for thirst.
- Reduce unnecessary environmental stimuli.
- Orient as needed.
- Provide a safe environment.
- Institute seizure precautions as needed.
- Give prescribed drugs.

Drug therapy

○ Demeclocycline or lithium for long-term treatment
○ Loop diuretics if fluid overload, history of heart failure, or resistance to treatment
○ 3% sodium chloride solution if serum sodium level is less than 120 or if the patient is seizing

▼ **ALERT** *Monitor the patient carefully when giving hypertonic saline solutions. They may cause water to shift out of cells, and lead to intravascular volume overload and serious brain damage.*

Monitoring

○ Breath sounds
○ Changes in level of consciousness
○ Daily weight
○ Heart sounds
○ Intake and output
○ Neurologic checks
○ Response to treatment
○ Serum electrolytes, especially sodium
○ Vital signs

▼ **ALERT** *Watch closely for signs and symptoms of heart failure, which may occur because of fluid overload.*

Patient teaching

Be sure to cover:
○ the disorder, diagnosis, and treatment
○ fluid restriction
○ methods to decrease discomfort from thirst
○ prescribed drugs, dosages, administration, and possible adverse effects
○ self-monitoring techniques for fluid retention, such as daily weight
○ signs and symptoms that require immediate medical intervention.

Discharge planning

○ Refer the patient to an endocrinologist for outpatient follow-up.
○ Refer the patient to a nutritionist to review the components of a high-salt, high-protein diet, as needed.

Thyrotoxicosis

Overview

Description

○ A metabolic imbalance caused by excess thyroid hormone
○ Also called hyperthyroidism

Pathophysiology

○ The thyroid gland, part of the endocrine system, is located in the neck.
○ It produces several hormones that regulate growth, digestion, and metabolism.
○ The thyroid gland responds to complex mechanisms that control the rates of hormone secretion.
○ Thyrotoxicosis results from excess quantities of thyroid hormone.

Causes

○ Graves' disease
○ Inflammation
○ Ingestion of excessive amounts of iodine
○ Ingestion of excessive amounts of thyroid hormone
○ Tumors of the thyroid gland, pituitary gland, testes, or ovaries

Prevalence

○ Affects 1 in 1,000 people
○ 85% of cases caused by Graves' disease

Massive goiter

Massive multinodular goiter causes gross distention and swelling of the neck.

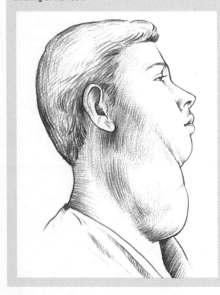

✷ *AGE AWARE Graves' disease is most common among people ages 30 to 40. Only 5% of patients with hyperthyroidism are younger than 15.*

Complications

○ Heart failure
○ Osteoporosis
○ Thyroid crisis or storm

▼ *ALERT Thyroid crisis or storm is an acute worsening of the symptoms of thyrotoxicosis that can occur with stress or infection. It's a medical emergency that can lead to life-threatening cardiac, hepatic, or renal failure.*

Assessment

History

○ Difficulty sleeping
○ Fatigue
○ Heat intolerance
○ Increased appetite
○ Increased sweating
○ Irregular or absent menstrual cycles in women
○ Muscle cramps
○ Nausea and vomiting
○ Palpitations
○ Pruritus
○ Thirst
○ Weight loss

Physical assessment

○ Bounding pulse
○ Clammy skin
○ Exophthalmos
○ Gynecomastia
○ Hypertension
○ Muscle weakness and atrophy
○ Nervousness
○ Pallor
○ Possible enlarged thyroid or goiter (See *Massive goiter.*)
○ Restlessness
○ Skin changes (abnormally dark or light)
○ Uncoordinated movements

Test results

Laboratory

○ Decreased serum thyroid-stimulating hormone (TSH) level
○ Elevated serum T_3 and T_4 levels
○ Increased thyroid resin uptake
○ Positive result in thyroid-releasing hormone (TRH) stimulation test (TSH level fails to rise within 30 minutes after TRH administration.)

Imaging

○ Thyroid scan reveals increased uptake of radioactive iodine (^{131}I).

ALERT *A thyroid scan is contraindicated during pregnancy.*

○ Ultrasonography confirms subclinical ophthalmopathy.

Diagnostic procedures
○ Electrocardiography may reveal paroxysmal supraventricular tachycardia or atrial fibrillation

Nursing diagnoses

○ Ineffective coping mechanisms
○ Ineffective tissue perfusion: cerebral

Key outcomes
The patient will:
○ maintain hemodynamic stability
○ remain alert and oriented
○ use coping mechanisms to deal with stress.

Interventions

General
○ Surgical partial thyroidectomy
○ Bed rest
○ A well-balanced diet with frequent small meals
○ Sunglasses or eye patches for exophthalmos
○ Minimal palpation of the thyroid gland to avoid provoking thyroid storm

Nursing
○ Keep the patient's room cool, quiet, and dark.
○ Provide emotional support, especially related to altered body image.
○ Give prescribed drugs.
○ Mix iodine with milk, juice, or water to prevent gastrointestinal distress. Give it with a straw to avoid staining the patient's teeth.

Drug therapy
○ Antithyroid drugs
○ Beta blockers
○ Isotonic eye drops
○ Radioactive iodine

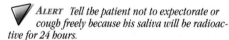 **ALERT** *Tell the patient not to expectorate or cough freely because his saliva will be radioactive for 24 hours.*

Thyroid storm
○ Corticosteroids
○ I.V. fluids
○ Nutrients and vitamins
○ Sedatives

Monitoring
○ Cardiac status
○ Daily weight
○ Glucose level

○ Intake and output
○ Serum electrolytes
○ Signs or symptoms of thyroid storm
○ Vital signs

Patient teaching

Be sure to cover:
○ the diagnosis, prognosis, and treatment
○ signs and symptoms of infection
○ ways to prevent infection
○ preoperative and postoperative thyroidectomy teaching, if appropriate
○ teaching before and after use of ^{131}I, if appropriate
○ the importance of follow-up care
○ signs and symptoms of thyroid crisis or storm, when to call the doctor, and when to go to the hospital
○ prescribed drugs, dosages, administration, and possible adverse effects
○ eye care.

Discharge planning

○ Refer the patient to a center for stress reduction techniques.
○ Refer the patient to an endocrinologist for follow-up.
○ Refer the patient to a nutritionist.

Toxic shock syndrome

Overview

Description
- An inflammatory response syndrome linked to bacterial infection
- An acute, life-threatening condition
- Commonly called TSS

Pathophysiology
- Toxic exoproteins are produced by infective organisms.
- TSST-1 is the most common toxin; staphylococcal enterotoxin B is the second most common.
- For illness to develop, the patient must be infected with a toxigenic strain of *Staphylococcus aureus* and lack antibodies to that strain.

Causes
- Penicillin-resistant *S. aureus*
- Tampon use
- Varicella infection
- Streptococcal pharyngitis

Prevalence
- Affects 1 in 100,000 people
- Affects mainly young people

 AGE AWARE *Toxic shock syndrome affects mainly menstruating women younger than age 30.*

- No menstruation in half of cases
- Affects both sexes and all ages

Guidelines for diagnosing toxic shock syndrome

Toxic shock syndrome is typically diagnosed based on the following criteria.
- Fever 104° F (40° C) or higher
- Diffuse macular erythrodermal rash (sunburn rash)
- Hypotension (systolic blood pressure 90 mm Hg or less in adults or below the 5th percentile for age)
- Involvement of at least three organ systems:
  – Gastrointestinal (vomiting, diarrhea)
  – Muscular (myalgias or liver function test at least twice the upper limit of normal)
  – Mucous membrane hyperemia (conjunctiva, vagina, oropharyngeal)
  – Renal (blood urea nitrogen or creatinine level at least twice normal upper limit, or pyuria)
  – Hepatic (total serum bilirubin or aminotransferase level twice normal level)
  – Hematologic (thrombocytopenia)
  – Central nervous system (disorientation or change in level of consciousness)
- Desquamation, especially of palms and soles, 1 or 2 weeks after onset of illness
- Other conditions ruled out

Complications
- Acute respiratory distress syndrome
- Desquamation of the skin
- Muscle weakness
- Musculoskeletal and respiratory infections
- Neuropsychiatric dysfunction
- Peripheral gangrene
- Renal and myocardial dysfunction
- Septic abortion
- Staphylococcal bacteremia

Assessment

History
- Diarrhea
- Dizziness
- Headache
- Intense myalgia
- Nausea and vomiting
- Possible recent streptococcal infection
- Possible tampon use or menstruation
- Sore throat

Physical assessment
- Altered mental status
- Fever (104° F [40° C] or higher)
- Hypotension
- Macular erythroderma (generalized or local)
- Peripheral edema
- Pharyngeal infection
- Purulent vaginal discharge
- Strawberry tongue
- Vaginal hyperemia

Test results
Laboratory
- Isolation of *S. aureus* from vaginal discharge or infection site (See *Guidelines for diagnosing toxic shock syndrome.*)
- Pyuria
- Azotemia
- Decreased serum albumin level
- Decreased serum calcium level
- Decreased serum phosphorus level
- Leukocytosis or leukopenia
- Thrombocytopenia
- Increased serum creatinine level

Nursing diagnoses
- Decreased cardiac output
- Deficient fluid volume
- Impaired tissue perfusion: peripheral
- Ineffective thermoregulation

Key outcomes
The patient will:
- maintain collateral circulation

- attain and maintain hemodynamic stability
- maintain adequate cardiac output
- remain afebrile
- have an adequate fluid volume.

Interventions

General

- Aggressive fluid resuscitation
- Correction of electrolyte imbalances
- Supportive treatment, possibly including ventilatory support
- Identification and decontamination of toxin production site
- Bed rest until acute phase resolves
- Examination and irrigation of recent surgical wounds

Nursing

- Give prescribed drugs.
- Assess fluid balance.
- Replace fluids I.V., as needed.
- Reorient as needed.
- Implement appropriate safety measures to prevent injury.
- Use standard precautions for any vaginal discharge and lesion drainage.

Drug therapy

- Antibiotics
- Antipyretics
- Inotropics
- I.V. fluids
- I.V. immunoglobulin
- Vasopressors

Monitoring

- Cardiovascular status
- Complications
- Fluid and electrolyte status
- Neurologic status
- Pulmonary status
- Response to treatment
- Vital signs

Patient teaching

Be sure to cover:
- the disorder, diagnosis, and treatment
- the need to avoid using tampons, especially superabsorbent ones, because of the risk of recurrence
- TSS prevention.

Discharge planning

- Refer the patient to a gynecologist for outpatient follow-up and teaching as needed.

Tuberculosis

Overview

Description

- Acute or chronic lung infection characterized by pulmonary infiltrates and the formation of granulomas with caseation, fibrosis, and cavitation
- Excellent prognosis with proper treatment and compliance
- Primary infection in the lungs, but mycobacteria common in other parts of the body
- Also known as TB

Pathophysiology

- Multiplication of the bacillus *Mycobacterium tuberculosis* causes an inflammatory process where deposited.
- A cell-mediated immune response follows, usually containing the infection in 4 to 6 weeks.
- The T-cell response results in formation of granulomas around the bacilli, making them dormant. This confers immunity to subsequent infection.
- Bacilli in granulomas may remain viable for many years, resulting in a positive purified protein derivative or other skin test for TB.
- Active disease develops in 5% to 15% of those infected.
- Transmission occurs when an infected person coughs or sneezes.

Risk factors

- Close contact with newly diagnosed TB patient
- Drug and alcohol abuse
- Gastrectomy
- History of silicosis, diabetes, malnutrition, cancer, Hodgkin's disease, or leukemia
- History of TB exposure
- Homelessness
- Immunosuppression and use of corticosteroids
- Multiple sexual partners
- Recent immigration from Africa, Asia, Mexico, or South America
- Residence in nursing home, mental health facility, or prison

Causes

- Exposure to *M. tuberculosis*
- Sometimes, exposure to other strains of mycobacteria

Prevalence

- Increasing in the United States because of homelessness, drug abuse, and HIV infection
- Globally, the leading cause of illness and death
- 8 to 20 million new cases yearly worldwide
- Twice as common in men as in women
- Four times as common in nonwhites as in whites
- More common in Black and Hispanic men ages 25 to 44
- Most common in people who live in crowded, poorly ventilated, unsanitary conditions

Complications

- Bronchopleural fistulas
- Infection of other body organs by small mycobacterial foci
- Liver involvement secondary to drug therapy
- Massive pulmonary tissue damage
- Pleural effusion
- Pneumonia
- Pneumothorax
- Respiratory failure

Assessment

History

Primary infection
- Anorexia, weight loss
- Low-grade fever
- May be asymptomatic after a 4- to 8-week incubation period
- Night sweats
- Weakness and fatigue

Reactivated infection
- Chest pain
- Cough that produces blood, mucopurulent sputum, or blood-tinged sputum
- Low-grade fever

Physical assessment

- Bronchial breath sounds
- Crepitant crackles
- Dullness over the affected area
- Wheezes
- Whispered pectoriloquy

Test results

Laboratory
- Positive tuberculin skin test in active and inactive TB
- Heat-sensitive, nonmotile, aerobic, acid-fast bacilli in stains and cultures of sputum, cerebrospinal fluid, urine, abscess drainage, or pleural fluid

Imaging
- Chest X-rays show nodular lesions, patchy infiltrates, cavity formation, scar tissue, and calcium deposits.
- Computed tomography or magnetic resonance imaging shows presence and extent of lung damage.

Diagnostic procedures
- Bronchoscopy specimens show heat-sensitive, nonmotile, aerobic, acid-fast bacilli in specimens.

Nursing diagnoses

○ Deficient knowledge (disease process)
○ Fatigue
○ Ineffective coping
○ Impaired spontaneous ventilation
○ Ineffective tissue perfusion: cardiopulmonary
○ Risk for infection

Key outcomes

The patient will:
○ maintain adequate ventilation
○ use support systems to assist with coping
○ identify measures to prevent or reduce fatigue
○ express an understanding of the illness
○ demonstrate infection-control precautions
○ comply with treatment regimen.

Interventions

General

○ Resumption of normal activities with continued drug therapy after 2 to 4 weeks, when disease is no longer infectious
○ Well-balanced, high-calorie diet in small, frequent meals
○ Rest, initially; activity as tolerated
○ Surgery for some complications

Nursing

○ Give prescribed drugs.
○ Monitor patient for drug reactions.
○ Isolate the patient in a quiet, properly ventilated room, and maintain tuberculosis precautions.
○ Provide diversional activities.
○ Properly dispose of secretions.
○ Provide adequate rest periods.
○ Provide well-balanced, high-calorie foods.
○ Provide small, frequent meals.
○ Consult with dietitian if oral supplements are needed.
○ Perform chest physiotherapy.
○ Provide supportive care.
○ Include the patient in decisions about his care.

Drug therapy

○ Daily oral doses for at least 6 months of antitubercular drugs
  – isoniazid
  – pyrazinamide
  – rifampin
  – ethambutol (sometimes)
○ Second-line drugs if needed
  – aminosalicylic acid (para-aminosalicylic acid)
  – capreomycin
  – cycloserine
  – pyrazinamide
  – streptomycin
○ Pyridoxine

Preventing tuberculosis

Explain respiratory and standard precautions to a hospitalized patient with tuberculosis. Before discharge, tell him that he must take precautions to prevent spreading the disease, such as wearing a mask around others, until his doctor tells him he's no longer contagious. He should tell all health care providers he sees, including his dentist and eye doctor, that he has tuberculosis so that they can institute infection-control precautions.

Teach the patient other specific precautions to avoid spreading the infection. Tell him to cough and sneeze into tissues and to dispose of the tissues properly. Stress the importance of washing his hands thoroughly in hot, soapy water after handling his own secretions. Also instruct him to wash his eating utensils separately in hot, soapy water.

Monitoring

○ Adverse reactions
○ Complications
○ Daily weight
○ Intake and output
○ Liver and kidney function tests
○ Visual acuity if taking ethambutol
○ Vital signs

Patient teaching

Be sure to cover:
○ the disorder, diagnosis, and treatment
○ prescribed drugs, dosages, administration, and possible adverse effects
○ when to consult the doctor
○ need for isolation
○ postural drainage and chest percussion
○ coughing and deep-breathing exercises
○ regular follow-up examinations
○ signs and symptoms of recurring TB
○ possible decreased hormonal contraceptive effectiveness while taking rifampin
○ need for a high-calorie, high-protein, balanced diet
○ TB prevention. (See *Preventing tuberculosis*.)

Discharge planning

○ Refer anyone exposed to an infected patient for testing and follow-up.
○ Refer the patient to a support group, such as the American Lung Association.
○ Refer the patient to a smoking-cessation program if indicated.

Vasculitis

Overview

Description

- Autoimmune disorder
- Includes many conditions characterized by blood vessel inflammation and necrosis
- Clinical effects reflect the vessels involved and tissue ischemia caused by obstructed blood flow

Pathophysiology

- Excessive amounts of circulating antigen trigger formation of soluble antigen-antibody complexes.
- The reticuloendothelial system can't clear these complexes effectively, and they're deposited in blood vessel walls.
- Increased vascular permeability from release of vasoactive amines by platelets and basophils enhances this deposition.
- Deposited complexes activate the complement cascade and cause chemotaxis of neutrophils, which release lysosomal enzymes.
- Vessel damage and necrosis develop.

Causes

- Several theories
  - Follows serious infectious disease and may be related to high doses of antibiotics
  - Formation of autoantibodies directed at the body's own cellular and extracellular proteins, which can activate inflammatory cells or cytotoxicity
  - Cell-mediated (T-cell) immune response
  - In atopic people, exposure to allergens

Prevalence

- Affects all ages (except mucocutaneous lymph node syndrome, which affects only children)

Complications

- Cerebrovascular accident
- Fibrous scarring of lung tissue
- Gastrointestinal bleeding
- Glomerulitis
- Intestinal obstruction
- Myocardial infarction
- Pericarditis
- Renal failure
- Renal hypertension
- Rupture of mesenteric aneurysm

Assessment

History

- A serious infectious disease treated with high-dose antibiotic therapy
- Varied findings based on blood vessels involved

Polyarteritis nodosa
- Abdominal pain
- Fever
- Headache
- Malaise
- Myalgias
- Weight loss

Physical assessment

Polyarteritis nodosa (depends on body system)
- Altered mental status and seizures (central nervous system)
- Arthritic changes (musculoskeletal)
- Hypertension (renal)
- Rash, purpura, nodules, and cutaneous infarcts (skin)
- Respiratory distress, peripheral edema, hepatomegaly, peripheral vasoconstriction (cardiovascular)

Test results

Diagnostic procedures
- Not all vasculitis disorders can be diagnosed definitively through specific tests. The most useful general diagnostic procedure is biopsy of the affected vessel.

Nursing diagnoses

- Acute pain
- Ineffective spontaneous ventilation
- Ineffective tissue perfusion: cardiopulmonary
- Risk for injury
- Situational low self-esteem

Key outcomes

The patient will:
- express feelings of increased comfort and decreased pain
- express positive feelings about self
- attain hemodynamic stability
- demonstrate adequate ventilation
- avoid complications.

Interventions

General

- Avoidance of antigenic drugs
- Avoidance of antigenic foods
- Avoidance of anti-inflammatory drugs and immunosuppressants
- Avoidance of offending environmental substances

Nursing

- Assess the patient for dry nasal mucosa. Instill nose drops to lubricate the mucosa and minimize crusting; irrigate nasal passages with warm normal saline solution.

- Keep the patient well hydrated with about 3 qt (3 L) of fluid daily.
- Make sure that a patient with decreased visual acuity has a safe environment.
- Regulate the room temperature to prevent additional vasoconstriction caused by cold.
- Provide emotional support to the patient and family.

Drug therapy
- Analgesics
- Antihypertensives
- Antineoplastics
- Corticosteroids
- Immunosuppressants

Monitoring
- Daily weight
- Gastrointestinal disturbances
- Intake and output
- Laboratory values, especially white blood cell count for leukopenia
- Neurologic status
- Renal function tests
- Signs and symptoms of organ involvement
- Vital signs

Patient teaching

Be sure to cover:
- the disorder, diagnosis, and treatment
- need to recognize adverse effects of drug therapy, watch for signs of bleeding, and report any of these findings to the doctor
- the importance of wearing warm clothes and gloves when going outside in cold weather.

Discharge planning

- Refer the patient to a smoking-cessation program if appropriate.

Vesicoureteral reflux

Overview

Description
- A genitourinary condition in which urine flows from the bladder back into the ureters and eventually into the renal pelvis or parenchyma
- Possible urinary tract infection (UTI) because the bladder empties poorly, which may lead to acute or chronic pyelonephritis with renal damage

Pathophysiology
- Incompetence of the ureterovesical junction and shortening of intravesical ureteral musculature allow backflow of urine into the ureter when the bladder contracts during voiding.

Causes
- Acquired diverticulum (from outlet obstruction)
- Congenital anomalies of the ureters or bladder
- Cystitis
- Flaccid neurogenic bladder
- High intravesical pressure from outlet obstruction
- Inadequate detrusor muscle buttress in the bladder from congenital paraureteral bladder diverticulum
- May be unknown

Prevalence

AGE AWARE Vesicoureteral reflux is most common during infancy in boys and during early childhood (ages 3 to 7) in girls.

- Primary vesicoureteral reflux from congenital anomaly: most common in females and rare in Blacks
- Occurs in up to 25% of asymptomatic siblings of children with diagnosed primary vesicoureteral reflux

Complications
- Renal impairment
- UTI

Assessment

History
- Burning on urination
- Urinary frequency and urgency
- With upper urinary tract involvement: high fever, chills, flank pain, vomiting, malaise

Physical assessment
- In infants, hematuria or strong-smelling urine
- Hard, thickened bladder (hard mass deep in the pelvis) if posterior urethral valves are causing an obstruction in male infants
- Signs and symptoms of UTI

- Dark, concentrated urine
- With upper urinary tract involvement: high fever, chills, flank pain, vomiting, and malaise

ALERT In children, fever, nonspecific abdominal pain, and diarrhea may be the only clinical effects. Rarely, children with minimal symptoms remain undiagnosed until puberty or later, when they begin to exhibit clear signs of renal impairment (anemia, hypertension, and lethargy).

Test results
Laboratory
- Bacterial count greater than 100,000/µl in clean-catch urine specimen
- Possibly white blood cells, red blood cells, and an increased pH in urine in the presence of infection.
- Specific gravity less than 1.010, showing an inability to concentrate urine
- Elevated creatinine levels (more than 1.2 mg/dl) in advanced renal dysfunction
- Elevated blood urea nitrogen levels (more than 18 mg/dl) in advanced renal dysfunction

Diagnostic procedures
- Cystoscopy, with instillation of a solution containing methylene blue or indigo carmine dye, may confirm the diagnosis.
- Excretory urography may show a dilated lower ureter, ureter visible for its entire length, hydronephrosis, calyceal distortion, and renal scarring.
- Voiding cystourethrography (fluoroscopic or radionuclide) identifies and determines the degree of reflux, shows when reflux occurs, and may pinpoint the cause.
- Nuclear cystography and renal ultrasound may detect reflux.
- Catheterization of the bladder after the patient voids determines the amount of residual urine.

Nursing diagnoses

- Risk for imbalanced fluid volume
- Risk for infection

Key outcomes
The patient will:
- return to normal urinary function
- remain free from infection
- develop no complications from this disorder
- maintain fluid volume balance.

Interventions

General
- Increased fluid intake
- Surgery
  - Vesicoureteral reimplantation for UTI that recurs despite adequate prophylactic antibiotic therapy

    − If a patient with bladder outlet obstruction in neurogenic bladder has renal dysfunction

Nursing

○ Encourage one of the parents to stay with children during all procedures.
○ Explain the procedures to the parents and to the child if he's old enough to understand.
○ Give prescribed drugs.
○ Make sure catheters are patent and draining well.
○ Maintain sterile technique during catheter care.

Drug therapy

○ Antibiotics

Monitoring

○ Comfort level
○ Intake and output
○ Serum creatinine level
○ Vital signs
○ White blood cell count

Patient teaching

Be sure to cover:
○ the disorder, diagnosis, and treatment
○ ensuring bladder emptying by double voiding (voiding once, waiting a few minutes, and trying again) each time the patient urinates
○ voiding every 2 to 3 hours whether or not the urge exists
○ recognizing and reporting recurring signs of UTI (painful, frequent, burning urination; foul-smelling urine)
○ the importance of completing the prescribed therapy or maintaining low-dose antibiotic prophylaxis.

Discharge planning

○ After surgery, close medical follow-up is needed even if symptoms haven't recurred.

Common fluid and electrolyte imbalances in pediatric patients

Imbalance	Causes	Signs and symptoms	Treatment
Hypovolemia (fluid volume deficit)	Dehydration, vomiting, diarrhea, decreased oral intake, and excessive fluid loss	Thirst, oliguria or anuria, dry mucous membranes, weight loss, sunken eyes, decreased tears, depressed fontanels (in infants), tachycardia, and altered level of consciousness	Oral rehydration (in mild to moderate dehydration), I.V. fluid administration (in severe dehydration), or electrolyte replacement
Hypernatremia (serum sodium level > 145 mEq/L [> 145 mmol/L])	Water loss in excess of sodium loss, diabetes insipidus (insufficient antidiuretic hormone [ADH] production or reduced response to ADH), insufficient water intake, diarrhea, vomiting, fever, renal disease, and hyperglycemia	Decreased skin turgor; tachycardia; flushed skin; intense thirst; dry, sticky mucous membranes; hoarseness; nausea; vomiting; decreased blood pressure; confusion; and seizures	Gradual replacement of water (in excess of sodium) or ADH replacement or vasopressin administration (for patients with diabetes insipidus)
Hyponatremia (serum sodium level < 138 mEq/L [< 138 mmol/L])	Syndrome of inappropriate antidiuretic hormone secretion, edema (from cardiac failure), hypotonic fluid replacement (for diarrhea), cystic fibrosis, malnutrition, fever, and excess sweating	Dehydration, dizziness, nausea, abdominal cramps, and apprehension	Sodium replacement, water restriction, diuretic administration, or fluid replacement (with ongoing fluid loss, such as with diarrhea)
Hyperkalemia (serum potassium level > 5 mEq/L [> 5 mmol/L])	Acute acidosis, hemolysis, rhabdomyolysis, renal failure, excessive administration of I.V. potassium supplement, and Addison's disease	Arrhythmias, weakness, paresthesia, electrocardiogram (ECG) changes (tall, tented T waves; ST-segment depression; prolonged PR interval and QRS complex; and absent P waves), nausea, vomiting, hoarseness, flushed skin, intense thirst, and dry, sticky mucous membranes	Dialysis (for renal failure), sodium polystyrene (Kayexalate) (to remove potassium via the gastrointestinal tract), I.V. calcium gluconate (antagonizes cardiac abnormalities), I.V. insulin or hypertonic dextrose solution (shifts potassium into the cells), bicarbonate (for acidosis), or restricted potassium intake
Hypokalemia (serum potassium level < 3.5 mEq/L [< 3.5 mmol/L	Vomiting, diarrhea, nasogastric suctioning, diuretic use, acute alkalosis, kidney disease, starvation, and malabsorption	Fatigue, muscle weakness, muscle cramping, paralysis, hyporeflexia, hypotension, tachycardia or bradycardia, apathy, drowsiness, irritability, decreased bowel motility, and ECG changes (flattened or inverted T waves, presence of U waves, and ST-segment depression)	Oral or I.V. potassium administration (I.V. infusions must be diluted and given slowly)

Common fluid and electrolyte imbalances in elderly patients

Imbalance	Causes	Signs and symptoms	Treatment
Hypervolemia (fluid volume excess)	Renal failure, heart failure, cirrhosis, increased oral or I.V. sodium intake, mental confusion, seizures, and coma	Edema, weight gain, jugular vein distention, crackles, shortness of breath, bounding pulse, elevated blood pressure, and increased central venous pressure	Diuretics, fluid restriction (< 1 quart [1 L]/day), or hemodialysis (for patients with renal failure)
Hypovolemia (fluid volume deficit)	Dehydration, vomiting, diarrhea, fever, polyuria, chronic kidney disease, diabetes mellitus, diuretic use, hot weather, and decreased oral intake secondary to anorexia, nausea, diminished thirst mechanism, or inadequate water intake (common in nursing-home patients)	Dry mucous membranes; oliguria or concentrated urine; anuria; postural hypotension; dizziness; weakness; confusion or altered mental status; possible severe hypotension, increased hemoglobin, hematocrit, blood urea nitrogen, and serum creatinine levels	Fluid administration (may be oral or I.V., depending on degree of deficit and patient's response; urine output of 30 to 50 ml/hour usually signals adequate renal perfusion)
Hypernatremia (serum sodium > 145 mEq/L [> 145 mmol/L])	Water deprivation, hypertonic tube feedings without adequate water replacement, diarrhea, and low body weight	Dry mucous membranes, restlessness, irritability, weakness, lethargy, hyperreflexia, seizures, hallucinations, and coma	Gradual infusion of hypotonic electrolyte solution or isotonic saline solution
Hyponatremia (serum sodium < 138 mEq/L [< 138 mmol/L])	Diuretics, loss of gastrointestinal (GI) fluids, kidney disease, excessive water intake, and excessive I.V. fluids or parenteral feedings	Nausea and vomiting, lethargy, confusion, muscle cramps, diarrhea, delirium, weakness, seizures, coma	Gradual sodium replacement, water restriction (1 to 1.5 L/day), or discontinuation of diuretic therapy (if ordered)
Hyperkalemia (serum potassium > 5 mEq/L [> 5 mmol/L])	Renal failure, impaired tubular function, potassium-conserving diuretic use (in patients with renal insufficiency), rapid I.V. potassium administration, metabolic acidosis, and diabetic ketoacidosis	Arrhythmias, weakness, paresthesias, electrocardiogram (ECG) changes (tall, tented T waves; ST-segment depression; prolonged PR interval and QRS complex; shortened QT interval, absent P waves)	Dialysis (for patients with renal failure), sodium polystyrene (Kayexalate) (to remove potassium via the GI tract), I.V. calcium gluconate (antagonizes cardiac abnormalities), I.V. insulin or hypertonic dextrose solution (shifts potassium into the cells), bicarbonate (for patients with acidosis), or potassium intake restriction
Hypokalemia (serum potassium < 3.5 mEq/L [< 3.5 mmol/L])	Vomiting, diarrhea, nasogastric suction, diuretic use, digoxin toxicity, and decreased potassium intake	Fatigue, weakness, confusion, muscle cramps, decreased bowel motility, ECG changes (flattened T waves, presence of U waves, ST-segment depression, prolonged PR interval), ventricular tachycardia or fibrillation	Oral or I.V. potassium administration (I.V. infusions must be diluted and given slowly)

NANDA taxonomy II codes

The taxonomy listed below represents the currently accepted classification system for nursing diagnoses. Six new nursing diagnoses have been approved for 2005: energy field disturbance, impaired religiosity, readiness for enhanced religiosity, risk for dysfunctional grieving, risk for impaired religiosity, and sedentary lifestyle.

Nursing diagnosis	Taxonomy II code	Nursing diagnosis	Taxonomy II code
Imbalanced nutrition: More than body requirements	00001	Urinary retention	00023
Imbalanced nutrition: Less than body requirements	00002	Ineffective tissue perfusion (specify type: renal, cerebral, cardiopulmonary, gastrointestinal, peripheral)	00024
Risk for imbalanced nutrition: More than body requirements	00003	Risk for imbalanced fluid volume	00025
Risk for infection	00004	Excess fluid volume	00026
Risk for imbalanced body temperature	00005	Deficient fluid volume	00027
Hypothermia	00006	Risk for deficient fluid volume	00028
Hyperthermia	00007	Decreased cardiac output	00029
Ineffective thermoregulation	00008	Impaired gas exchange	00030
Autonomic dysreflexia	00009	Ineffective airway clearance	00031
Risk for autonomic dysreflexia	00010	Ineffective breathing pattern	00032
Constipation	00011	Impaired spontaneous ventilation	00033
Perceived constipation	00012	Dysfunctional ventilatory weaning response	00034
Diarrhea	00013	Risk for injury	00035
Bowel incontinence	00014	Risk for suffocation	00036
Risk for constipation	00015	Risk for poisoning	00037
Impaired urinary elimination	00016	Risk for trauma	00038
Stress urinary incontinence	00017	Risk for aspiration	00039
Reflex urinary incontinence	00018	Risk for disuse syndrome	00040
Urge urinary incontinence	00019	Latex allergy response	00041
Functional urinary incontinence	00020	Risk for latex allergy response	00042
Total urinary incontinence	00021	Ineffective protection	00043
Risk for urge urinary incontinence	00022	Impaired tissue integrity	00044
		Impaired oral mucous membrane	00045

Nursing diagnosis	Taxonomy II code	Nursing diagnosis	Taxonomy II code
Impaired skin integrity	00046	Ineffective community therapeutic regimen management	00081
Risk for impaired skin integrity	00047		
Impaired dentition	00048	Effective therapeutic regimen management	00082
Decreased intracranial adaptive capacity	00049	Decisional conflict (specify)	00083
Disturbed energy field	00050	Health-seeking behaviors (specify)	00084
Impaired verbal communication	00051	Impaired physical mobility	00085
Impaired social interaction	00052	Risk for peripheral neurovascular dysfunction	00086
Social isolation	00053		
Risk for loneliness	00054	Risk for perioperative-positioning injury	00087
Ineffective role performance	00055	Impaired walking	00088
Impaired parenting	00056	Impaired wheelchair mobility	00089
Risk for impaired parenting	00057	Impaired transfer ability	00090
Risk for impaired parent/infant/child attachment	00058	Impaired bed mobility	00091
		Activity intolerance	00092
Sexual dysfunction	00059	Fatigue	00093
Interrupted family processes	00060	Risk for activity intolerance	00094
Caregiver role strain	00061	Disturbed sleep pattern	00095
Risk for caregiver role strain	00062	Sleep deprivation	00096
Dysfunctional family processes: Alcoholism	00063	Deficient diversional activity	00097
Parental role conflict	00064	Impaired home maintenance	00098
Ineffective sexuality patterns	00065	Ineffective health maintenance	00099
Spiritual distress	00066	Delayed surgical recovery	00100
Risk for spiritual distress	00067	Adult failure to thrive	00101
Readiness for enhanced spiritual well-being	00068	Feeding self-care deficit	00102
Ineffective coping	00069	Impaired swallowing	00103
Impaired adjustment	00070	Ineffective breast-feeding	00104
Defensive coping	00071	Interrupted breast-feeding	00150
Ineffective denial	00072	Effective breast-feeding	00106
Disabled family coping	00073	Ineffective infant feeding pattern	00107
Compromised family coping	00074	Bathing or hygiene self-care deficit	00108
Readiness for enhanced family coping	00075	Dressing or grooming self-care deficit	00109
Readiness for enhanced community coping	00076	Toileting self-care deficit	00110
Ineffective community coping	00077	Delayed growth and development	00111
Ineffective therapeutic regimen management	00078	Risk for delayed development	00112
Noncompliance (specify)	00079	Risk for disproportionate growth	00113
Ineffective family therapeutic regimen management	00080	Relocation stress syndrome	00114
		Risk for disorganized infant behavior	00115
		Disorganized infant behavior	00116

Nursing diagnosis	Taxonomy II code	Nursing diagnosis	Taxonomy II code
Readiness for enhanced organized infant behavior	00117	Risk for powerlessness	00152
		Risk for situational low self-esteem	00153
Disturbed body image	00118	Wandering	00154
Chronic low self-esteem	00119	Risk for falls	00155
Situational low self-esteem	00120	Risk for sudden infant death syndrome	00156
Disturbed personal identity	00121	Readiness for enhanced communication	00157
Disturbed sensory perception (specify: visual, auditory, kinesthetic, gustatory, tactile, olfactory)	00122	Readiness for enhanced coping	00158
		Readiness for enhanced family processes	00159
Unilateral neglect	00123	Readiness for enhanced fluid balance	00160
Hopelessness	00124	Readiness for enhanced knowledge (specify)	00161
Powerlessness	00125	Readiness for enhanced management of therapeutic regimen	00162
Deficient knowledge (specify)	00126		
Impaired environmental interpretation syndrome	00127	Readiness for enhanced nutrition	00163
		Readiness for enhanced parenting	00164
Acute confusion	00128	Readiness for enhanced sleep	00165
Chronic confusion	00129	Readiness for enhanced urinary elimination	00166
Disturbed thought processes	00130	Readiness for enhanced self-concept	00167
Impaired memory	00131		
Acute pain	00132		
Chronic pain	00133		
Nausea	00134		
Dysfunctional grieving	00135		
Anticipatory grieving	00136		
Chronic sorrow	00137		
Risk for other-directed violence	00138		
Risk for self-mutilation	00139		
Risk for self-directed violence	00140		
Posttrauma syndrome	00141		
Rape-trauma syndrome	00142		
Rape-trauma syndrome: Compound reaction	00143		
Rape-trauma syndrome: Silent reaction	00144		
Risk for posttrauma syndrome	00145		
Anxiety	00146		
Death anxiety	00147		
Fear	00148		
Risk for relocation stress syndrome	00149		
Risk for suicide	00150		
Self-mutilation	00151		

Herbs that affect fluids and electrolytes

Aloe

Reported uses

- For burns, insect bites, and scrapes
- For promotion of wound healing
- For analgesic, anti-inflammatory, and antipruritic effects
- For emollient effects
- For cathartic, laxative effects

Nursing considerations

- Laxative effects occur within 16 hours of ingestion.

✳ *AGE AWARE If the patient ingests aloe, watch for signs of dehydration, especially if the patient is elderly.*

- Monitor electrolyte levels, especially potassium, after long-term use.
- Monitor wound healing with topical use.

Patient teaching

- Urge the patient to consult a health care provider if he takes prescribed drugs, especially digoxin, diuretics, or corticosteroids.

Angelica

Reported uses

- For diuretic effects
- For kidney, urinary, gastrointestinal, and respiratory tract conditions
- For rheumatic and arthritic symptoms

Nursing considerations

- Monitor the patient for persistent diarrhea.
- Assess the patient for dermatologic reactions.
- Photodermatosis is possible after contact with the plant juice or extract.

Patient teaching

- Urge the patient to consult a health care provider, particularly if the patient is pregnant or takes a gastric acid blocker or anticoagulant.
- Advise the patient to seek medical treatment if a rash develops.

Cranberry

Reported uses

- For urinary tract infection (UTI)
- For renal calculi
- For asthma
- For fever

Nursing considerations

- Tinctures may contain up to 45% alcohol.
- Cranberry is safe for use in pregnancy and by breast-feeding patients.
- When used regularly, it may reduce the frequency of bacteriuria with pyuria in women with recurrent UTI.

Patient teaching

- Advise the use of appropriate antibiotics to treat UTI.
- Warn diabetics that cranberry juice contains sugar and that sugar-free cranberry juice or supplements are available.
- Explain that the unsweetened, unprocessed form of cranberry juice is effective in preventing bacteria from adhering to the bladder wall.

Green tea

Reported uses

- For prevention of cancer, hyperlipidemia, atherosclerosis, dental caries, and headaches
- For treatment of wounds, skin disorders, stomach disorders, and infectious diarrhea
- For central nervous system stimulant, mild diuretic, antibacterial, and topical astringent effects

Nursing considerations

○ Daily consumption should be less than 5 cups or the equivalent of 300 mg of caffeine.
○ Adverse effects of chlorogenic acid and tannins can be avoided by adding milk to tea.
○ The first signs of toxic reaction are vomiting and abdominal cramps.

Patient teaching

○ Warn the patient about toxic reactions.
○ Explain that heavy consumption may increase the risk of esophageal cancer.
○ Caution that green tea interferes with absorption of iron supplements.

Horse chestnut

Reported uses

○ For chronic venous insufficiency, varicose veins, phlebitis, leg pain, tiredness, tension, and leg swelling
○ For lymphedema, hemorrhoids, and enlarged prostate
○ For analgesic, anticoagulant, antipyretic, astringent, expectorant, and tonic effects
○ For skin ulcers, cough, and diarrhea

Nursing considerations

▼ **ALERT** *The roots, seeds, twigs, sprouts, and leaves of horse chestnut are poisonous and can be lethal.*

○ Signs and symptoms of toxicity include loss of coordination, salivation, hemolysis, headache, seizures, vomiting, diarrhea, dilated pupils, muscle twitching, depression, paralysis, respiratory and cardiac failure, and death.

Patient teaching

○ Explain that this herb is classified by the Food and Drug Administration as unsafe.

✳ **AGE AWARE** *Warn that, in a child, consumption of leaves, twigs, and seeds equaling 1% of body weight may be lethal.*

Kava

Reported uses

○ For anxiety, stress, and restlessness
○ For wound healing, headaches, seizure disorders, upper respiratory tract infection, tuberculosis and rheumatism, and skin disease
○ For urogenital infection, menstrual problems, and vaginal prolapse
○ For intestinal problems, otitis, and abscesses

Nursing considerations

○ Periodically monitor the patient's liver function tests and complete blood count.
○ Toxic amounts can cause progressive ataxia, muscle weakness, and ascending paralysis.

▼ **ALERT** *The Food and Drug Administration has reported a link between kava and such liver problems as cirrhosis, hepatitis, and liver failure.*

Patient teaching

○ Caution that this herb may be habit-forming if taken for longer than 3 months.
○ Explain that kava shouldn't be taken with sedative-hypnotics, psychotropic drugs, levodopa, or antiplatelet drugs.
○ Warn the patient to avoid alcohol while taking this herb.
○ Monitor the patient for evidence of liver disease.

Nettle

Reported uses

○ For allergic rhinitis, osteoarthritis, rheumatoid arthritis, renal calculi, asthma, and benign prostatic hyperplasia
○ For diuretic, expectorant, general health tonic, blood builder and purifier, pain reliever and anti-inflammatory effects
○ For lung tonic effects in ex-smokers
○ For eczema, hives, bursitis, tendinitis, laryngitis, sciatica, and premenstrual syndrome

Nursing considerations

○ This herb is reported to be an abortifacient and may affect the menstrual cycle.
○ Allergic adverse reactions from internal use are uncommon.

Patient teaching

○ Recommend caution if the patient takes an antihypertensive or antidiabetic.
○ Warn the patient that skin contact may cause adverse reactions, such as burning and stinging, that may last 12 hours or longer.
○ Explain that capsules and extracts should be stored at room temperature, protected from heat and direct light.
○ Instruct women taking this herb to report planned, suspected, or known pregnancy.
○ Advise patients not to breast-feed while taking this herb.

Saw palmetto

Reported uses

○ For symptoms of benign prostatic hyperplasia, cough, and congestion

○ For mild diuretic, urinary antiseptic, and astringent effects

Nursing considerations

○ If the patient takes saw palmetto for benign prostatic hyperplasia, obtain a baseline prostate-specific antigen value because the herb may cause a false-negative test result.
○ Laboratory values didn't change significantly in clinical trials of people taking 160 mg to 320 mg daily.

Patient teaching

○ Urge the patient to seek medical advice before taking saw palmetto for prostate or bladder symptoms.
○ Tell the patient to take this herb with food to minimize gastrointestinal effects.
○ Caution the patient to avoid this herb if pregnant, planning a pregnancy, or breast-feeding.

St. John's wort

Reported uses

○ For moderate depression, anxiety, sciatica, and viral infections
○ For bronchitis, asthma, gallbladder disease, nocturnal enuresis, gout, and rheumatism

Nursing considerations

▼ **ALERT** *If symptoms of depression continue after 6 weeks of taking St. John's wort, a different therapy should be considered.*

○ Monitor the patient's response to this herb.
○ St. John's wort decreases the effects of certain prescribed drugs and may increase the risk of toxicity if the herb is stopped abruptly.

Patient teaching

○ Advise the patient to avoid this herb if planning pregnancy (both men and women).
○ Explain that St. John's wort may cause increased sensitivity to direct sunlight.

Selected references

Alexander, M., and Corrigan, A.M. *Core Curriculum for Infusion Nursing,* 3rd ed. Philadelphia: Lippincott Williams & Wilkins, 2003.

Allison, S.P. and Lobo, D.N. "Fluid and Electrolytes in the Elderly," *Current Opinion in Clinical Nutrition and Metabolic Care* 7(1):27–38, January 2004.

Amoore, J., and Adamson, L. "Infusion Devices: Characteristics, Limitations and Risk Management," *Nursing Standard* 17(28):45–52, March–April 2003.

Becker, K.L., et al. *Principles and Practice of Endocrinology and Metabolism,* 3rd ed. Philadelphia: Lippincott Williams & Wilkins, 2003.

Bockenkamp, B., and Vyas, H. "Understanding and Managing Acute Fluid and Electrolyte Disturbances," *Current Practices* 13(7):520–28, 2003.

Braunwald, E., et al. *Harrison's Principles of Internal Medicine,* 15th ed. New York: McGraw-Hill Book Co., 2001.

Cartotto, R., et al. "A Prospective Study on the Implications of a Base Deficit During Fluid Resuscitation," *Journal of Burn Care and Rehabilitation* 24(2):75–84, March–April 2003.

Cohen, M.R. "Medication Errors. I.V. Fluid Evaporation: Working Up A Sweat," *Nursing2002* 32(10):14, October 2002.

Cook, L.S. "I.V. Fluid Resuscitation," *Journal of Infusion Nursing* 26(5):296–303, September–October 2003.

Critical Care Challenges: Disorders, Treatments, and Procedures. Philadelphia: Lippincott Williams & Wilkins, 2003.

Critical Care Nursing Made Incredibly Easy! Philadelphia: Lippincott Williams & Wilkins, 2004.

Davidhizar, R., Dunn, C.L., and Hart, A.N. "A Review of the Literature on How Important Water Is to The World's Elderly Population," *International Nursing Review* 51(3):159–66, September 2004.

Dudek, S.G. *Nutrition Essentials for Nursing Practice,* 5th ed. Philadelphia: Lippincott Williams & Wilkins, 2005.

Eaton, J. "Detection of Hyponatremia in the PACU," *Journal of Perianesthesia Nursing* 18(6):392–7, December 2003.

Fluid and Electrolytes Made Incredibly Easy!, 3rd ed. Philadelphia: Lippincott Williams & Wilkins, 2005.

Ford, N.A., Drott, H.R., and Cieplinski-Robertson, J.A. "Administration of I.V. Medications Via Soluset," *Pediatric Nursing* 29(4):283–6, 319, July–August 2003.

Hadaway, L.C. "Delivering Multiple Medications via Backpriming," *Nursing2004* 34(3):24, 26, March 2004.

Hadaway, L.C. "Infusing Without Infecting," *Nursing2003* 33(10):58–63, October 2003.

Heitz, U., and Horne, M.M. *Pocket Guide to Fluid, Electrolyte, and Acid-Base Balance,* 5th ed. St. Louis: Mosby, Inc., 2005.

Ignatavicius, D.D., and Workman, M.L. *Medical-Surgical Nursing: Critical Thinking for Collaborative Care,* 4th ed. Philadelphia: W.B. Saunders, 2002.

Infusion Nurses Society, Alexander, M., and Corrigan, A.M. *Core Curriculum for Infusion Nursing,* 3rd ed. Philadelphia: Lippincott Williams & Wilkins, 2003.

I.V. Therapy Made Incredibly Easy!, 3rd ed. Springhouse, Pa.: Lippincott Williams & Wilkins, 2005.

Johnson, R.J., and Feehally, J. *Comprehensive Clinical Nephrology,* 2nd ed. St. Louis: Mosby–Year Book, 2003.

Just the Facts: Fluids and Electrolytes. Springhouse, Pa.: Lippincott Williams & Wilkins, 2004.

Khanna, A., and Kurtzman, N.A. "Metabolic Alkalosis." *Respiratory Care* 46(4):354–65, April 2001.

LeFever Kee, J., Paulanka, B.J., and Purnell, L. *Handbook of Fluid, Electrolytes, and Acid-Base Imbalances,* 2nd ed. Clifton Park, N.Y.: Delmar Publishers, 2004.

Mims, B.C. et al, *Critical Care Skills, 2nd Edition — A Clinical Handbook,* Philadelphia: W. B. Saunders, 2004.

Morgera, S., et al. "Renal Replacement Therapy with High-Cutoff Hemofilters: Impact of Convection and Diffusion on Cytokine Clearances and Protein Status." *American Journal of Kidney Disease* 43(3):444–53, 2004.

Nursing2005 Drug Handbook, 25th ed. Philadelphia: Lippincott Williams & Wilkins, 2004.

Potter, P.A., and Perry, A.G. *Fundamentals of Nursing,* 6th ed. St. Louis: Mosby, Inc., 2005.

Puglise, K. "Test Your Knowledge: Fluids and Electrolytes," *Journal of Infusion Nursing* 26(3):127–8, May–June 2003.

Schrier, R.W. *Manual of Nephrology: Diagnosis and Therapy,* 6th ed. Philadelphia: Lippincott Williams & Wilkins, 2004.

Schrier, R.W. *Renal and Electrolyte Disorders,* 6th ed. Philadelphia: Lippincott Williams & Wilkins, 2002.

Smeltzer, S., and Bare, B. *Brunner & Suddarth's Textbook of Medical-Surgical Nursing,* 10th ed. Philadelphia: Lippincott Williams & Wilkins, 2004.

Suhayda, R., and Walton, J.C. "Preventing and Managing Dehydration," *Medsurg Nursing* 11(6):267–78, December 2002.

Swartz, R, et al. "Improving the Delivery of Continuous Renal Replacement Therapy Using Regional Citrate Anticoagulation," *Clinical Nephrology* 61(2):134–43, 2004.

Teehan, G.S., et al. "Update on Dialytic Management of Acute Renal Failure," *Journal of Intensive Care Medicine* 18(3):130–38, 2003.

Trimble, T. "Peripheral I.V. Starts: Insertion Tips," *Nursing2003* 33(8):17, August 2003.

Trimble, T. "Peripheral I.V. Starts: Securing and Removing the Catheter," *Nursing2003* 33(9):26, September 2003.

Index

A

Abdominal aortic aneurysm, 64-65
Abdominal X-rays
  in abdominal aortic aneurysm, 64
  in cirrhosis, 100
  in pancreatitis, 206
  in peritonitis, 210
  in poisoning, 216
ABO blood group, 30, 31i
Acetate as total parenteral nutrition additive, 32
Acid-base balance, 26-27
  chloride regulation and, 24, 24i
  in diabetic ketoacidosis, 114
  effect of hyperkalemia on, 156t
  regulatory systems for, 26-27
  role of potassium in, 14i, 15
Acidosis. *See also* Metabolic acidosis *and* Respiratory acidosis.
  pH level and, 26
  potassium balance and, 14i, 15
Acids, 26
Activated partial thromboplastin time in disseminated intravascular coagulation, 116
Active transport, fluid movement and, 4, 5i
Acute glomerulonephritis, 44-45
Acute hematopoietic radiation toxicity, 232
Acute infective tubulointerstitial nephritis, 46-47
Acute poststreptococcal glomerulonephritis, 44-45
Acute pyelonephritis, 46-47
Acute renal failure, 238-239
  classifying, 238
  phases of, 238
Acute respiratory distress syndrome, 48-49
  stages of, 48
Acute respiratory failure, 50-51
Acute tubular necrosis, 52-53
  preventing, 239
Acute tubulointerstitial nephritis, 52-53
Addisonian crisis, 54
Addison's disease, 54-55
Adenosine triphosphate, active transport and, 4, 5i
ADH. *See* Antidiuretic hormone.
Adrenal crisis, 54
Adrenal hormone level in Sheehan's syndrome, 260
Adrenal hypofunction, 54-55

Adrenal virilism, 56-57
Adrenocorticotropic hormone level in Cushing's syndrome, 104
Adrenogenital syndrome, 56-57
Adult respiratory distress syndrome, 48-49
Age as factor
  in Addison's disease diagnosis, 54
  in adrenal hypofunction, 56
  in aloe ingestion, 291
  in Alport's syndrome, 58
  in anorexia nervosa, 70
  in aortic stenosis, 74
  in bulimia, 88
  in congenital adrenal hyperplasia, 56
  in Cushing's syndrome, 104
  in cystic fibrosis, 106
  in cystinuria, 108
  in diabetes insipidus, 110
  in diabetes mellitus, 112
  in diabetic ketoacidosis, 114
  in dialysis, 241
  in electrolyte levels, 22-23, 182
  in Fanconi's syndrome, 124
  in fluid distribution, 3
  in fluid loss, 6
  in hemolytic uremic syndrome, 144
  in hypervolemia, 10
  in hypochloremia, 172
  in hypoparathyroidism, 180
  in kidney cancer, 184
  in liver failure, 188
  in lung cancer, 190
  in magnesium levels, 18
  in medullary sponge kidney, 192
  in metabolic alkalosis, 196
  in myasthenia gravis, 200
  in near drowning, 202
  in nephrotic syndrome, 204
  in pericarditis, 208
  in pheochromocytoma, 212
  in poisoning, 216
  in pregnancy-induced hypertension, 222
  in psychogenic polydipsia, 226
  in rapidly progressing glomerulonephritis, 234
  in regulating acid-base balance, 27

i refers to an illustration; t refers to a table.

i refers to an illustration; t refers to a table.

i refers to an illustration; t refers to a table.

i refers to an illustration; t refers to a table.

i refers to an illustration; t refers to a table.

Diabetic ketoacidosis, 114-115
  distinguishing, from hyperosmolar hyperglycemic
    nonketotic syndrome, 163i
Dialysis. *See* Hemodialysis *and* Peritoneal dialysis.
DIC, 116-117
Diffusion, fluid movement and, 4, 4i
Dilated cardiomyopathy, 92-93
  assessment findings in, 93t
  pathophysiology of, 92i
Disseminated intravascular coagulation, 116-117
Diuretics, chloride deficiency and, 24

E

Echocardiography
  in abdominal aortic aneurysm, 64
  in aortic insufficiency, 72
  in aortic stenosis, 74
  in cardiogenic shock, 262
  in cardiomyopathy, 92, 94
  in pericarditis, 208
  in thoracic aortic aneurysm, 66
  in ventricular aneurysm, 68
Eclampsia, 222-223
Edema, evaluating, 10i
Elderly patients, fluid and electrolyte imbalances in, 287t
Electric shock, 118-119
  classifying, 118
Electrocardiography
  in acute renal failure, 239
  in acute respiratory failure, 50
  in acute tubular necrosis, 52
  in anorexia nervosa, 71
  in aortic insufficiency, 72
  in aortic stenosis, 74
  in burns, 90
  in cardiogenic shock, 262
  in chronic bronchitis, 86
  in diabetic ketoacidosis, 114
  in electric shock, 118
  in emphysema, 120
  in heart failure, 140
  in hypercalcemia, 152
  in hyperkalemia, 156
  in hypermagnesemia, 158
  in hypertension, 169
  in hypokalemia, 174
  in hypomagnesemia, 176
  in hypoparathyroidism, 180
  in metabolic acidosis, 194
  in metabolic alkalosis, 196
  in near drowning, 202
  in pericarditis, 208
  in poisoning, 216
  in pulmonary edema, 228
  in pulmonary embolism, 230

Electrocardiography *(continued)*
  in respiratory alkalosis, 248
  in rhabdomyolysis, 255
  in sarcoidosis, 258
  in septic shock, 266
  in thyrotoxicosis, 275
  in ventricular aneurysm, 68
Electroencephalography in chronic renal failure, 240
Electrolyte levels
  in acute poststreptococcal glomerulonephritis, 44
  in acute renal failure, 238
  in acute respiratory failure, 50
  in acute tubular necrosis, 52
  in adrenal hypofunction, 55
  in anorexia nervosa, 70
  in bulimina nervosa, 89
  in burns, 90
  in chronic glomerulonephritis, 98
  in chronic renal failure, 240
  in cirrhosis, 100
  in Crohn's disease, 102
  in Cushing's syndrome, 104
  in cystic fibrosis, 107
  in diabetes insipidus, 110
  in diabetic ketoacidosis, 114
  in Fanconi's syndrome, 124
  in heat syndrome, 142, 143
  in hepatorenal syndrome, 146
  in hyperaldosteronism, 150
  in hyperosmolar hyperglycemic nonketotic
    syndrome, 162
  in hyperparathyroidism, 164
  in hypertension, 168
  in hypomagnesemia, 176
  in hypoparathyroidism, 180
  in hypovolemic shock, 264
  in kidney cancer, 184
  in Legionnaires' disease, 186
  in liver failure, 188
  in metabolic acidosis, 194
  in metabolic alkalosis, 196
  in near drowning, 202
  in pancreatitis, 206
  in poisoning, 216
  in psychogenic polydipsia, 226
  in radiation exposure, 232
  in rapidly progressing glomerulonephritis, 234
  in renal tubular acidosis, 242
  in rhabdomyolysis, 254
  in septic shock, 266
  in syndrome of inappropriate antidiuretic hormone
    secretion, 272
  in toxic shock syndrome, 276

i refers to an illustration; t refers to a table.

Electrolytes. *See also* Electrolyte levels *and specific*
     electrolyte.
   charges and, 12
   extracellular, 12-13, 12i
   intracellular, 12i, 13
   measurement of, 13
   movement and balance of, 13
   as component of total parenteral nutrition solution, 32
Electromyography in Guillain-Barré syndrome, 138
Electroneutrality, 12
Electron microscopy
   in Alport's syndrome, 58
   in amyloidosis, 60
Emphysema, 120-121
   pathophysiology of, 120, 121i
Empyema, 214-215
Endoscopic retrograde cholangiopancreatography in
     pancreatitis, 206
Enterocolitis, 256-257
Epidemic cholera, 96-97
Erythrocyte sedimentation rate
   in acute pyelonephritis, 46
   in anorexia nervosa, 70
   in Crohn's disease, 102
   in Legionnaires' disease, 186
   in multiple myeloma, 198
   in pericarditis, 208
   in sickle cell anemia, 269
Esophageal cancer, 122-123
Esophageal X-rays in esophageal cancer, 122
Esophagogastroduodenoscopy in cirrhosis, 101
Esophagoscopy in esophageal cancer, 122
Evans formula for fluid replacement, 91
Excretory urography
   in acute pyelonephritis, 46
   in chronic renal failure, 240
   in cystinuria, 108
   in hypertension, 169
   in medullary sponge kidney, 192
   in polycystic kidney disease, 220
   in renal calculi, 236
   in renal vein thrombosis, 244
   in vesicoureteral reflux, 282
Extracellular fluid, 3, 3i
Exudative effusion, 214

F

Factor VIII, 31
Fanconi's syndrome, 124-125
Fecal occult blood test
   in Crohn's disease, 102
   in gastritis, 128
Femoral vein catheterization, vascular access and, 34i
Fibrin degradation products, level of
   in acute poststreptococcal glomerulonephritis, 44
   in disseminated intravascular coagulation, 116

Fibrinogen level
   in blood transfusion reaction, 84
   in disseminated intravascular coagulation, 116
Fluid
   daily intake and output of, 6, 6i
   distribution of, 2-3, 3i
     age as factor in, 3
   movement of, 4-5, 4i, 5i
   types of, 2, 2i, 28-29, 28i
Fluid and electrolyte imbalances, disorders related
     to, 44-283
Fluid and electrolyte replacement, 28-29
   after burn, 91
Fluid balance, 6-7, 6i, 7i
   sodium regulation and, 16, 16i
Fluid loss, types of, 6, 6i
Fluid shifts, 2, 5
Focal glomerulosclerosis, 204
Food poisoning, 130-131
Fresh frozen plasma, 30-31

G

Gallium scan in dilated cardiomyopathy, 92
Gastric acid stimulation test in gastric cancer, 126
Gastric cancer, 126-127
   classifying, 126
Gastritis, 128-129
Gastroenteritis, 130-131
Gastrointestinal effects
   of hypercalcemia, 153t
   of hyperkalemia, 156t
   of hypernatremia, 161t
Gastrointestinal radiation toxicity, 232
Gastrointestinal system
   chloride balance and, 24
   magnesium balance and, 18
   phosphorus balance and, 22
Gastroscopy in gastric cancer, 126
Genitourinary effects
   of hyperkalemia, 156t
   of hypernatremia, 161t
Glomerular filtration rate, 6
   in hydronephrosis, 148
Glomerulonephritis
   acute poststreptococcal, 44-45
   chronic, 98-99
   membranoproliferative, 204
   rapidly progressing, 234-235
Glucose level
   in adrenal hypofunction, 55
   in anorexia nervosa, 70
   in burns, 90
   in chronic renal failure, 240
   in Cushing's syndrome, 104
   in diabetes mellitus, 112-113
   in diabetic ketoacidosis, 114

i refers to an illustration; t refers to a table.

i refers to an illustration; t refers to a table.

i refers to an illustration; t refers to a table.

Liver enzyme levels. *See also specific enzyme.*
  in cardiogenic shock, 262
  in cystic fibrosis, 107
  in liver failure, 188
Liver failure, 188-189
Liver function studies in gastric cancer, 126
Liver scan in cirrhosis, 100
Liver transplant rejection, assessment findings in, 136
Lung biopsy in Goodpasture's syndrome, 132
Lung cancer, 190-191
  types of, 190

M
Macronodular cirrhosis, 100-101
Magnesium, 18-19
  balance of, 18
  deficiency of, 176-177
  dietary sources of, 18-19
  excess of, 158-159
  functions of, 18
  measurement of, 18
  normal levels of, 18
  recommended daily requirement for, 18-19
  relationship of, to albumin levels, 18
Magnetic resonance imaging
  in Cushing's syndrome, 104
  in esophageal cancer, 122
  in pericarditis, 208
  in pheochromocytoma, 212
  in polycystic kidney disease, 220
  in thoracic aortic aneurysm, 66
  in tuberculosis, 278
Malignant hypertension, 168
Malignant plasmacytoma, 198-199
Medullary sponge kidney, 192-193
Membranoproliferative glomerulonephritis, 204
Mesothelioma, 76-77
Metabolic acidosis, 194-195. *See also* Acidosis.
  anion gap and, 154
  as hyperkalemia complication, 156
Metabolic alkalosis, 196-197. *See also* Alkalosis.
  hypochloremia and, 172i
Micronodular cirrhosis, 100-101
Micronutrients as total parenteral nutrition additives, 32
Multinodular goiter, 274i
Multiple myeloma, 198-199
Murmur
  in aortic insufficiency, 72, 73i
  in aortic stenosis, 74, 75i
Muscular aortic stenosis, 94-95
Musculoskeletal effects
  of hypercalcemia, 153t
  of hyperkalemia, 156t
  of hypernatremia, 161t
Myasthenia gravis, 200-201
Myelomatosis, 198-199

N
NANDA taxonomy II codes, 288-290t
Native arteriovenous fistula, vascular access and, 34i
Near drowning, 202-203
  dry vs. wet, 202
Nephrocarcinoma, 184-185
Nephron, 6, 7i
Nephrotic syndrome, 204-205
  pathophysiology of, 204, 204i
Nerve conduction studies in Guillain-Barré syndrome, 138
Nettle, effect of, on fluids and electrolytes, 292
Neurologic effects
  of hypercalcemia, 153t
  of hyperkalemia, 156t
  of hypermagnesemia, 158t
  of hypernatremia, 161t
  of hypomagnesemia, 18t
Neuromuscular effects
  of hypermagnesemia, 158t
  of hypomagnesemia, 18t
Normal saline solution, 2, 28, 28i

O
Ophthalmoscopy
  in hypertension, 169
  in pregnancy-induced hypertension, 222
Organ rejection. *See* Graft rejection syndrome.
Osmosis, fluid movement and, 4, 4i

PQ
Packed red blood cells, 30
Pancreatitis, 206-207
Paracentesis in peritonitis, 210
Parathyroid hormone
  calcium balance and, 20
  deficient secretion of, 180-181
  phosphorus balance and, 22, 22i
Paratyphoid fever, 256-257
Parkland formula for fluid replacement, 91
Partial thromboplastin time in septic shock, 266
Passive transport, fluid movement and, 4, 4i
Patellar reflex, testing, 159i
Pediatric patients, fluid and electrolyte imbalances in, 286t
Perfluorocarbons, 30
Pericarditis, 208-209
Peritoneal dialysis
  contraindications and cautions for, 38
  documenting, 39
  equipment for, 38
  essential steps in, 38-39
  indications for, 38
  patient teaching for, 39
  setup for, 39i
  special considerations for, 39
Peritonitis, 210-211

i refers to an illustration; t refers to a table.

i refers to an illustration; t refers to a table.

Renal buffers, acid-base imbalances and, 27
Renal calculi, 236-237
Renal carcinoma, 184-185
Renal failure
    acute, 238-239
    chronic, 240-241
Renal system
    chloride balance and, 24
    fluid balance and, 6, 7i
    magnesium balance and, 18
    phosphorus balance and, 22
    potassium regulation and, 14
Renal tubular acidosis, 242-243
Renal vein thrombosis, 244-245
Renin-angiotensin-aldosterone system, fluid balance
    and, 7
Respiratory acidosis, 246-247. *See also* Acidosis.
Respiratory alkalosis, 248-249. *See also* Alkalosis.
Respiratory buffers, acid-base imbalances and, 26-27
Respiratory distress syndrome, 250-251
Respiratory effects of hypernatremia, 161t
Respiratory syncytial virus infection, 252-253
Reticulocyte count in hemolytic uremic syndrome, 144
Retrograde urography in polycystic kidney disease, 220
Rhabdomyolysis, 254-255
Rh factor, 30, 84
    sensitization to, 84
$Rh_o(D)$ immune globulin, Rh sensitization and, 84
Ringer's solution, 28

S

Salmonella infection, 256-257
    preventing, 257
Salt-losing congenital adrenal hyperplasia, 56-57
Sarcoidosis, 258-259
Saw palmetto, effect of, on fluids and electrolytes, 292-293
Sensible fluid loss, 6, 6i
Septic shock, 266-267
Sheehan's syndrome, 260-261
Shock
    cardiogenic, 262-263
    hypovolemic, 264-265, 265i
    septic, 266-267
Shock lung, 48-49
SIADH, 272-273
Sickle cell anemia, 268-269
Sigmoidoscopy in Crohn's disease, 102
Silicosis, 270-271
Small bowel X-ray in Crohn's disease, 102
Sodium, 16-17. *See also* Sodium-potassium pump.
    balance of, 16-17, 16i, 17i
    deficiency of, 178-179
    dietary sources of, 17
    excess of, 160-161
    functions of, 16

Sodium *(continued)*
    measurement of, 16
    normal levels of, 16
    recommended daily requirement for, 17
Sodium-potassium pump, 4, 14, 17, 17i
Solute, 2
Spinal X-ray in near drowning, 202
Sputum culture
    in acute respiratory distress syndrome, 49
    in acute respiratory failure, 50
    in chronic bronchitis, 86
    in cystic fibrosis, 107
Stiff lung, 48-49
St. John's wort, effect of, on fluids and electrolytes, 293
Stool examination
    in cholera, 96
    in cystic fibrosis, 107
    in gastroenteritis, 130
    in salmonella infection, 256
Subclavian vein catheterization, vascular access and, 34i
Swan's neck deformity, 124
Sweat test in cystic fibrosis, 107
Syndrome of inappropriate antidiuretic hormone
    secretion, 272-273
Synovial fluid analysis in gout, 135

T

Tensilon test in myasthenia gravis, 200
Thallium scan in hypertrophic cardiomyopathy, 94
Thirst mechanism, fluid balance and, 7
Thoracic aortic aneurysm, 66-67
Thrombin time in disseminated intravascular
    coagulation, 116
Thyroid hormone level
    in anorexia nervosa, 70
    in Sheehan's syndrome, 260
    in thyrotoxicosis, 274
Thyroid-releasing hormone stimulation test in
    thyrotoxicosis, 274
Thyroid resin uptake in thyrotoxicosis, 274
Thyroid scan in thyrotoxicosis, 274-275
Thyroid-stimulating hormone level in thyrotoxicosis, 274
Thyroid storm, 274, 275
Thyrotoxicosis, 274-275
Total parenteral nutrition, 32-33
    adverse reactions to, 32-33
    lipid emulsions and, 32
    solution components for, 32
Toxicology tests
    in acute respiratory distress syndrome, 49
    in asphyxia, 78
    in respiratory alkalosis, 248
Toxic shock syndrome, 276-277
    diagnostic criteria for, 276
TPN. *See* Total parenteral nutrition.

i refers to an illustration; t refers to a table.

Transcellular fluid, 3
Transesophageal echocardiography in thoracic aortic
    aneurysm, 66
Transudative effusion, 214
Transvenous endomyocardial biopsy in dilated
    cardiomyopathy, 92
Traveler's diarrhea, 130-131
  preventing, 130
Triglyceride level
  in chronic renal failure, 240
  in nephrotic syndrome, 205
Troponin level in cardiogenic shock, 262
Trousseau's sign, eliciting, 170i
Tuberculin skin test
  in asthma, 81
  in pericarditis, 208
  in pleural effusion, 214
  in tuberculosis, 278
Tuberculosis, 278-279
  preventing, 279
Typhoid fever, 256-257

U

Ultrasonography
  in abdominal aortic aneurysm, 64
  in chronic glomerulonephritis, 98
  in Cushing's syndome, 104
  in esophageal cancer, 122
  in pancreatitis, 206
  in renal calculi, 236
Universal donors, 30
Universal recipients, 30
Upper gastrointestinal endoscopy in gastritis, 128
Urea breath test in gastritis, 128
Uric acid level
  in anorexia nervosa, 70
  in gout, 134
Urinalysis
  in acute poststreptococcal glomerulonephritis, 44
  in acute pyelonephritis, 46
  in acute renal failure, 238
  in acute tubular necrosis, 52
  in Alport's syndrome, 58
  in amyloidosis, 60
  in blood transfusion reaction, 84
  in burns, 90
  in chronic glomerulonephritis, 98
  in chronic renal failure, 240
  in Cushing's syndrome, 104
  in cystinuria, 108
  in diabetes insipidus, 110
  in diabetes mellitus, 113
  in diabetic ketoacidosis, 114
  in Goodpasture's syndrome, 132
  in heat syndrome, 143

Urinalysis *(continued)*
  in hemolytic uremic syndrome, 144
  in hepatorenal syndrome, 146
  in hydronephrosis, 148
  in hyperosmolar hyperglycemic nonketotic
    syndrome, 162
  in hypertension, 168
  in near drowning, 202
  in nephrotic syndrome, 205
  in polycystic kidney disease, 220
  in rapidly progressing glomerulonephritis, 234
  in renal vein thrombosis, 244
  in rhabdomyolysis, 254
  in vesicoureteral reflux, 282
Urine formation and excretion, 6, 7i
Urine specific gravity
  in acute pyelonephritis, 46
  in acute renal failure, 238
  in acute tubular necrosis, 52
  in chronic renal failure, 240
  in diabetes insipidus, 110
  in hyperosmolar hyperglycemic nonketotic
    syndrome, 162
  in hyponatremia, 178
  in hypovolemic shock, 264
  in psychogenic polydipsia, 226
  in renal calculi, 236
  in renal tubular acidosis, 242
  in septic shock, 266
  in vesicoureteral reflux, 282
Urine studies. *See also specific test.*
  in multiple myeloma, 198
  in pheochromocytoma, 212
  in pregnancy-induced hypertension, 222
  in psychogenic polydipsia, 226
  in renal calculi, 236
Urobilinogen level in cirrhosis, 100

V

Vasculitis, 280-281
Vasopressin. *See* Antidiuretic hormone.
Ventilation as factor in acid-base balance, 26-27
Ventilation perfusion scan in pulmonary embolism, 230
Ventricular aneurysm, 68-69
Ventriculography in ventricular aneurysm, 68
Vesicoureteral reflux, 282-283
Viral enteritis, 130-131
Vitamin D, calcium balance and, 20
Vitamin deficiency
  in cirrhosis, 100
  in Crohn's disease, 102
Vitamins as component of total parenteral nutrition
    solution, 32
Voiding cystourethrography in vesicoureteral reflux, 282

i refers to an illustration; t refers to a table.

W

Water deprivation test in psychogenic polydipsia, 226
Wet lung, 48-49
White blood cell count
  in acute pyelonephritis, 46
  in acute respiratory failure, 50
  in adrenal hypofunction, 55
  in anorexia nervosa, 70
  in asthma, 81
  in Crohn's disease, 102
  in cystinuria, 108
  in diabetic ketoacidosis, 114
  in empyema, 214
  in gout, 134
  in near drowning, 202
  in pancreatitis, 206
  in pericarditis, 208
  in radiation exposure, 232
  in sickle cell anemia, 269
White blood cell differential in multiple myeloma, 198
White blood cell transfusion, 30
White lung, 48-49
Whole blood, 30
Widal's test in salmonella infection, 256

XYZ

X-ray. *See also specific type.*
  in gout, 134
  in hyperparathyroidism, 164
  in hyperphosphatemia, 166
  in hypoparathyroidism, 180
  in multiple myeloma, 198
  in radiation exposure, 232

i refers to an illustration; t refers to a table.